Health Informatics

More information about this series at http://www.springer.com/series/1114

Thomas Wetter

Consumer Health Informatics

New Services, Roles, and Responsibilities

With contributions by
George Demiris, Amanda K. Hall, Andrea Hartzler,
Jina Huh, Georgios Raptis and Lisa M. Vizer

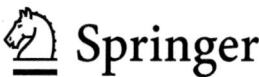
Springer

Thomas Wetter
Institute for Medical Biometry
  and Informatics
University of Heidelberg
Heidelberg, Germany

Department of Biomedical
  Informatics and Medical Education
University of Washington School of Medicine
Seattle, WA, USA

ISSN 1431-1917   ISSN 2197-3741   (electronic)
Health Informatics
ISBN 978-3-319-19589-6   ISBN 978-3-319-19590-2   (eBook)
DOI 10.1007/978-3-319-19590-2

Library of Congress Control Number: 2015942896

Springer Cham Heidelberg New York Dordrecht London
© Springer International Publishing Switzerland 2016
This work is subject to copyright. All rights are reserved by the Publisher, whether the whole or part of the material is concerned, specifically the rights of translation, reprinting, reuse of illustrations, recitation, broadcasting, reproduction on microfilms or in any other physical way, and transmission or information storage and retrieval, electronic adaptation, computer software, or by similar or dissimilar methodology now known or hereafter developed.
The use of general descriptive names, registered names, trademarks, service marks, etc. in this publication does not imply, even in the absence of a specific statement, that such names are exempt from the relevant protective laws and regulations and therefore free for general use.
The publisher, the authors and the editors are safe to assume that the advice and information in this book are believed to be true and accurate at the date of publication. Neither the publisher nor the authors or the editors give a warranty, express or implied, with respect to the material contained herein or for any errors or omissions that may have been made.

Printed on acid-free paper

Springer International Publishing AG Switzerland is part of Springer Science+Business Media (www.springer.com)

Foreword

After years in the making, consumer health informatics is coming of age. People measure their physiological reactions, monitor their diets, network with others, track their physical activity, search the Internet, communicate with clinicians, and otherwise use information technologies to support taking care of themselves. Enthusiastic reports tout this key area of health informatics as the way to patient empowerment and improved health care. In this welcome and refreshingly balanced book, Thomas Wetter thoughtfully reflects on the promise and potential of these new technologies and examines attendant social changes and ethical considerations.

This book was some years in the making. Thomas had been working on it since before he asked me to participate in a panel at the 2013 American Medical Informatics Association (AMIA) Annual Symposium [1]. He became cochair of the International Medical Informatics Association's Working Group on Consumer Health Informatics in 2007 and chair in 2010. The group's focus on, in the 1996 words of the US General Accounting Office, "the use of modern computers and telecommunications to support consumers in obtaining information, analyzing unique health care needs and helping them make decisions about their own health" dates from its founding in 2000 [2]. AMIA's Consumer and Health Evaluation Working Group (renamed the "Consumer Health Informatics Working Group" and, most recently, the "Consumer and Pervasive Health Working Group") already was operating. Then-president Patricia Flatley Brennan asked me to head a Consumer Informatics Task Force to help guide AMIA more into this emerging area. The following year, AMIA's 2000 Spring Congress included a track on consumer health informatics. It was apparent that patients could be empowered and enlightened while forging new relationships with providers by using computers [3].

During the previous ten years, investigators had developed a variety of applications. They were for medication adherence, smoking cessation, appointment reminders, health behavior counseling, and more. By 2004, consumer health informatics was mature enough for Springer books highlighting the accomplishments. Springer published *Consumer Informatics: Applications and Strategies in Cyber Health Care*. Its preface credited pioneers of the previous decade, including Warner Slack and Thomas Ferguson, who presented a tutorial at the 1993 AMIA annual symposium. Tom Ferguson coined the term "consumer health informatics" [4]. *Consumer Health Informatics: Informing Consumers and Improving Health Care*, to which I contributed, came out the following year [5]. *Investing in eHealth: What It Takes to Sustain Consumer Health Informatics* followed soon after [6]. Such books included chapters on patient empowerment and collaborative health care, designing and delivering patient-centered information, home care technologies, patient perspectives and expectations, patient-patient and patient-provider communication, ethical issues, evaluation methods, privacy and security, implementation models, and case studies.

Interest kept growing and technologies kept developing. Companies and health care organizations set up patient portals, personal health records, and social networks among patients. More and more, people got and shared health information from the Internet and Web-based services. In the USA, the 2009 Health Information Technology for Economic and Clinical Health (HITECH) Act promoted electronic medical records. They were envisioned to be linked eventually to patient portals, personal health records, and other patient-provided information. Part of the Patient Protection and Affordable Care Act of 2010 established the Patient-Centered Outcomes Research Institute (PCORI) with a mandate "to improve the quality and relevance of evidence available to help patients, caregivers, clinicians, employers, insurers, and policy makers make informed health decisions." Patients were included in order to ensure that PCORI focused on questions and concerns patients considered most relevant [7]. Health-related smart phone applications and wearable devices became popular, and Springer published a recent volume on mHealth [8].

Consumer Health Informatics: New Services, Roles and Responsibilities reflects the burgeoning interest in meeting collaborative health information needs of consumers and providers. It admirably achieves several purposes. For those wanting an overview of consumer health informatics, it provides a helpful classification scheme based on the roles of consumer and clinician. It also gives a detailed accounting of numerous studies, products, applications, and trends that characterize the consumer health informatics landscape.

In addition, this book contributes to many areas laid out at early conferences and the founding of the IMIA and AMIA Consumer Health Informatics Working Groups. Chapter after chapter, it addresses topics brought to attention then and still being discussed [3]. Thomas carefully tests and explores both visible and behind-the-scenes aspects of using the technologies. He skillfully dissects what consumers may not know about sources of information they are being provided, contracts to which they are agreeing, and potential effects of applications they are using. He provides pointers to improve usability. As a result, readers can make wiser decisions about the whats and hows of the range of applications and technological platforms. Thomas's careful and insightful work provides a model for others.

But this book does far more by interweaving a constant thread of ethics into the discussion. Thomas starts with his concern for patients and what will become of them as an aging population faces a shortage of in-person care. His underlying compassion and patient-centeredness permeate this book. He explores social, ethical, and legal issues together with health consequences in consumer health informatics. He laudably goes beyond the more common topics of privacy, licensure, and regulation, though they, too, are well discussed. For Thomas, patients come first. Their feelings, capabilities, needs, opportunities, achievements, and outcomes are paramount while he also highlights potential risks and limitations of the ways the technologies can be used. I became more sensitive to these concerns when interviewing participants in a trial involving a patient-facing application [9, 10]. I believe them pressing enough to have since reviewed general ethical issues as well as legal ones [11–13]. Thomas's thoughtful tempered analysis is an important contribution to these growing areas of health information technology ethics.

This volume not only fills a gap in the literature but also lays out ways to think about issues in health informatics. These issues come to the fore in consumer health informatics, but need to be addressed more generally. I know readers will find, as I do, that this comprehensive and useful book is a valuable addition to our field.

New Haven, CT, USA   Bonnie Kaplan, PhD, FACMI
2015   Yale University

References

1. Wetter T, van Voorhees B, Kaplan B, DeMuro PR, Waldo AB. Ethical, legal, and policy barriers to unleashing the full power of consumer health informatics for care delivery. In: American medical informatics association annual symposium, Washington, DC, Nov 2013. Available at http://knowledge.amia.org.
2. http://www.imia-medinfo.org/new2/GA/2012beijing/1210GA-beijing%20-vp-wgsig-reports.pdf. Accessed 19 June 2015.
3. Kaplan B, Brennan PF. Consumer informatics supporting patients as co-producers of quality. JAMIA (J Am Med Inform Assoc). 2001;8(4):309–16.
4. Nelson R, Ball M, editors. Consumer informatics: applications and strategies in cyber health care (health informatics). Berlin/Heidelberg: Springer; 2004.
5. Lewis D, Eysenbach G, Kukafka R, Stavri PZ, Jimison H, editors. Consumer health informatics: informing consumers and improving health care. Berlin/Heidelberg: Springer; 2005.
6. Gustafson DH, Brennan PF, Hawkins RP, editors. Investing in eHealth: what it takes to sustain consumer health informatics. Berlin/Heidelberg: Springer; 2007.
7. http://www.pcori.org/about-us. Accessed 20 June 2015.
8. Malvey D, Slovensky DJ. mHealth: transforming healthcare. Berlin/Heidelberg: Springer; 2014.
9. Kaplan B, Farzanfar R, Friedman RH. Research and ethical issues arising from ethnographic interviews of patients' reactions to an intelligent interactive telephone health behavior advisor system. In: Ngwenyama O, Introna L, Myers M, DeGross JI, editors. New information technologies in organizational processes: field studies and theoretical reflections on the future of work. Boston: Kluwer Academic; 1999.
10. Kaplan B, Farzanfar R, Friedman RH. Personal relationships with an intelligent interactive telephone health behavior advisor system: a multimethod study using surveys and ethnographic interviews. Int J Med Inform. 2003;71(1):33–41.
11. Kaplan B, Litewka S. Ethical challenges of telemedicine and telehealth. Camb Q Healthcare Ethics. 2008;17(4):401–16.
12. Kaplan B, Selling health data: de-identification, privacy, and speech. Camb Q Healthcare Ethics. 2015;24(3):256–71.
13. Kaplan B. How should health data be used? Privacy, secondary use, and big data sales. Camb Q Healthcare Ethics. (in press).

Preface

When I had joined Heidelberg University in 1997 and had developed the classes I was supposed to teach, I started looking around for a long-term challenge that should guide my efforts for the next couple of years. It was the time when large companies sent best agers in droves into early retirement because so many young applicants would fill the ranks and cost less salary. It was, however, also the time of the first reports, e.g., by OECD, that warned of a thinning workforce and an avalanche of retirees. Being in health care and knowing that the avalanche of retirees meant an avalanche of patients, I came to the conclusion that "Affordable Health for Aging Societies" should be my mission. AHAS was written in block letters on my white board to always remind me.

But how to proceed? Before it had taken concrete shape on my mind, I attended a health IT conference in Portland (OR) and heard Enrico Coiera give a keynote address that mounted to the conclusion that, to let the health care system survive the avalanche, 80 % of medical care would have to be self-service medicine in 2020.

Well, keynote is keynote. But Enrico's central idea was crystal clear to me immediately: My mission would be employing ICT to enable the patient to actively play a safe role in his health care. This is what had been coined Consumer Health Informatics a few years before.

Meanwhile, Consumer Health Informatics is coming of age. Being twenty-some years old it should find its place in health care not too far in the future. I dearly hope that this volume will be instrumental to that end because I believe that from the facts and conclusions about the diminishing future health care workforce, a moral obligation for health professionals to pursue Consumer Health Informatics can be deduced. Following a keynote that Ted Shortliffe gave at the AMIA Annual Symposium 2013 "Informatics Is a Health Profession": We as a health information profession are not marginal but central to this end. The moral obligation that I feel has been among my personal motives to keep pushing for quite a while to finish this book. It is summarized in the very last section of the book (Sect. 17.12). It builds on progress and consolidation in many fields also covered in this volume.

I believe that this is a necessary book because the field still is in a chaotic state. This is evident from Sect. 1.6 and from countless partially contradictory examples.

Well, chaos is not bad in its own right. Great ideas can emerge from chaos. However, when it becomes serious in terms of patient safety, we should at least understand, better, control the chaos. The field is not only at chaos but also wildly dispersed. This relates to the journals where scholarly articles are published (cf. Sect. 1.6.4) and also to numerous underwhelming funding and business models, while the preferred stakeholders (health plans or governments, depending on model of health care finance) are reluctant to commit themselves.

Despite all these concerns it seems doable. So many experiments presented in this volume show promising results, and our understanding of how to address risks grows (cf. Sect. 17.11). And there are great opportunities beyond attenuating the effects of the future health care workforce shortage. Rather than just offering approved knowledge and supporting approved procedures, Consumer Health Informatics sets out to become an independent source of new knowledge (cf. Sects. 6.3.3 and 9.10.3).

A book like this cannot be written in one year. It actually took more than five years, with some on and off due to other obligations that a full professor has. That seems to imply that some parts are five years old, some five days. This is true and false at the same time. It is true that some chapters were conceived five years ago and some three months ago. That seems to imply that some chapters are outdated, while others are up to date. This, again, is true and false at the same time. It is true that not each and every paragraph reflects the absolutely newest state. Rather did we, my coauthors and myself, do our best to write a principled account of the field. We developed arguments about opportunities and risks, methods for safety, effectiveness, human comprehension and literacy, etc. and identified examples that would underline our arguments and illustrate our methods. Some examples indeed vanished while we wrote whereas others came into existence. But the principles and methods do not expire within a pentad. We hope that ours hold for a decade (or so). If that is the case the book will have its value for another five years (or so). The reader can bring up his own new examples and match them against the arguments and methods. As time passes he will find examples that no longer match. That is why we as authors should start now with the next edition. If our spouses allow.

A book like this cannot be written without many people's help and backing up. First of all I have a great publisher. Early on Grant Weston has given me the confidence that I can concentrate to write a nice book and that Springer would make it look nice. Which saved me days, if not weeks, to tweak out millimeters and points to squeeze content on a page. Grant has also given well-appreciated advice where to allocate and where to withdraw effort. And his patience with my ongoing delays was incredible.

I had numerous people who gave their advice in various forms, many serving as critical chapter readers or pointing me to priceless resources. They are (in alphabetical order, and I dearly hope that I do not miss anybody):

- Michael Ashton
- Axel Bauer
- Leslie Berger

Preface

- Mike Conway
- Paul Fearn
- Sebastian Grommes
- Marten van der Heijden
- Konstantin Kinzel
- Tugba Kutun
- Marion and Joachim Lammarsch
- Tom Moore
- Peter Nawroth
- Alexander Rieß
- Lou Ann Scarton
- Ulla Wetter
- Gaby Wildenbos
- Thomas Willert

Furthermore I received wonderful feedback and challenges from the students in my classes that I taught in Salt Lake City, Amsterdam, Brisbane, Seattle, and Heidelberg.

My two academic homes also contributed magnificently. I had and still have wonderful discussions with my colleagues in Seattle with Wanda Pratt and Andrea Hartzler giving the most inspired impulse. I also found many articles in the UW electronic library that were nowhere else at my disposal. My colleagues in Heidelberg and Heilbronn tolerated delays and timeouts that I took to an extent that went far beyond what can be expected. Our department head Petra Knaup kept encouraging me and mildly pushing me and never lost her patience.

But above and before all, my family has tolerated my mental absenteeism with unbelievable patience. My parents Paul and Irmgard Wetter, nee Michels, passed away too early to see it finished. They would have been so proud. My grandchildren Josua, Daniel, and Timon probably do not remember at all that there was a time when grandpa was *not* writing a book. My children Anne-Mareike, Miriam, Marius, and Daria do remember, but they, too often, did not dare ask or involve me in activities that took more than a couple of hours.

Comes my beloved wife of nearly forty years, Angelika. For her, I was next door and still far away half an eternity. She has kept things going and has backed me up where I was in charge and whenever I felt really bad comforted me "We'll do it after the book."

Angelika, thank you a thousand times.

Heidelberg, Germany
March 28, 2015

Thomas Wetter

Contents

Part I Introducing the Domain and Levels of Service

1 Character of Domain and Organization of Book 3
    1.1   Introduction 3
            1.1.1   Pioneers 3
            1.1.2   An Inspiration 4
    1.2   Consumer Health Informatics as a Discipline 5
            1.2.1   What Defines Consumer Health
                      Informatics? Helpful Terms 5
            1.2.2   Consumer Health Informatics as
                      a Scientific Discipline 6
            1.2.3   Consumer Health Informatics as Range
                      of Phenomena 7
    1.3   Core Methodology 11
            1.3.1   Search Support 11
            1.3.2   Data Sharing 11
            1.3.3   Interface Design 12
            1.3.4   User Assessment and Personalization 13
            1.3.5   End User Participation 14
    1.4   Supportive Methodology 14
            1.4.1   Evaluation 14
            1.4.2   Going Life 16
    1.5   Hardware 17
            1.5.1   Voice and Sound 17
            1.5.2   Biosignals 17
            1.5.3   Pointing and Virtual Space 17
            1.5.4   Positioning 18
            1.5.5   Smart Phones 18
    1.6   Where in the Literature is Consumer Health Informatics? 19
            1.6.1   Fruitless Search for MeSH Keywords 19
            1.6.2   Opportunistic Search in PubMed 20

		1.6.3	Estimated Growth Rates	20
		1.6.4	Scatter Across Media	22
	1.7	Aims of This Volume		24
		1.7.1	Positive Attitude: We Need It	24
		1.7.2	Wide Perspective: It Can Be Done	25
		1.7.3	Sound Methodology: How It Should Be Done	25
	1.8	Organization of the Book in Detail		26
		1.8.1	Organization of the Book: Part I	26
		1.8.2	Organization of the Book: Part II	27
		1.8.3	Organization of the Book: Part III	28
	1.9	Additional Topics Worth Individual Chapters Under the Viewpoint Taken		28
		1.9.1	Scalability	29
		1.9.2	Disparity	29
		1.9.3	Public Health	29
		1.9.4	Rare Diseases	29
		1.9.5	Applications	30
	1.10	Alternative Viewpoints		30
		1.10.1	Transient Stimuli and Funding Programs	30
		1.10.2	Devices	31
		1.10.3	User Centeredness	35
	References			37
2	**Economy 1: Immanent Mismatch Between Demand and Supply of Health Care Workforce**			39
	2.1	Introduction		39
	2.2	Methodological Considerations		40
		2.2.1	Criteria to Select Variables	40
		2.2.2	Criteria to Select Nations	41
		2.2.3	Criteria to Select Information Resources	41
		2.2.4	Base Figures and Derived Indicators of Health Care Demand and Supply	42
		2.2.5	The "Best Case" Strategy of Selection	44
	2.3	Sources and Results		45
		2.3.1	The USA	45
		2.3.2	Germany	46
		2.3.3	US: German Differences	49
		2.3.4	Challenging the Assumptions	50
	2.4	Options to Match Supply and Demand		52
		2.4.1	Rationing	53
		2.4.2	Volume Increase at Equal Cost, with Quality at Risk	54
		2.4.3	Reduced Effort per Case Through Quality Improvement	54

		2.4.4	Growth	55
		2.4.5	Diversification of Delivery	56
	2.5	Benefits from Growth in Other Industries and Segments		57
	References			58
3	**Level 0: Searching – Finding – Trusting – Acting – Risking One's Life?**			61
	3.1	Introduction		61
	3.2	Facts and Behaviors		61
		3.2.1	Trends of Utilization of the Internet and Other Media	61
		3.2.2	Increasing Compliance Meets Declining Comprehension	62
	3.3	Effects, Risks, and Adverse Effects		63
		3.3.1	Searching: Finding?	63
		3.3.2	True Risks	71
	3.4	Trust		73
		3.4.1	Trust as a Basic Human Notion	73
		3.4.2	Innate Instincts and Their Reincarnation in the Digital Age	73
		3.4.3	Trustmarks	75
	3.5	Trustworthy Providers: More or Less		76
		3.5.1	NIH and Its Organisations	76
		3.5.2	Wikipedia's and MedlinePlus's Contents	78
	3.6	A Short Note on apps		79
	References			80
4	**Level 1: Enhancing the Provider – Client Relation Through IT**			83
	4.1	Introduction		83
	4.2	Level 1 Consumer Health Informatics Versus Telemedicine		84
	4.3	Incorporating New Media into Patient-Physician Communication		84
		4.3.1	E-Mail	84
		4.3.2	Social Networks	86
		4.3.3	Electronic Health Records	88
	4.4	Condition Specific Services		90
		4.4.1	Discharge Management and Follow-Up Care	90
		4.4.2	Managing Chronic Diseases	92
	4.5	A Short Note on apps		96
		4.5.1	Customer Relationship apps	96
		4.5.2	Condition Specific apps	97
	References			98

5	**Level 2: Services Without In-Person Contact Between Provider and Client**		101
	5.1	Introduction	101
	5.2	Examples	102
		5.2.1 Health Awareness	102
		5.2.2 Mental Health Coaching	103
		5.2.3 Somatic Diseases	110
		5.2.4 Online Pharmacies	114
		5.2.5 Online Counseling	118
	5.3	A Short Note on apps	124
		5.3.1 Information Broker apps	124
		5.3.2 Logistics Support apps	125
		5.3.3 Reminders	125
		5.3.4 Condition Specific apps	126
	5.4	Variety of Service Characteristics	130
	5.5	Considerations on Scaling Up	131
	References		133
6	**Level 3: Patient Power on the Web: The Multifaceted Role of Personal Health Wisdom**		135
	6.1	Conceptualizing the Wisdom of Patients: A Unique Value Proposition	135
	6.2	Exchanging Patient Wisdom Online: An Evolving Landscape of Social Media	136
		6.2.1 Interacting Through Internet Forums	137
		6.2.2 Capturing Knowledge Through Blogs	137
		6.2.3 Building Collective Wisdom Through Wikis	138
		6.2.4 Collaborating Through Social Networking Tools	139
	6.3	Leveraging Patient Wisdom: Varied Levels of Use Among Individuals, Groups, and Crowds	140
		6.3.1 Individual Level: From Foraging Alone to Shared Experience	141
		6.3.2 Group Level: From Shared Experience to Collaborative Bricolage	142
		6.3.3 Crowd Level: From Collaborative Bricolage to Collective Discovery	143
	6.4	Conclusion	144
	References		144
7	**Distinctive Features of Services Conveyed Through Mobile Apps**		147
	7.1	Introduction	147
	7.2	Values Added Through the Technology	147
	7.3	Distributors' Take on Medical Quality	149
	7.4	Clients' Traps and Barriers in Checking Quality	151

	7.5	Further Necessary Precautions When It Becomes Serious Medicine...	152
	References...		154

Part II Building Safety Nets Around the Active Client

8 Dimensions of Patient Risks and Requirements for Patient Safety ... 157
- 8.1 The Client as Resource 157
- 8.2 High Stakes and High Demands 158
- 8.3 Outline of the Assessment Scheme 159
- 8.4 Overview of Assessment Dimensions 163
  - 8.4.1 Medical Risk 163
  - 8.4.2 Personality 167
  - 8.4.3 Cognition... 171
  - 8.4.4 Identity and Authentication 183
- 8.5 Further Reading 186
- References... 186

9 Services for All Stages of the Metabolic Syndrome and Its Consequences 189
- 9.1 Introduction 189
- 9.2 Diabetes Pioneers: The IDEATel Project 189
- 9.3 Outline of Chapter 190
- 9.4 Risk Awareness and Primary Prevention 191
  - 9.4.1 Fostering Awareness 191
  - 9.4.2 Turning Awareness into Risk Avoiding Behavior 193
- 9.5 Treatment Support and Coaching 200
  - 9.5.1 Simple Tight Medical Guidance 200
  - 9.5.2 Medical Guidance and Tailored Behavioral Information.. 200
  - 9.5.3 Tight Medical Guidance and Behavioral Coaching 202
  - 9.5.4 On the Way to Automated Insulin Dosing.............. 203
- 9.6 Fostering Self Management 205
  - 9.6.1 In Search of Factors for Services to Last 206
  - 9.6.2 Building a Service That Reflects Own Experiences.... 207
  - 9.6.3 Exploring the Consequences of Smart Phone Ubiquity 209
- 9.7 Complications Management....................................... 210
- 9.8 Attenuation of Comorbidities 211
- 9.9 Adding Level 3 Self Support 212
- 9.10 Concluding Remarks... 213
  - 9.10.1 Collateral Benefits 213
  - 9.10.2 New Options on the Horizon 213
  - 9.10.3 Visitors and Responders: Research Questions.......... 213
- References... 214

10 Basic Services Reach Out Towards Under-Served Populations 217
- 10.1 Introduction 217
- 10.2 Short Text Based Messages: SMS 217
  - 10.2.1 Public Health Outreach 218
  - 10.2.2 Unidirectional Behavioral Stimuli 220
  - 10.2.3 Client Initiated Request Processing 224
  - 10.2.4 Closed Loop Services 226
  - 10.2.5 Enhancing Complex Therapies 227
  - 10.2.6 Delivery of Test Results 228
- 10.3 Interactive Voice Response: IVR 229
  - 10.3.1 Public Health Outreach 229
  - 10.3.2 Enhancing Complex Therapies 230
  - 10.3.3 Cognitive Assessment 231
- 10.4 A Closer Look at Effectivity 232
  - 10.4.1 Intervention vs. Other Factors 232
  - 10.4.2 Behavioral vs. Clinical Effect 232
  - 10.4.3 Size and Format of the Intervention Effort 235
- 10.5 Expanding the Scope 237
  - 10.5.1 Enhancing the Technology 237
  - 10.5.2 Involving Clients' Peers 239
- References 242

11 Smart Homes: Empowering the Patient Till the End 245
- 11.1 Overview 245
- 11.2 Smart Home Functionalities 249
- 11.3 Acceptance 249
- 11.4 Ethical Considerations 250
- 11.5 The Evidence for Smart Homes 251
- 11.6 Future Trends 252
- References 252

12 Partial Solutions for Patient Safety 255
- 12.1 Introduction 255
- 12.2 Medical Risk 255
  - 12.2.1 Medical State and History 255
  - 12.2.2 Identification of Familial Risk 259
- 12.3 Personality 263
  - 12.3.1 Personality Traits 264
  - 12.3.2 Mental Healthiness 265
  - 12.3.3 Interfering Attitudes 266
- 12.4 Cognition 266
- 12.5 Identify and Authentication 267
- References 268

Part III Additional Methodology

13 Privacy and Data Protection: Mission Impossible? 273
- 13.1 Protection of Your Data: Why?...................................... 273
- 13.2 What Data Should Be Protected? 273
- 13.3 What Kind of Protection Do We Need? How Can Protection Be Achieved? 274
- 13.4 How Health Data and Services Should Be Protected? 275
- 13.5 The Bottom Line for Companies Running Health Services 277
- 13.6 Know Your Enemy... 277
- 13.7 Protection of Your Data: Can I Trust Health Services? 278
- References... 279

14 The Patient-Centered Electronic Health Record and Patient Portals 281
- 14.1 Introduction 282
  - 14.1.1 Evolution of Patient-Centered Health Information Systems in the USA....................... 282
- 14.2 PHR and Patient Portal Components............................. 283
  - 14.2.1 Data... 284
  - 14.2.2 Functionality 286
- 14.3 PHRs and Patient Portals in Context............................. 287
  - 14.3.1 Political Forces and Meaningful Use 287
  - 14.3.2 Access 289
  - 14.3.3 Use and Usability 289
  - 14.3.4 Liability, Reliability, and Accuracy 291
- 14.4 Conclusion 292
- References... 292

15 Scrutinized Proof of Effectiveness or Cost Effectiveness Regarding Patient Reported Outcomes 295
- 15.1 Introduction 295
- 15.2 Awareness and Precautions Prior to Beginning a Trial............ 296
  - 15.2.1 Nature of the "Active Agent"........................... 296
  - 15.2.2 Change Within and Around 297
  - 15.2.3 Clients' Behavioral Patterns............................ 298
  - 15.2.4 Control of the Test Setting............................. 304
- 15.3 Historical Comparisons.. 305
- 15.4 Randomized Controlled Trials 307
  - 15.4.1 Effectiveness Trials 308
  - 15.4.2 Cost-Effectiveness Trials 312
- 15.5 Noninferiority Trials 314
- 15.6 Definite Evidence from Non-randomized Trials 316
- 15.7 Cochrane: Supreme Evidence Fading............................. 320

	15.8	After the Trial: Does It Still Work?	321
		15.8.1 Non-representative Study Samples	321
		15.8.2 Prohibitive Effort to Maintain Service Level	322
		15.8.3 Arguable Cost-Effect Relation	322
		15.8.4 Carving Active Agents	322
		15.8.5 Stakeholder Influence	323
	15.9	Further Reading	323
	References		324

16 Economy 2: Economic Subsistence of Services When Research Funding Ends 327

- 16.1 Introduction 327
- 16.2 Client Membership Fees 327
  - 16.2.1 Apps 328
  - 16.2.2 Internet 329
- 16.3 Client Fees for Service 329
  - 16.3.1 Apps 329
  - 16.3.2 Internet 330
- 16.4 Heterogeneous Co-branding 331
- 16.5 Service-Device Bundles 332
- 16.6 Providers' Customer Relationship Services 333
- 16.7 Online Pharmacies 334
- 16.8 Employer Sponsorship 335
- 16.9 Third Party Entrepreneurship 335
- 16.10 Charity 336
- 16.11 Government Organisations 336
- 16.12 Health Insurance Coverage 337
- References 338

17 Towards Future Consumer Health Informatics Adapted Health Care Legislation 339

- 17.1 Introduction 339
- 17.2 Frames of Reference 339
- 17.3 Legislation, Ethics and Research 341
- 17.4 Present Regulations 342
  - 17.4.1 Structures and Resources in the USA 343
  - 17.4.2 Structures and Resources in Germany 348
- 17.5 Practice of Medicine, Provision of Information, or Business? 352
  - 17.5.1 Criteria for Practice of Medicine 353
  - 17.5.2 Criteria for Business 354
- 17.6 Present Legislation Meets Present Practice 355
  - 17.6.1 US: German Commonalities and Differences 355
  - 17.6.2 Legal Assessment of Present Approaches 356
- 17.7 Side Entries 365
  - 17.7.1 Well-Being 365
  - 17.7.2 C-Referral 366

17.8	Transactions Across Borders		366
17.9	Health Informatics Professionals Ethics		368
17.10	Research Under Ethical Supervision		369
17.11	Ethical Considerations for Future Consumer Health Informatics Legislation		370
	17.11.1	Moral Behavior	370
	17.11.2	Behavioral Codes	371
	17.11.3	Principles Underlying Medical Professional Codes	371
	17.11.4	Respect for Autonomy	373
	17.11.5	Nonmaleficence	375
	17.11.6	Beneficence	377
	17.11.7	Distributive Justice	380
	17.11.8	Consumer Health Informatics in Utilitarian and Other Theories of Justice	381
17.12	Directions for Legislation		383
References			384

Trademarks 387

Nomenclature 389

General Index 393

Index of Services 415

Part I
Introducing the Domain and Levels of Service

Chapter 1
Character of Domain and Organization of Book

1.1 Introduction

In this chapter we will lead the reader into the field of Consumer Health Informatics as we see it. Starting from some pioneers and sources of inspiration we will draw a map of the volume to come. The map will identify some white spots: topics that should be in the map but are not because they exceed the scope that can be covered in one volume on Consumer Health Informatics. Some adjacent topics will be described: perspectives different from the one we take, with clear other merits.

1.1.1 Pioneers

Three projects, all initiated before the turn of the millennium, all demonstrating different aspects of Consumer Health Informatics that have set trends will first be introduced.

1.1.1.1 Baby CareLink

A group at Beth Israel Deaconess Medical Center in Boston established an at that time pioneering communication facility that allowed parents of pre-term newborns to "see" their baby in the NICU from home and to communicate with staff at the hospital (cf. [6]). This gave parents the opportunity to get acquainted with the situation and to have a matured feeling about their baby's behavior when they finally got him or her home. In an RCT parents in the experimental Baby CareLink arm were more satisfied and secure about the situation. More babies in that arm could be discharged directly to the family home as opposed to community hospital.

Baby CareLink has typical elements of Consumer Health Informatics that we will return to. It enables the parents to take a more active part. It enhances the communication with staff and it provides convenience, 24/7 video presence, as opposed to limited and nervous visit hours. And, like the following, it targets a vulnerable population.

1.1.1.2 IDEATel

IDEATel is an equally pioneering Consumer Health Informatics service for diabetics in "federally designated medically underserved" areas in New York state [10, 11]. Different communication channels (including slow videoconferencing and data upload facilities) connect them to their care providers. Details can be found in Sect. 9.2. Typical again is the increased capacity of patients to care for themselves and the convenience to do it from home. IDEATel also demonstrates that such comprehensive services can be maintained for more than 15 years and reach and positively impact large patient groups.

1.1.1.3 PCASSO

Masys and coworkers [8] have pioneered the patient experience with electronic medical records made available to them by and large unfiltered. In contrast to the former two their patients were well educated and not so severely ill which qualified them as subjects that would give a clear account of their experiences. These were primarily positive. "Information toxity", i.e. adverse effects of intimidating findings communicated unbolstered did not materialize in this relatively healthy cohort. Other clearly trend-setting elements should be mentioned: different security levels that could be assigned to pieces of information and the methods to protect privacy – a private key infrastructure with patient keys residing on diskettes that had to be presented to get access – appear archaic through the type of token but are absolutely up to date what the concepts are concerned (cf. Chap. 13).

1.1.2 An Inspiration

While these services evolved – hardly noticed as can be seen from the figures in Sect. 1.6.1 – Enrico Coiera wrote a visionary article in BMJ [2]. He pointed to early signs of a developing shortage of the health care workforce and envisioned how delivery of health care would have to develop to cope with the expected strain. Two major themes are that it does not suffice to design technologies but rather sociotechnical systems and that patients will be much more active, if not the driver, of their care processes, supported through brokers that locate required resources.

At a conference in Portland (OR) in the same year Coiera formulated that "in 2010 80 % of medicine will be self service". A strong impulse to consider how the patient can be given the means to play that role.

1.2 Consumer Health Informatics as a Discipline

It is among the aims of this volume to contribute to a more systematic and rigorous perspective on Consumer Health Informatics. It is not meant as a collection or digest of projects or schools although it draws a lot on real examples. It rather tries to be a methodology that reaches from a medical problem to routine use of a service seamlessly integrated with or productively complementing existing delivery of care. In this introductory chapter directions towards this aim will be outlined.

1.2.1 What Defines Consumer Health Informatics? Helpful Terms

1.2.1.1 Definition

We will regard Consumer Health Informatics as a discipline of

> **Take Home**
> Information and communication technology based methods, services, and equipment that enable the lay citizen to safely play an active role in his health and preventive care.

Such medical, public health, nursing or preventive services conveyed or enhanced by technologies such as internet, cell phone, etc. will be covered where the patient has some agent as opposed to a mere recipient role.

1.2.1.2 Client, Subject, User: New Names for New Patient Roles

Terms to denote the individual that uses a Consumer Health Informatics service are somewhat misleading. According to Webster[1] a patient is "1. a person undergoing treatment for disease or injury or 2. anything passively affected ... as opposed

---

[1] Webster's Comprehensive Dictionary of the English Language 2003.

to agent". A consumer is "1. one who consumes ... or 2. uses up an article of exchangeable value". "Patient" freezes the traditional passive role which is congruent with a paternalistic self image of the physician. "Consumer" suggests that health can be purchased, tried and thrown away, with physicians in a merchant role. To emphasize serious search for authentic advice we will preferably use "client" instead, i.e. "2. one who engages the services of any professional advisor" (Webster). Although originating from law "client" generally suggests the specific character of the need and the binding character of the service while upholding an active client role. The latter is also heralded through the programmatic "patient empowerment", an umbrella term for technical and other advances to upgrade the patient's active contribution.

In some places client behavior is regarded through the perspective of psychology or sociology. In those places we will use "subject", i.e. "3. something upon which thought ... is employed ... a theme of consideration" (Webster). This should not be mistaken for a passive role as a person in need of health related advice. It rather is a study target role where capabilities or limitations of playing an active role in one's health care are being investigated. Finally we will employ "user" when it is about the spontaneous interaction of a person with computational or communication devices.

1.2.1.3 Telemedicine Patients Versus Consumer Health Informatics Clients

Telemedicine is a commonly used term for implementing medical treatment from a distance through information and communication technology. Telemedicine is a valuable contribution to medical care that has developed into a discipline of its own. It is, though, not a core topic here because it sees the patient in a passive role. Technology is a conveyor of classical physician initiated action rather than an enabler of active client contribution.

> **Take Home**
> As opposed to telemedicine where *patients* passively receive treatment we often speak of *clients* who seek advice, *users* of software and devices, or *subjects* in trials.

1.2.2 Consumer Health Informatics as a Scientific Discipline

From a theory of science perspective it may not appear appealing to the reader to characterize the discipline as a set of services, as we will try to maintain. Traditionally, disciplines can define themselves through phenomena, problems, or artefacts. Physics, e.g., assembles observations and models to provide explanations of phenomena encountered in the world of matter. The same applies to the humanities, with observations and models now being about the world of human experience. Medicine defines itself through diseases, i.e. problems to be solved. Its methods vary widely, from molecular to epidemiological and public health. Artifacts are central to all engineering disciplines, with the methods varying again: In civil engineering it reaches from chemistry and material science to psychology and usability of buildings.

Consumer Health Informatics has something of all this. Like the humanities it observes and models the phenomena of humans using information technology for health purposes. Like medicine it seeks for care and cure for all kinds of diseases. Like engineering it builds artifacts. Neither can live without the other. Full coverage of Consumer Health Informatics as a phenomenon even goes beyond: for services to go live they require legal approval and to survive they need sustainable funding. Therefore, business administration and law are contributing factors, too. This will now be further outlined to conclude that regarding Consumer Health Informatics as a set of services is productive for a systematic treatment. In this volume we regard "service" pragmatically. Readers interested in an in-depth sociological analysis of offering medical services to the patient's home are referred to [1].

> **Take Home**
> Consumer Health Informatics has elements from the natural sciences, humanities, medicine, and engineering, but none of these perspectives are as productive as regarding Consumer Health Informatics as a set of services.

1.2.3 Consumer Health Informatics as Range of Phenomena

While keeping the "service" perspective in mind we will now take a first quick look at the large variety of phenomena and scenarios where individuals are enabled through technology to safely play an active role in their health care.

1.2.3.1 Searching and Finding: Transient Encounters

Valuable advice can be gained through finding a specific piece of information as a result of a phone call, Internet search, or visit to a health kiosk. Finding out that a skin sign resembles a photograph of a beginning melanoma may lead to the decision to see a dermatologist and consequently have one's life saved through early surgical intervention. A minor single incidental encounter has major consequences. Encounters where search leads to content which enables decision making, or the respective services, will later be called Level 0 services.

Countless medical web sites are visited by scores of individuals every day, seeking advice on a plethora of signs, conditions, or therapies. Estimates have it that one-third of Internet searches target medical content. Providers range from highly respected institutions such as the National Library of Medicine to self-appointed experts on some niche problems. Information found can be as life saving as life threatening. This is a mass phenomenon and therefore a must in a book on Consumer Health Informatics although the service nature of just publishing on the internet is somewhat blurred.

Some of the available information takes a neutral stance, leaving it to the reader to draw his[2] own conclusions. This contrasts to offerings that try to bluntly persuade the reader toward some attitude or behavior. http://www.cbn.com/cbnnews/healthscience/2012/December/Starving-Cancer-Ketogenic-Diet-a-Key-to-Recovery/ is a fully arbitrary example and not meant to specifically blame its providers. It proclaims that cancer can be starved by carbohydrate free diet. Episodic evidence such as heart breaking personal testimonies, surrogate proof of authority of the authors, good graphical elements etc. persuade the reader toward behaviors without warrant.

Clients locate such resources by entering terms (such as "cancer diet" for the above example) into search engines. Using search engines such as http://google.com^{TM} delivers myriads of results (295 mio for "cancer diet"). To make searches more efficient and at the same time to focus on approved quality is a type of Consumer Health Informatics service for clients with instantaneous and transient information needs.

1.2.3.2 Awareness, Assessment and Screening

Part of the information seeking behavior of the broad public is to assess ones individual risk of having or being about to develop a certain condition. Many people know the BMI calculator: measuring one aspect of overweight tells its user how much his risk for diabetes or cardiovascular conditions is increased above the normal value. Add some questions about relatives with diabetes and some behavioral questions and out comes an elaborate approach to individual risk assessment. The stance is that a client with a primary awareness provides some data about himself and is helped to get focused whether he should follow up.

Screening is a type of assessment. Respective services combine the analysis of individual odds for a condition with recommendations for professional medical evaluation. Assisting with rational decisions to not follow up or to follow up appropriately is a somewhat farther reaching Consumer Health Informatics service. It moderates actions that the client can take and may even offer personalized logistics support by identifying nearby providers. Service provider responsibility now goes beyond accuracy of information. It includes not to tempt hypochondriac

---

[2]For the purpose of readability we will use male forms throughout the book unless – like in conditions such as breast cancer – women are the only or clearly major client group of a service.

clients to overreact in response to marginally increased risks and not to lull clients at significantly increased risk.

1.2.3.3 Technology Enhanced Treatment: Adding Channels of Communication

Many Consumer Health Informatics approaches offer complementary or follow-up care in conjunction with a traditional medical encounter. Telephone calls to the doctor or reminders from some community health services are forerunners of this kind of service. Exchanging e-mail with ones physician, although rarely used for reasons that are still being investigated, takes this to another level. Beyond e-mail there is a wide variety of sophisticated web, mobile phone, or ambient sensor technology based Consumer Health Informatics services that share a common feature: a classical medical case, treated classically through a healthcare professional or institution. Information or communication technology enhances the classical service. The Consumer Health Informatics service begins and ends approximately at the same time when the classical service begins and ends. Baby CareLink is a typical example of this type that is briefly described in the Pioneers section (Sect. 1.1.1.1).

Follow-up care after minor surgery may take days, while a contract with an asthma patient may last a lifetime. Classical providers may at the same time be Consumer Health Informatics service providers who also deliver the contents, such as the Mayo Clinic, cf. Sect. 4.5.1. Or they contract with third party offerings provided by patient self support groups or charities, cf. Sect. 5.2.3.3.

Recently ConsHI services have started to be offered without a classical provider–patient contact. These will later be called Level 2 services while those extending classical services will be called Level 1. Concerning duration they do not principally differ. However, of course, a legal framework, rules for accountability, etc. have to be found for Level 2.

1.2.3.4 Lifelong Resource: Fostering Client Ownership

The longitudinal, all encompassing electronic patient record has been championed by authorities and visionary clinicians for decades. Ideally, it can start with heritable diseases diagnosed in the family or own prenatal diagnostics, with the circumstances of conception and birth, and include all medical or nursing encounters as well as allowing the client to contribute observations of his own. Given such a resource any search result, assessment, or treatment has a backbone against which to interpret findings. For instance might the skin sign be more alarming when found in a person where a relative has already been diagnosed with melanoma. A Consumer Health Informatics service can offer considerable added value when present conclusions about new signs are substantiated through recurrence to case history or genetic disposition.

1.2.3.5 Lifelong Attitude: Fostering Client Commitment

While in the first place a longitudinal electronic record is just there for everybody to use it can also be a mediator for the patient to turn into a client, who takes responsibility for a complete record, adds own observations, learns, and manages situations for which he used to require professional services. For centuries, a paternalistic attitude has governed medical care. The care giver decides and the patient accepts and complies – or does not comply. Recently, evidence of improved outcomes has advocated for a more empowered patient. The hope is that a more active and conscious contribution to decisions fosters better contribution to the process of care. In Shared Decision Making this is conceived as a negotiation process between care giver and patient. The Informed Patient role rather assumes that the patient decides based on a wealth of information that the care provider has made available. Consumer Health Informatics is neutral concerning this distinction. It emphasizes the lifelong attitude of being an actor and contributor and introduces the longitudinal patient record as an enabling factor.

1.2.3.6 Sensor Rich Surveillance: Using the Physical Environment

Ambient sensors have already been mentioned. They form the major hardware asset of a more intrusive and immediate impact type of Consumer Health Informatics services. Ambient assisted living tries to be ubiquitous and all encompassing 24/7. Its farthest developed part, smart home technology, is intended for fragile individuals such as elderly in a low human surveillance nursing environment. For early detection of hazardous behaviors such as falls, ignition related events etc. tools scan the whole environment, by the same token violating all spontaneously felt privacy concerns, to aid in prevention and automatically detect suspected hazards and summon human assistance. Sensors can also play a role to detect deteriorating capacity of Consumer Health Informatics clients to play their role. They identify erratic rather than coordinated motion, nervosity etc.

1.2.3.7 Leveraging Client Wisdom: Using the Knowledge Environment

Helpful advice may also flow immediately between individuals who are members of a Consumer Health Informatics self support group. They are living with their disease and have their portfolio of coping with symptoms and treatment side effect, but also day to day management of practical problems, expertise that doctors do not necessarily possess. Getting the best of sharing such client wisdom is a growing strand within Consumer Health Informatics.

While this happens one on one between clients through altruistic attitude and behaviors, those pieces of advice confirmed or successfully replicated by other clients are the seed from which new general knowledge emerges; knowledge that cannot be created through consideration and planned experimentation alone. Client expertise is the core of Level 3 Consumer Health Informatics.

> **Take Home**
> Consumer Health Informatics covers a very wide range of phenomena, including:
> - Transient search encounters
> - Building awareness
> - Technology based or enhanced treatment
> - Healthy life companion
> - Sensor rich environment
> - Collection of crowd wisdom

1.3 Core Methodology

To develop the required software and technical infrastructures that underly Consumer Health Informatics services, the following is a brief introduction and selection of methods required.

1.3.1 Search Support

The example in Sect. 1.2.3.1 clearly shows that innocent search for health information using apparently meaningful queries and established search engines can have equally overwhelming and potentially harmful results. Therefore, better search engines, better use of the existing engines and better interpretation of search results are among the major success criteria for a safe and efficient entry into the world of Consumer Health Informatics. This includes unbiased assessment of the quality of renowned resources such as NLM's PubMed or Wikipedia, the investigation of trustmarks such as Health on the Net (HON), and of client heuristics.

1.3.2 Data Sharing

Data sharing, aka personal health record (PHR), is a necessary ingredient of most approaches with serious or continued impact on the client's health. It starts with a one-stop shop completion of a depression scale on the Internet: Data become shared between the visitor of the web site and – guess who? The need to protect privacy starts right here. Telephone lines can be tapped as can be Internet connections. Unless good provisions are taken to protect them, transmitted data are exposed to public intrusion. On the other hand longitudinal data are a key for successful management of chronic conditions. Granting the client access to his data improves his opportunities of empowerment and self initiated action when the data so advise. Therefore, methods to allow transparent access to data for those entitled and preventing access for those not entitled is a core technology in support of Consumer Health Informatics.

1.3.3 Interface Design

Regardless of search, data sharing or any other activity of the client using Consumer Health Informatics services, it happens through an interface between human and machine. Since client comprehension of content and client safety are indispensable criteria, the questions of what information can be shared safely and through what interfaces is key.

1.3.3.1 General Usability Heuristics

Methods and principles of the design of human – machine interfaces are a scientific discipline in their own right. Jakob Nielsen was one of the pioneers of the field who came up with ten principles summarized at www.nngroup.com/articles/ten-usability-heuristics/. Based on this Zhang and coworkers [13] added heuristics for medical devices. The heuristics include consistency, match between system and world, how to give the client the feeling that he is in control etc. Next we draw the attention to aspects that are specific for Consumer Health Informatics and not necessarily covered in the above heuristics.

1.3.3.2 Balancing Appeal, Change, and Core Content

Consumer Health Informatics interfaces face other challenges than interfaces for industrial workplaces. Interfaces to software in workplace settings are mandatory parts of many processes and users cannot opt out. In such cases efficiency and lack of change mostly satisfy users who want to have their jobs done fast and without errors. For this they are trained and even if interfaces are poor they have to find ways and can ask colleagues. Consumer Health Informatics clients use their service to their liking. Their inclination to pick up information, report behaviors or symptoms over extended periods of time correlates with the motive to visit the service's website or app. They will opt out from services with poor and opt in to services with appealing interface. On the long run, to maintain services attractive while at the same time preserving their core diagnostic or therapeutic concepts user interface considerations must inform a process of conservative change: change to maintain the clients' curiosity while preserving the medical core.

1.3.3.3 The Added Value of Multimedia

Although major parts of medical knowledge are still readily available as text multimedia gain ground and should be considered from two perspectives. Depending on the medical specialty they may be core assets such as images of skin signs for the client to compare to his own skin or staged virtual reality confrontations as therapy of phobias. Clients can take photos, voice or movie recordings of their signs with up to date tablet computers or smart phones. In all such cases the media enhanced content represents itself. The interface challenges are quality of the media and appropriate integration in other content and interactions, such as visibility of system state and match between system and world.

Media in form of icons, graphical owner manuals, flow charts etc. may, however, represent other content: text descriptions that are to hard to read and instructions that are hard to follow. This is one strand of research to overcome the problem of limited literacy addressed in the next section.

1.3.4 User Assessment and Personalization

1.3.4.1 Literacy

Historically, lots of valuable knowledge is still available as natural language text. This certainly holds for the abundance of specialty language articles, textbooks, guidelines etc. However, patient brochures from self support groups, public health authorities etc. have also tried to reach out to patients for quite a while. On the other hand, population statistics on literacy and even more so functional health literacy are alarming. A large share of the traditionally under-served parts of populations of rich nations such as the United States and Germany cannot draw the right conclusions from food labels, medication instructions, etc. Different native languages within one country (English or Spanish, German or Turkish) add to the challenge of not just sending but delivering the required information. Therefore, diagnosing literacy of a prospective client, adapting reading levels of presented text, using media other than text, minimalist triage type versions for clients without proven literacy, are methods of Consumer Health Informatics.

1.3.4.2 Client Personal Background

Even more subtle differences relate to different cultural backgrounds of the clients. While a certain recommendation may come natural and appealing for a Christian client it may appear strange for Muslims or Hindus. The need and processes of matching clients' capabilities to comprehend and willingness to cooperate with the material and advice offered by a Consumer Health Informatics service pose challenges of personalization.

1.3.4.3 Personalization

Many of the methods above are a types of personalization of services. Since many investigations show that context appropriate personalization in those or other ways is a high loading success factor, we mention it here separately.

1.3.5 End User Participation

In software engineering, it is approved practice to have future users participate in the design of software applications. Logistically it is feasible with an organization bringing in new software to identify employees who will be future users to sit on the development team for certain design considerations. Future clients of a Consumer Health Informatics application are harder to get one's hands on. A convenience sample of friends of the developers may not bring up the real issues. Volunteers who are healthy and are not affected by the problem are also of limited help (cf. Sect. 12.2.2.1 for an example). Persons who are presently affected want the service now and do not want to volunteer on a premature prototype in a process that will not deliver until several years down the road. General selection biases that mostly affect the volunteering (cf. Sect. 15.2.3.1) add to the problem.

> **Take Home**
> To substantiate a very wide range of phenomena a core methodology is required, including:
> - Search support
> - Data storage and sharing
> - Design of usable and appealing interfaces
> - Assessment of client capabilities
> - End user participation

1.4 Supportive Methodology

While the methods above emphasize the conception and creation of services we now turn to methods required to take a service into routine, metaphorically: "from bench to client's palm".

1.4.1 Evaluation

In the life cycle of a service at some time the contribution that it makes must be determined. This is evaluation in the literal sense of assigning value. We concentrate on the aspects of efficacy, safety and cost effectiveness.

1.4 Supportive Methodology

1.4.1.1 Trials

First and above all it cannot be the aim to widely distribute services that do not have the desired effect. If we parallel a (new) Consumer Health Informatics service with a new medical treatment we face agencies such as the FDA authorized to approve treatments for routine use. This normally requires a trial, preferably an RCT. Trials for Consumer Health Informatics services require additional sophistication because they cannot assume that the subject is a chemical processor of the therapeutic substance and at the same time part of a measuring device. The subject rather is and is meant to be an active client who behaves to his liking and whose reporting of signs and symptoms is affected through reflections on the experiment and his role. Coping with such factors and confounders is an essential part of the augmented trial methodology for Consumer Health Informatics services.

1.4.1.2 Client Safety Assessment

Alongside with investigating efficacy, attention must be paid whether clients are of sound mind and capable of trustworthy communication and action. Think of an asthma patient who receives aerosol dosage recommendations based on his self reported recent dosage and shortage of breath. Such clients may become a risk for themselves by concealing or under-reporting signs, faking compliance or just disorientation in time or space. Like the family physician Consumer Health Informatics services need "senses", "seismographs", methods to monitor plausibility and consistency of client behavior which initiate human fallback intervention before some catastrophic failure hits.

1.4.1.3 Cost Effectiveness Analysis

Whenever a research approach is about to become a routine offering funding becomes a core question. Therefore, investigations that seriously estimate efforts made and savings, effects, or utilities gained provide the ground for sustainable establishment of the respective service.

Cost-effectiveness assessment is not an easy topic. With cost spread across development, deployment, maintenance, legal, on the side of the provider and equipment on the side of the user, and with the users spreading across a nation or beyond, such investigations have to handle various unknowns and still make a convincing case. For many researchers in medical informatics and the disciplines that deliver the medical content and help tailor the interaction, content and design appear as the primary challenges that have to be mastered. However, if cost effectiveness is not proven as well, investors, health plans, employers etc will not buy in. If they do not buy in, efforts will not scale up and nationwide effects will not be achieved. In other words: If Consumer Health Informatics as a set of services is taken seriously, cost effectiveness is the ultimate criterion.

1.4.1.4 Non-inferiority

For a Consumer Health Informatics service we may face the situation that it is much cheaper, more convenient, not restricted through limited numbers of professionals, or other advantage that makes it worthwhile to consider routine use. If only we knew that it is not inferior in medical effect. For such situations a new class of trial designs has been developed in bio-statistics. Non-inferiority designs take the inferiority – i.e. a difference in effect – as null hypothesis. If this null hypothesis is refuted they conclude that the new treatment is significantly not inferior. Since this is a sound method of proof – as opposed to claiming equal effect if superiority could not be proven – we present it as part of the Consumer Health Informatics evaluation methodology.

1.4.2 Going Life

1.4.2.1 Legal and Ethical Analysis

Consumer Health Informatics resides in a common arena with practicing medicine, professional counseling, trade, (healthy) lifestyle, peer support, and freedom of speech. Criteria to classify a service as being one of the above determines whether it can be offered legally in some country or state. The intrinsic global nature of Consumer Health Informatics adds the dimension of complexity which legislation applies when Consumer Health Informatics service provider, contents author and client reside in different states and whether laws can be enforced regarding scattered affiliations of the stakeholders. It should be noted that these precautions and concerns relate to routine operation. They do not relate to IRB supervised Consumer Health Informatics research because IRB approval necessitates that stakeholders are clearly identified and accountable.

1.4.2.2 Sustained Funding

While researchers in Consumer Health Informatics can apply for grants for NIH, NSF etc. other resources must be found for the transition to and sustenance of routine operation. Client fees, business and health care partnerships, subsidizing through merchandize or pharmaceutical sales, employer health benefits and state and health plan programs are compared.

Take Home
For Consumer Health Informatics services to make it from full functionality to routine use, their added value, their legal nature and a source of continued funding must be secured.

1.5 Hardware

The following outline will demonstrate that the hardware used for Consumer Health Informatics services comes in a large variety. According to the "set of services" perspectives that this volume takes hardware will only be expanded when the comprehension of a described service calls for hardware details. A general observation, however, is that a distinction between consumer products and specialized sensory becomes less important.

1.5.1 Voice and Sound

Some telephone contact based services qualify for Consumer Health Informatics criteria, including the pioneer IDEATel (cf. [11]). Human voice comes to mind as the natural correspondent to classical landline telephony. However, voice now also comes through IP and telephones with special keys for disabled are also used for simple alerting mechanisms. Human voice also comes through cell phones, which, again, can also be used as sensors for heart beat sounds or to localize an individual in need through GPS positioning. In other words: voice is not phone and phone is not voice anymore. Rather will we point to special opportunities of the multivalent phone technology when a service depends on it.

1.5.2 Biosignals

Heart rate, ECG, spirometry, skin conductivity etc. have become mobile or available in the client's home. However, off the shelf consumer electronics can be reprogrammed to be biosignal detectors, like the cell phone based heart rate monitor in Sect. 1.5.1. Acceleration sensor devices have long been in use in aeronautics and control of vehicles of all kinds. Now they also help identify situations where a person may have fallen and come as specialized small tokens – like an amulet – or built into smart phones or tablets. Again distinctions between specialized sensory and consumer products blur. Non dedicated devices deliver dedicated information and dedicated devices deliver information they have not been invented for.

1.5.3 Pointing and Virtual Space

Pointing and clicking on a graphical computer display presently is the farthest spread metaphor for information exchange between humans and machines. Touchscreens are an easy extension of that metaphor. However, three-dimensional motion has become part of computer games such as Nintendo®'s Wii™ player. Why not use pointing or moving in 3D for measuring and training coordination, balance, or other medically relevant indicators? In combination with virtual reality enacted staged confrontations against phobias it is already in Consumer Health Informatics use, cf. Sect. 5.2.2.1. In other words: pointing persists as a metaphor that has gone far beyond graphical user interfaces of computer screens.

1.5.4 Positioning

Originating from military applications GPS has become widely available for civilian use since the year 2000, first through specialized navigation systems and fast progressing in consumer products such as navigation or activity tracking systems. Combined with digital maps it offers the opportunity to locate a device with an accuracy of appr. 1 meter, sufficient to assist the holder of the device in various ways. Applications for the client range from pure convenience functions such as identifying the nearest pharmacy to emergency rescue. Public health applications include tracking carriers of infectious diseases or refugee migration waves after natural disasters.

1.5.5 Smart Phones

Most of the above hardware features are now convening in the multi-talent "smart phone". Therefore, its role in Consumer Health Informatics is bound to grow although specific risks need attention and fall-backs when failure safe deployment of medical services is the agenda. As a successor of the classical mobile phone the smart phone is gaining ground so fast that it is covered in a dedicated chapter (cf. Chap. 7). In low and middle income countries broadband coverage is also increasing fast but smart phones are still in the minority. Therefore, voice, including IVR, and SMS exchange through client held phones still plays a role and proves efficient to foster treatment adherence in some cases.

> **Take Home**
> Although devices are necessary carriers of many services we mostly discuss them only to the extent that is required to understand their contribution to a service.

1.6 Where in the Literature is Consumer Health Informatics?

Consumer Health Informatics is a diverse field with a history of about 25 years. At the 2007 MedInfo conference in Brisbane where the author of this book gave a tutorial on Consumer Health Informatics and the plan for this book was born some 125 of the 715 contributions dealt with Consumer Health Informatics services, supportive methodologies, or evaluations. In the literature we find a growing number of endeavors and success stories. What we do not find yet is a comprehensive methodology, sustainable business models, and a genuine place in health care delivery.

Since Consumer Health Informatics is likely to be a forthcoming segment of the medical industry, its scientific progress should be covered in PubMed. To find it, however, the seeker has to be creative since it does not have a MeSH keyword. Search for partial strings of consumer health informatics creates mostly misleading concepts.

1.6.1 Fruitless Search for MeSH Keywords

Searching MeSH for Consumer Health returns Consumer Health Information = *Information intended for potential users of medical and health care services. There is an emphasis on self-care and preventive approaches as well as information for community-wide dissemination and use.* With the exception of *self care* this has the patient in a passive role only.

Consumer Health Information is subsumed in MeSH under Health education, which also subsumes Health Education, Dental; Health Fairs; Patient Education as Topic and Sex Education. With the exception of health fairs, there is an overlap but again the underlying perspective is one way: the client is a passive recipient.

Health informatics is expanded as Medical Informatics which is much too wide and Public Health Informatics = *The systematic application of information and computer sciences to public health practice, research, and learning. It is the discipline that integrates public health with information technology. The development of this field and dissemination of informatics knowledge and expertise to public health professionals is the key to unlocking the potential of information systems to improve the health of the nation.* This focuses on authorities that are officially in charge of public health. Consumer Informatics does not retrieve a MeSH term at all.

To conclude, information content is covered through the above MeSH keywords. However, how it is conveyed legally and safely in a comprehensive service where the client actively contributes is not covered. It is not covered, either, how to evaluate whether the client enjoys some benefit to his health or to his health related quality of life through subscribing to a service, how to implement a service in a sustainable scalable way when a trial has proved its value, how to finance without conflict of interest, how to maintain the character of the service when the knowledge changes, and cross-border delivery of medical services, to mention just a few.

1.6.2 Opportunistic Search in PubMed

For the following observations numerous MeSH keywords and boolean combinations of keywords were tentatively used to get an impression of their specificity. Most were discarded because less than 3 % of retrieved articles found in small samples each addressed Consumer Health Informatics services. Samples were too small and scrutiny of the investigation was not meant to be sufficient to claim this as a scientific result. However, to systematically achieve specificity above 1/3 likely target scenarios of Consumer Health Informatics services such as Health Promotion[MeSH], Health Knowledge, Attitudes, Practice[MeSH], Patient Education[MeSH], Patient Advocacy [MeSH], Peer Group[MeSH] or medical problems that suggest Consumer Health Informatics such as Smoking Cessation[MeSH] had to be combined with matching keywords denoting use of information and communication technology such as User-Computer Interface[MeSH], Internet[MeSH], Text Messaging[MeSH], Telephone[MeSH], Medical Informatics [MeSH] and a variety of others to eventually achieve a sufficient yield of pertinent articles.

1.6.3 Estimated Growth Rates

For combinations of one keyword denoting a type of service with one or several keywords denoting an informatics method of delivery specificities were roughly estimated based on small samples of 20 articles each. Development of publication numbers over time were then estimated based on automated PubMed queries for five four year intervals from 1994 to 2013. The figures in the curves each denote articles found times estimated specificity of a keyword combination boolean. Those combinations were included where specificities were above 0.6. Some of them are very general, such as Patient Education [MeSH] while others are very specific, such as Agoraphobia[MeSH] OR Phobic Disorders[MeSH]. For ((Smoking[MeSH] OR Smoking-Cessation[MeSH]) AND Internet

1.6 Where in the Literature is Consumer Health Informatics?

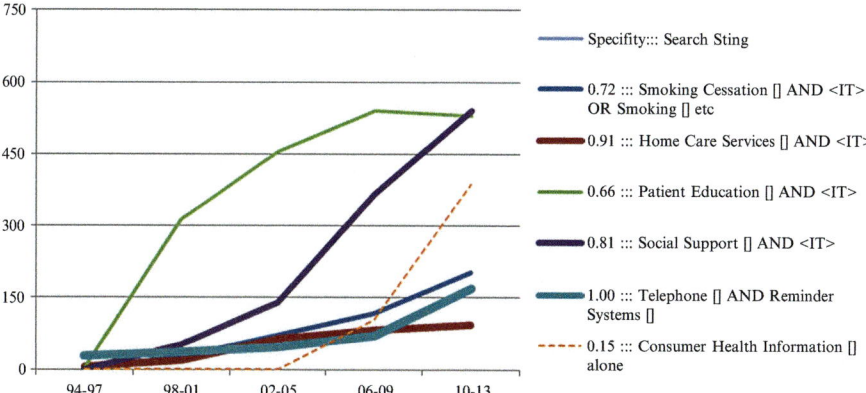

Fig. 1.1 Growth of literature on Consumer Health Informatics: General terms

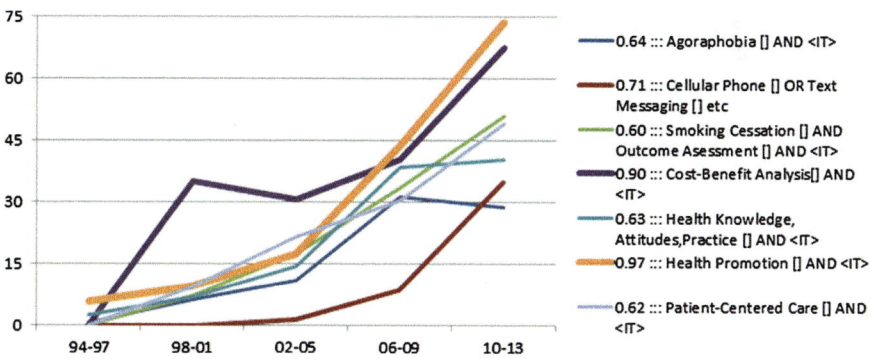

Fig. 1.2 Growth of literature on Consumer Health Informatics: Specific terms

[MeSH]) where both specificity and absolute numbers were among the largest, a conjunction with Outcome Assessment [MeSH] was also tested. Cellular Phone [MeSH] OR Text Messaging [MeSH] alone delivered sufficient return in the most recent time periods if AND Patients [MeSH] was added; so it was included as well. Furthermore, the apparently best matching keyword, Consumer Health Information was included although its specificity was only 0.15.

A first observation is that it is not at all a straightforward approach. It rather requires experience with both the field of Consumer Health Informatics and with MeSH to achieve reasonable search results. These are subsequently presented in two figures. Figure 1.1 displays results with high yield search strings that rendered between estimated 261 and 1841 results in the past 20 years, while Fig. 1.2 covers the smaller more specific part with between 45 and 174 articles. Legends show estimated specificity ::: service type [] AND <IT>, where <IT> denotes a keyword for information or communication technology. The thickness of a line points to the specificity of the respective search string.

The keywords selected for demonstration led to 5236 hits in 20 years, more than 40 % of which appeared in 2010 to 2013. It should be noted that these are not 5236 distinct articles, since there is a small overlap between the yields from different searches. However, when submitting the disjunction of all included search strings as one query the yield is 4558.[3] Therefore, the used keywords induce an overlap of only appr. 15 %. This underlines the above observation that readers will not find their articles by using just some keywords and hoping for collateral hits. It does not help either to rely on `Consumer Health Information`: it only contributes 491 or appr 10 % of the overall yield.

For most search strings and intervals we find increase and often accelerated increase, although there are noteworthy exceptions. An exception for which there is no explanation at hand is the third interval decline of `Cost-Benefit Analysis [MeSH] ...` and the last interval one of `Agoraphobia [MeSH] ....`. Declines or flattening increases in some of the other such as `Social Support [MeSH] ... Health Knowledge, Attitudes, Practice [MeSH] ...` and most obvious `Patient Education [MeSH] ...` are likely owed to the increase in `Consumer Health Information` in precisely the same period.

1.6.4 Scatter Across Media

As we already saw search for Consumer Health Informatics articles goes through numerous MeSH keywords, with moderate specificity at best. But articles are also scattered across numerous scientific journals. The 4700 distinct articles retrieved for the calendar years 1994 through 2013 are scattered across 1221 different journals. To some extent this reflects that Consumer Health Informatics has been tried for nearly every medical discipline. Therefore, articles with sufficient medical substance have partially reached medical specialty journals rather than journals devoted to the methodology of Consumer Health Informatics. There are actually many journals that have just one of the 4700 hits in 20 years. Zooming in to the more pertinent journals we find 301 with at least three articles in 20 years and 97 with at least eight. Finally, 22 journals collect more than 20 articles each, at least one per year. They have all been retrieved from PubMed i.e. are to some extent pertinent to medicine and delivery of health care. However, nine do not have a JCR impact factor. The remaining 13 are displayed in Fig. 1.3. They are ordered by numbers of articles found, and impact factors also displayed. As one would expect the "Journal of Medical Internet Research" (JMIR) is the leader – by a small margin – over "Patient

---

[3] At 1pm on July 1, 2014; at 6pm the yield was 4700, which are used for the analysis in Sect. 1.6.4.

1.6 Where in the Literature is Consumer Health Informatics?

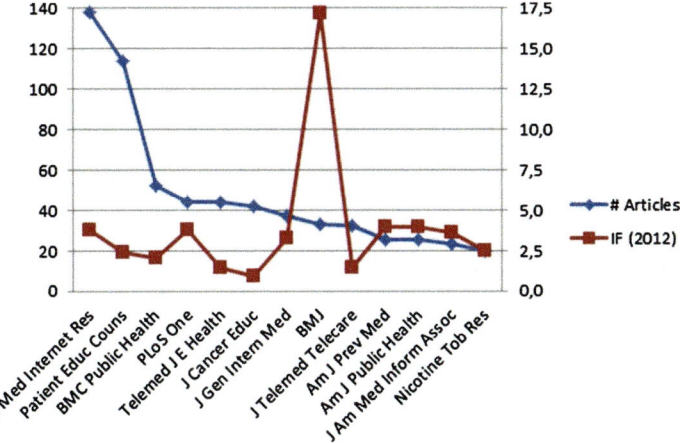

Fig. 1.3 Journals covering the largest volume of Consumer Health Informatics articles

Education and Counseling". The true margin in favor of JMIR is larger, since JMIR started in 1999 as opposed to 1990 for Patient Education and Counseling. Generally, the top 13 that have a JCR impact factor include core medical journals such as the impact factor leader "British Medical Journal" or "Nicotine and Tobacco Research". They also include others that are related to patient education dedicated in a medical domain such as "Journal of Cancer Education". This is where more articles would certainly be retrieved had we applied MeSH keywords throughout the medical specialties and sub-specialties. Finally, the top 13 include delivery of care journals such as "BMC Public Health" or "American Journal of Preventive Medicine" and informatics methods such as "Telemedicine Journal and e-Health" or "Journal of the American Medical Informatics Association". This appears appropriate regarding the multifaceted nature of Consumer Health Informatics. However, from the perspective of the researcher or practitioner who wants to keep himself up to date, it is a substantial logistics barrier. Few institutions will have subscriptions for all the journals listed.

As a side note, some of the non-JCR listed journals achieved high coverage with "Journal of Health Communication" scoring highest, 182 articles since its onset in 1996 and "Studies in Health Technology and Information" second, 80 articles, in the 20 years analyzed.

JMIR suggests to be a core journal and focal point in the field. With 1149 articles in the years 1999 through 2013 it offers a high volume combined with a high impact factor in comparison with other journals analyzed here. A closer look reveals some necessary distinctions. First, only 138 of the 1149 JMIR articles were retrieved through the search terms that underlie this bibliographic analysis. On a small sample of articles arbitrarily taken from the year 2012 a few reasons become visible immediately. The largest number of articles in JMIR that were rightly not retrieved through our keywords were Internet or mobile services that were not meant for patients but for health care professionals, such as Internet-based textbooks or CME (7/15). Five of 15 articles should have been retrieved. They were not because the MeSH keywords used for these articles were very specific in terms of the medical problems addressed or the delivery of care supported. This latter observation reemphasizes the fact that the lack of a dedicated keyword for services that assign active roles to patients in their health or preventive care is urgently needed to foster coherent communication in the field.

Take Home

Consumer Health Informatics is a fast growing field with an equally fast growing literature. However, to gain insights into the state of the art a seeker of pertinent articles must be extremely creative and extremely well endowed:

- Very few boolean combinations of MeSH terms achieve specificities above 0.6.
- The apparent MeSH term of choice `Consumer Health Information` achieves ~0.15.
- Articles are scattered across more than 1200 scientific journals.
- As many as 22 journals publish one ore more articles per year.

Therefore, a researcher who needs an overview, will spend a lot of time on search and a lot of money on purchasing from journals that his institution has not subscribed.

1.7 Aims of This Volume

1.7.1 Positive Attitude: We Need It

Most Western societies feel similar stress on their health care systems. Medical progress and aging societies create the impression that the cost of health care is continually rising. It may be asked whether the cost per unit care delivered really rises or whether we rather have an imbalance between growing demand by more persons in need for more advanced available treatments, and funds for the medical industry not growing.

But money is the smaller problem. Little attention has been paid so far to the fact that we are also facing a growing imbalance between the working generation a proportion of which is the medical workforce and the retirement age population that needs services over-proportionally. With an increasing number of elderly and also with an increasing number of lifestyle related chronic conditions already occurring at a relatively young age, the imbalance between care providers and care receivers will continue to deteriorate. Unless we accept denial of many services to many in need we either require a substantially increased medical workforce or new ways of

1.7 Aims of This Volume

delivery of medical services. This book will try to make the case that Consumer Health Informatics suggests itself as one such way.

1.7.2 Wide Perspective: It Can Be Done

To make this case the book will among others draw on numerous examples. They include:

- Teaching clients to assess the trustworthiness of medical websites (Sect. 3.5.1)
- Internet delivered chronic pain management (Sect. 4.4.2)
- Internet delivered depression treatment (Sect. 5.2.2.3)
- An app for diabetic kids and their parents to advise on glucose uptake and insulin dosage (Sect. 5.3.4.4)
- An app to analyze photos of suspicious skin regions for melanoma (Sect. 5.3.4.5)
- Internet pharmacies (Sect. 5.4)
- Smart home environments where sensors monitor for clients' safety and convenience (Sect. 11.2)
- New knowledge being discovered from text mining patient self help social media (Sect. 6.3.3)
- SMS encouragement to seek skilled birth attendants' service in Tanzania (Sect. 10.2.2.1.2)

Not all these services are laudable. But they demonstrate that no age group, no region, no medical domain, no sector of IT or CT is missing.

1.7.3 Sound Methodology: How It Should Be Done

The number and variety of examples create a feeling of feasibility in their own right. Some, however, will also arouse a feeling of doubt whether the presented Consumer Health Informatics service is medically safe, legal, technically reliable, manageable through the client etc. The major research and educational contribution of this book is to provide methods and mental tools to assess existing or to plan future Consumer Health Informatics services, to identify risks and whether they can be curbed, to establish efficacy, to understand the legal nature and if need be ethical foundations to advance legislation, and to plan a service as a business, including cost-effectiveness and funding models. Assessing all these aspects before starting to build something should enable the reader to check upfront whether a planned service has a fair chance to succeed or whether it would be a responsible decision not to develop or deploy the service.

> **Take Home**
> For demographic reasons our societies need Consumer Health Informatics. Consumer Health Informatics is happening in many experiments and few routine services all around us. A methodology is evolving. It is the aim of this volume to substantiate all these assertions.

1.8 Organization of the Book in Detail

The book has three major parts and various appendices. These parts are devoted to a systematic entry into the field, to selected aggregations of examples, and to supportive methodology.

1.8.1 Organization of the Book: Part I

Part I, "Introducing the domain and levels of service", first introduces the field as a whole and some of its pioneering services. After the present chapter with its more in-depth introductory remarks we have a detailed analysis and models that substantiate the claim that we are absolutely running short in supply of health care personnel in not more than 15 years and that, therefore, Consumer Health Informatics may play an important role in taking workload off the human delivered medical care (Chap. 2).

The four next chapters are each devoted to one level of Consumer Health Informatics services. Each comes with the characteristics of the level and various examples. The levels are one of the most important new mental tools to bring order to the overwhelming variety, not to say chaos, of Consumer Health Informatics ventures. Level 0, which carries the number 0 because the service nature is only marginal here, is the arena of the Internet, the Play and App Stores, etc where providers advertise themselves, where clients seek and sometimes find. Legally it mostly is the arena of the First amendment of the US constitution or the German Recht der freien Meinungsäußerung. Therefore, evidence free unwarranted personal opinion finds itself next to highly serious well researched articles or apps. Provider side quality and client side sophistication of search raise the odds that he who searches finds appropriate information (Chap. 3). Level 1 Consumer Health Informatics services enhance an existing provider – client relation through methods and devices of ICT. Examples include enhanced discharge management, management of chronic diseases such as chronic pain, asthma, rheumatism, but also mental diseases such as depression. Phone calls between physician and patient that have been made for decades also fall under Level 1. Numerous means other than synchronous landline telephony are now available. Their use is to some extent covered through AMA policies and corresponding corpora in other countries. However, physicians face farther ranging responsibility and accountability depending on the data shared and the media used (Chap. 4). Level 2 Consumer Health Informatics services abstain from face-to-face initiation of the provider – client relation, they are virtual only. Examples include all conditions above but also various risk awareness, screening, and preventive services. We also encounter logistics support – physician locator and scoring systems, Internet pharmacies etc. Level 2 offers great opportunities in terms of effective service that would scale up easily. However, Level 2 services that present as practicing medicine rather than just delivering information of all kinds, are illegal. Therefore, besides the full range of medical, technical, financial, etc challenges the design of Level 2 service must also be very well considered legally (Chap. 5). In Level 3 Consumer Health Informatics services roles change again: Rather than professionals as providers, patients offer their advice and experience in self-support groups. Such groups mushroom for conditions such as breast cancer, diabetes, hypertension, etc. Most material provided is meant seriously and at least subjectively true. Moderators may have an eye on totally off the mark contributions. However, contents of self-support media have proved so valuable and objectively true that new off-label indications for pharmaceuticals or new side effects of chemo-therapies could be discovered (Chap. 6). Legally, Level 3 Consumer Health Informatics services are covered through freedom of speech. Only if physicians assume a one-on-one counselor role with individual clients Level 2 legal analysis may apply.

While considerations above are mostly independent of whether the Internet or mobile apps are the underlying carrier technology, Part I concludes with one chapter on specific aspects of mobile apps. It addresses simplicity, ubiquity, and the fun effect as enablers of broad acceptance. It also notes the lack of any medical quality assurance on the part of the distributors (e.g. Apple, Google^{TM}, Amazon$^{®}$) and that even well informed clients may have hard times to verify quality themselves. It furthermore notes new dependencies and incurred risks for sustained delivery of Consumer Health Informatics services through apps (Chap. 7).

1.8.2 Organization of the Book: Part II

Part II, "Building safety nets around the active client", devotes the first and the last chapter to the client and his interests, capabilities, limitations and incurred risks. The client has been termed the least utilized and at the same time most vulnerable resource in his own health care. To get our hands on vulnerabilities we first introduce dimensions of risk leading to an assessment scheme. They include predispositions for diseases that would modify advice delivered such as screening intervals for breast cancer. They also include limitations on the client's part to cooperate with the service, such as adverse attitudes, emotional lability, or insufficient literacy. Finally we address the necessity to authenticate actors who cooperate with Consumer Health Informatics services. The first chapter of Part II names and motivates the dimensions of risk and makes strong claims that it is the responsibility of a

Consumer Health Informatics service provider to assess and control risks pertinent to the specific service (Chap. 8). In the last chapter in Part II selected technical solutions to satisfy the raised claims are presented (Chap. 12).

In between we present various example domains – for their own sake but also to deliver contexts to discuss the risk management solutions. The first application chapter is medically motivated. We walk through the metabolic syndrome from primary prevention through management of diabetes to attenuation of comorbidities. Consumer Health Informatics services from all levels have been selected to demonstrate the diversity in approach and effectiveness (Chap. 9). The second application chapter is motivated through a basic technology – mobile phones with their capacity of voice and text communication – and the consequential opportunity to also reach typically under-served populations and populations in 3rd world countries. The third application chapter is motivated by a scenario: frail persons wishing to live independently as long as possible. Smart home functionalities are introduced and analyzed from an acceptance and ethics perspective (Chap. 11).

1.8.3 Organization of the Book: Part III

Part III, "Additional methodology", addresses topics that may not come to mind immediately but support necessary steps to take Consumer Health Informatics "from bench to palmtop". First we analyze what privacy, authenticity, integrity and other requirements exist for data used in Consumer Health Informatics services and how these requirements can be satisfied. Next we analyze and compare the options of longitudinal electronic records of clients' health histories to be maintained by providers ("Patient Portal") or by the clients themselves ("Personal Health Records") and how this relates to Meaningful Use (MU). The following chapter is devoted to method to prove effectiveness, cost-effectiveness, non-inferiority, i.e. the value added through new a Consumer Health Informatics service. Special emphasis is given to the fact that active client contributions are central to Consumer Health Informatics and that therefore all kinds of clients' reflections, second thoughts, and agendas interfere with a treatment effect. Once proven effective services leave the arena of research funding and enter the field of regular business and health care. The next chapter analyzes models how to fund Consumer Health Informatics services in routine use. Finally, we deliver a detailed analysis and a wide range of ethics arguments whether services are still legal when no longer safeguarded through IRB approved precautions of a trial and how societies can and should get prepared to legalize approved and safe services.

1.9 Additional Topics Worth Individual Chapters Under the Viewpoint Taken

When the services perspective on Consumer Health Informatics is taken various topics would deserve chapters but go beyond the scope of this volume.

1.9 Additional Topics Worth Individual Chapters Under the Viewpoint Taken

1.9.1 Scalability

One of the claims of this whole approach to Consumer Health Informatics is that it delivers care at nearly the same level as humans would, however for growing populations without need to increase the workforce at the same proportion as the client base. This is the question or challenge of scalability. It is only briefly and anecdotally addressed in Sect. 5.5.

1.9.2 Disparity

It is a common expectation towards health care delivery that it each reaches all in equal need equally. This includes the theoretical challenges addressed in Sect. 17.11.7 to specify "equal", "equally" and to set up procedures to practically determine a justified need. In practice we face the problem over again that Consumer Health Informatics services primarily serve the rich, the well educated, the non-minorities, with few notable exceptions that use the basic technology of Chap. 10 (Sects. 10.2.4 and 10.2.3). Therefore the present patterns and degree of disparity and methods to reduce it deserve more attention than they have in this volume.

1.9.3 Public Health

In terms of benefits for whole societies public health surveillance and outreach are very worthwhile applications for Consumer Health Informatics. Just a few examples are included (cf. Sects. 10.2.1 and 10.3.1). Basic principles of designing campaigns in the light of new logistic options but also related privacy concerns should be addressed more basically.

1.9.4 Rare Diseases

Bringing together the widely geographically scattered knowledge of patients suffering from a rare disease benefits utmost from virtual vicinity in Internet based self support groups. The potential and dynamics of such groups in general are the topic of Chap. 6. To bring the technical opportunities to bear problems such as a common language or translation functions in international groups have to be addressed.

1.9.5 Applications

Since medical applications are used throughout and give rise to three chapters in Part II there is no chapter for applications as such. Rather are all medical or delivery of care applications searchable through an index point "application, <type of application>".

1.10 Alternative Viewpoints

Consumer Health Informatics with all is aspects is by far too large to be fully covered in one book. In the following sections we mention some directions that can legitimately be considered to be part of or even to constitute Consumer Health Informatics. For these we argue how they relate to the perspective taken here and why we have not chosen to put them center stage.

1.10.1 Transient Stimuli and Funding Programs

Much has been moved in the US since the release of the Meaningful Use (www.healthit.gov/policy-researchers-implementers/meaningful-use-regulations) and the Health IT Strategic Planning (www.healthit.gov/policy-researchers-implementers/health-it-strategic-planning) programs in the years 2009 and 2011. The Meaningful Use campaign has directed money and hence attention towards upgrading the EHR, at Stage 1 by data quality and coverage of the clinical encounter, at Stage 2 towards exchange of information and care coordination and at Stage 3 to demonstrate that outcomes improve. Stage 2 includes the request to the provider to make data available to the patient electronically in a timely manner and communicate with him through secure electronic media. This certainly contributes to but it should not be equated with Consumer Health Informatics. It requests technical solutions and secure processes of information sharing but does not address whether the patient can meaningfully use the revealed information. It does not care about client literacy, has no safeguard against irrational reactions to alarming data, let alone concise planned utilization in Consumer Health Informatics Level 1 or Level 2 services. Finally Meaningful Use Stage 3 outcomes are not health outcomes but structure and process quality outcomes such as equal coverage of under-served populations or that patients participate in shared decision making. To summarize: Meaningful Use is likely to foster Consumer Health Informatics but it is not Consumer Health Informatics .

The Health IT Strategic Planning starts with Stage 3 of Meaningful Use and sets performance goals on top, relating to health care cost, health outcome, trust into, and adoption of health IT. Goal IV is to "Empower Individuals with Health

IT to Improve their Health and the Health Care System". In its rationale it argues that a "public that has a voice in designing ... IT policies and programs ... can be a powerful driver ...". If the right public actually raises that voice this may come true. The question, however, is whether healthy volunteers are the right public and, if not, if patients with a severe condition are willing to serve as volunteers. Looking deeper into Goal IV it requests to "integrate patient-generated health information and consumer health IT with clinical application to support patient-centered care." This comes closest to what this volume is about. It should be noted that in the Health IT Strategic Planning consumer health IT is regarded as an industry and a market with no mention who pays for its products and services. The program repeatedly writes of consumer health IT applications and never of services. This seems to take for granted that an application is good and safe when it is functional, like in Sect. 1.10.3. This premise is challenged in Chaps. 8 and 12 of this volume.

> **Take Home**
> The Meaningful Use (MU) program has directed a lot of attention and funding to functions in health IT that are or come close to Consumer Health Informatics. Three major differences are
>
> - MU formulates requirements while Consumer Health Informatics develops and deploys solutions.
> - MU requests functionality of applications while Consumer Health Informatics regards applications as parts of services and focuses on the end-to-end service quality.
> - MU is US based while Consumer Health Informatics is universal.

1.10.2 Devices

1.10.2.1 Quantified Self

Quantified Self, also known as Personal Analytics or through various other terms, is a vibrant movement where all kind of gadgetry in consumers' hands – mostly, actually, in consumers' pockets or around consumers' wrists or chests – measure vital signs that would have been regarded part of the holy medical grail one generation earlier. Off the shelf products[4] record and communicate to smart phones cardiovascular, sleep, and all kinds of motion parameters. More advanced devices from emerging other manufacturers cover breathing, muscle tone, skin conductivity

---

[4]According to www.mobihealthnews.com/28825/fitbit-jawbone-nike-had-97-percent-of-fitness-tracker-retail-sales-in-2013/ Fitbit®, Jawbone®, Nike™ together had a market share of 97 % in 2013.

and many more. At the core Quantified Self is individuals tracking themselves, for health, narcissistic, psychotic or other reason and interpreting signs and trends with respect to some medical or not so medical theory. The subjective motive and motivation can be improving health through health awareness. But if misguided it may cause harm by taking basically healthy behaviors too far or by seeking behavioral cures where medical interventions are due.

Quantified Self makes its way through numerous web site and app store finds. Millions of hits show when searching Google™ for `quantified self`. Scholarly writing is rare if not absent and there is no MeSH keyword. Bookshelves are dominated by the writings of apostles of the movement.

If made available as part of a well considered and safe service, self quantified data can be valuable in different ways:

- individually: to provide a history that precedes or overlaps with a newly diagnosed disease. Good data may inform a more targeted treatment.
- as a group experience: to share obstacles mastered and achievements made with peers. Advice from persons in equal situations may be more trustworthy and convincing than abstract advice from textbooks or programs.
- for society: to substantiate new research through pooled data from self quantifier peer groups. For other types of data the emergence of new insights from mass client data is discussed in Chap. 6.

Therefore, self quantifying can contribute to Consumer Health Informatics and it definitely has the client in the central agent role. However, if not embedded in a service with a diagnostic or therapeutic concept and with safeguards against the consequences of inappropriate use it is not Consumer Health Informatics.

1.10.2.2 Medical Devices

Quantified Self resides in the realm of well-being and better life and the consumer has convenient access to data recorded for inspection, monitoring, goal setting, and sharing with peers. Quantified Self does not claim to diagnose, let alone cure, diseases. Therefore, regulation only applies to electrically safe function as it would for other consumer electronics products. Opposed to that medical devices are a genuine part of medical procedures, some fundamentally supporting patient survival, such as implanted insulin pumps or cardiac pacemakers. Somewhere in the middle is medical software that includes control of such devices, decision support, collection and presentation of data etc. `Medical devices` is not a MeSH keyword, however, `Equipment and supplies` seems to cover historically while `Medical device legislation` was not introduced until 2013, more than 20 years later than the pertinent legislation outlined below. There are, though, numerous textbooks that instruct on procedures to take medical devices to market.

The approach to legally using devices and software for genuinely medical purposes differs between the European Union (EU) and the USA.

1.10 Alternative Viewpoints

US legislation introduces Medical Devices in the 1976 amendment [12] to the 1938 FD&C (Federal Food, Drug, and Cosmetic Act). In the 1938 law the Secretary of Agriculture is named as the executive force to implement and control the subsequent regulations but has for long delegated to the FDA which outlines the present procedures at http://www.fda.gov/MedicalDevices/DeviceRegulationandGuidance/Overview/default.htm. Its major ingredients are risk classes I, II, and III with class number increasing device intrusiveness and autonomy. It requests general controls for class I, performance standards for class II, and premarket approval for class III. In the most recent amendment the "Safe Medical Devices Act of 1990" [9] a strong element of tracing devices in use has been added. Adverse event reporting and policies to react and to retract if need be are provided.

Simply speaking, class I devices are matters that are attached externally to the body without interactivity with the patient, such as earphone cushions of audiometers, air or water caloric stimulators or battery-powered external artificial larynxes. Class II devices include potentially powered devices that perform according to settings made by a specialist user and do not behave autonomically. Examples are transcutaneous air conduction hearing aid systems that amplify sound to compensate for impaired hearing or electroglottographs, AC-powered measuring devices of the performance of the larynx. Class III devices, finally, exert autonomous action such as a suction antichoke devices to automatically suck objects from an obstructed airway or cardiovascular pacemakers (all examples from http://www.fda.gov/MedicalDevices/DeviceRegulationandGuidance/Overview/ClassifyYourDevice/ucm051530.htm).

The examples have been selected to demonstrate a common principle of the still prevailing medical devices legislation which is implicitly present everywhere. The 1976 amendment for class III premarket approval requests to "determine() the safety and effectiveness ... with respect to the persons ... and the conditions of use" and that the "effectiveness ... be determined ... by experts qualified by training and experience" ([12], Sec 513 (a)(2)–(3)) Although never mentioned explicitly the whole spirit is that clinicians apply and patients undergo the use of devices. Patients as accountable users are not covered yet although the need is obvious from many places in this volume.

At about the time of the Safe Medical Devices Act of 1990 the European Union has created a common abstract framework for medical devices called Directive 93/42/EEC in 1993 which has been turned into national legislations in the subsequent years. Judging from the German implementation we find the same basic ideas as in the USA: Increasing classes of risk call for more scrutinized procedures to demonstrate safe use. Noteworthy differences in detail are:

- The duration of applying a device to the patient's body plays an important role in the EU.
- Rather than just II Europe has two risk classes IIa and IIb that differ in the duration of application or degree of invasiveness or criticality of targeted organs.

- For the highest risk class III the directive encourages providers to build and get approval for an all encompassing quality assurance system in which case they need not seek external approval for devices to be brought to market.
- Software is explicitly mentioned as a device in its own right or as part of a device. Validation according to the principles of the software industry is requested. Software alone is assigned a risk class in application of the same rules as for devices while software that is part of a device inherits the risk class of the device.

Although only marginally mentioned in the EU directive it is clearly meant for medical devices to be applied to patients through clinicians. US legislation and EU directive share the "blind" spot of not regulating devices for the hands of accountable clients.

To summarize, the field of devices for health purposes is split into a consumer segment and a professional segment. The consumer segment is only regulated to the extent that electrical devices are. Such gadgets are fully in the client's responsibility and clinicians are not legitimized to prescribe the use or incorporate collected data into their decision making because they would rely on functionality for which there exists no proof. The professional segment perfectly fits into a paternalistic conception of medicine where maxims of nonmaleficence and benevolence make the clinician fully accountable towards the patient and where he needs security that devices he uses are as effective and safe as can reasonably be assured. Consumer Health Informatics in the sense of this volume requests end-to-end provider responsibility. Though fostering client agent-ship a provider assumes the role of safeguarding client cooperation. Such Consumer Health Informatics requires features from both devices segments: that use of devices is safe, that they are incorporated in comprehensive services, and that clients are actively involved whenever appropriate. The devices market is not yet prepared for that.

Since software plays an ever growing role in both clinical care and Consumer Health Informatics the following spotlight on legislation of medical devices software demonstrates controversy and need for action here as well. Approaches differ strongly between the USA and Europe.

In the United States the regulation of software has been debated for long. A legislative initiative around the year 2000 to establish FDA approval of software under an amendment of the Federal Food, Drug, and Cosmetic Act ("FD&C Act") was countered by informatics professional associations which rather suggested to establish local Software Oversight Committees. More recently, in 2014 Congress representatives introduced the PROTECT initiative[5] which suggests that most medical and health software be exempt from FDA regulation. The legislative initiative is driven by an open market spirit: that the fast growing market of clinical and health software not be impeded by slow regulation. It covers software that supports

---

[5] Available at http://www.fischer.senate.gov/public/_cache/files/7b25f3a3-2d8b-4638-aba9-b12cc68fde0d/tam14031.pdf

health care providers in a health care setting ("clinical") from administrative or operational software outside immediate delivery of care ("health"). This definition presumably covers all hospital based or personalized electronic health records which active Consumer Health Informatics often assumes as a passive resource in the background. The definition excludes software that "directly diagnose(s) a patient ...without the intervention of a health care professional" or that is integral part or component of a (physical) device. So for the most advanced uses of devices in Consumer Health Informatics services we are thrown back to the "devices in the hands of clinicians" stalemate. Only recently have first advances been made by the FDA where guidance is provided what kinds of mobile health apps need or do not need regulation ([5][6]).

In Europe the situation is reverse in some sense. While the US trend is towards less regulation the European is towards more. In its Directive 2007/47/EC [4] the European Union unmistakably declared that software for medical purposes fully falls under the regulations that already hold for medical devices. National legislations were put into place in the subsequent years which turn out as a major obstacle for professional software, let alone the fast market of consumer software and apps.

> **Take Home**
> The Consumer Health Informatics related devices arena is not precisely circumscribed and in flux. The border between well-being, lifestyle and home electronics, quantified self on the one and medical devices on the other end is not clearly drawn. For devices deemed medical in the USA and Europe we have different risk classes. Especially for software regarded as a medical device a liberal attitude dominates in the USA, to exempt software from regulation in the best interest of an impediment free development and use. By contrast the EU has recently subsumed medical software under devices and enforced a process of national legislations to handle software accordingly.

1.10.3 User Centeredness

A survey by Hesse and Shneiderman [7] comes close in analysis. The authors report about the enormous progress in terms of computers and Internet access, the growth of health related information and the high and broad consumer interest in medical topics such as cancer. However, they write, "(w)hat people often found online, though, was a cacophony of mixed messages and information sites of

---

[6]FDA released an update under the same URL that came too late to be incorporated into this edition.

unequal quality and usefulness" and "credibility differences between physician and Internet may be widening, with trust in physicians trending upwards and trust in the Internet trending downwards". In line with requests made by the IOM [3] they raise demands towards safety, effectiveness, patient-centeredness and timeliness, which are partially congruent with the approach that we take in this volume but often do not "go the extra mile" that we believe needs to be gone. For safety they assign a role to the client's environment – as we do – and advocate for foolproof systems to be achieved by consistent, predictable, controllable interfaces. They neglect risks we see that the user may not be consistent, predictable and in control of his behavior at some point in time. Their effectiveness demand burns down to making that which is known available as fast and as pervasively and intellegibly as possible through good interfaces. They want evidence visibly built into the system. Our notion of effectiveness rather is that evidence be delivered whether a whole Consumer Health Informatics service is superior to delivering the same service through human beings, or at least non inferior and lower in effort. Hesse and Shneiderman consider patient-centeredness as taking the biological and the communicational nature of the patient into account. They demand for biological pathways and pharmacogenetics adapted advice, as we do. As to communication they advocate a "principle of universal design" and virtual "curb cuts": design principles that enable equitable access for all and e.g. the use of text-reading software for the visually impaired. Their anticipation that "plain language ... will help ensure that labels, instructions, ... are equally accessible to all" seems overoptimistic regarding the fact that more than 40 Mio US inhabitants presumable are functionally illiterate (cf. Sect. 8.4.3.2.1). Finally, their timeliness claim is very general, mainly pointing to the risks of multifaceted information systems with ads poping up and multiple layers of telephone answering functions standing in the way of immediate access to ones personally relevant information. Generally Hesse and Shneiderman's perspective of putting the user and his immediate environment center stage is in accordance with our approach. However, with more being known now than 2007 we have to take their steps somewhat farther.

> **Take Home**
> User centeredness in the way propagated in [7] emphasizes an important common element with Consumer Health Informatics: that diligence and clear principles are required to deploy information systems that users can handle easily and conveniently. We are less optimistic that this will guarantee communication without flaws, trustworthy behavior, clients' unblurred perception of data they record, and the huge in volume problem of illiteracy.

References

1. Chidzambwa L. The social considerations for moving health care services into the home: a telecare perspective. Health Policy Technol. 2013;2:10–25. doi: 10.1016/j.hlpt.2012.12.003.
2. Coiera E. Four rules for the reinvention of health care. BMJ. 2004;328:1197–9.
3. Institute of Medicine Committee on Quality of Health Care in America. Crossing the quality chasm: a new health system for the 21st century. Washington, DC: The National Academies Press; 2001.
4. EU. Directive 2007/47/ec of the European Parliament and of the Council. ec.europa.eu/consumers/archive/sectors/medical-devices/files/revision_docs/2007-47-en_en.pdf, Sept 2007.
5. FDA. Mobile medical applications. Guidance for industry and food and drug administration staff. http://www.fda.gov/downloads/MedicalDevices/.../UCM263366.pdf, Sept 2013.
6. Gray JE, Safran C, Davis RB, Pompilio-Weitzner G, Stewart JE, Zaccagnini L, Pursley D. Baby CareLink: using the internet and telemedicine to improve care for high-risk infants. Pediatrics. 2000;106(6):1318–24.
7. Hesse BW, Shneiderman B. eHealth research from the user's perspective. Am J Prev Med. 2007;32(5S):S97–103. doi: 10.1016/j.amepre.2007.01.019.
8. Masys D, Baker D, Butros A, Cowles KE. Giving patients access to their medical records via the internet: the PCASSO experiment. JAMIA. 2002;9(2):181–91. doi: 10.1197/jamia.M1005.
9. 101st Congress. Safe medical devices act of 1990. thomas.loc.gov/cgi-bin/query/z?c101:H.R. 3095:, Jan 1990.
10. Shea S, Kothari D, Teresi JA, Kong J, Eimicke JP, Lantigua RA, Palmas W, Weinstock RS. Social impact analysis of the effects of a telemedicine intervention to improve diabetes outcomes in an ethnically diverse, medically underserved population: findings from the IDEATel study. Am J Public Health. 2013;103:1888–94. doi: 10.2105/AJPH.2012.300909.
11. Shea S, Starren J, Weinstock RS, Knudson PE, Teresi J, Holmes D, Palmas W, Field L, Goland R, Tuck C, Hripcsak G, Capps L, Liss D. Columbia University's Informatics for Diabetes Education and Telemedicine (IDEATel) project: rationale and design. JAMIA. 2002;9(1):49–62.
12. 94th Congress. Medical Device Amendment of 1976. www.gpo.gov/fdsys/pkg/STATUTE-90/pdf/STATUTE-90-Pg539.pdf, May 1976.
13. Zhang J, Johnson TR, Patel VL, Paige DL, Kubose T. Using usability heuristics to evaluate patient safety of medical devices. J Biomed Inform. 2003;36(1):23–30. doi: 10.1016/S1532-0464(03)00060-1.

Chapter 2
Economy 1: Immanent Mismatch Between Demand and Supply of Health Care Workforce

2.1 Introduction

Developed mostly western countries have enjoyed more than six decades without major wars, epidemics, or famines. Populations get older in most of these countries. The phenomenon is almost universal, but its pace and shape differs across countries. With the exception of fading effects of World War Two still visible in 1960, the comparison between the 1960, the 2000 and the extrapolated 2040 age cohort pyramids suggest themselves as displaying intrinsic natural trends of populations in the absence disasters.

The years between 1950 and 1960 have been characterized as the baby boom. Birth rates were higher than death rates, reflecting optimism in a positive future on the one hand and continued medical progress on the other. After the baby boom came the baby bust and is here to stay. At the same time life expectancy has increased at a constant rate of 2 years per decade, with women always ahead half a decade of longer life expectancy for no known biological reason.

As a consequence it has become broadly acknowledged that population pyramides in developed societies are changing their shape. With proportions of older age groups increasing we are permanently confronted with dire prognosis about the funding of retirement pensions and of health care. This chapter will substantiate some of these demographic arguments by providing historical and recent figures and projections. It will, however, put more emphasis on work force than on finance. Concretely, we will analyze how populations have grown and will presumably keep growing or will decline, do the same for the whole work force and the health care work force and will come to observations and projections as to how many individuals in a population used to share, share now and will share in the foreseeable future the services of one physician, one nurse etc. i.e. we will explore several variants of the old age dependency ratio, resp. the more illustrative 1/old age dependency. Since utilization of health care resources is much higher at older ages leaving away young age dependency should not affect the validity of predicting health care services shortage too much. This is also underlined through a leaflet by the American Geriatrics Society at http://www.americangeriatrics.org/files/documents/Adv_Resources/PP_Priorities.pdf which contrasts the requirements for medical and nursing care of young and old people and through [6] which adds to the workload imposed upon the health care system through excess need of the chronically ill.

Under the assumptions that the population development continues along the lines of the past decades and that the organization of health care generally remains the same we will extrapolate that either health professionals will have to serve many more individuals or that a much larger proportion of the working population will have to work in the health care industry. Here finance will be back in the game: in that case a much larger part of the GDP will have to flow into health care.

> **Take Home**
> If populations in developed countries keep developing like in the past decades without any major disaster, a scarcity of the work force and primarily the health care workforce is immanent. Methods to substantiate and quantify this prognosis extrapolate from present population and medical industry statistics and census data.

2.2 Methodological Considerations

Regarding the sizes of the analyzed national economies, the immense variety of data being collected and published, and the inherent imprecision of census and population statistics selections have to be made and achieved results cannot claim to be more than orders of magnitudes and trends. Achieved projections will, however, demonstrate such a clear supply vs. demand deficit that some imprecision in the base data does not invalidate the drawn conclusions. Subsequently we outline and provide argument for the criteria applied to use some and not to use other data and how and why to combine them, trying to point to types of errors that the made choices may entail.

2.2.1 Criteria to Select Variables

Among the tremendous numbers of potentially useful variables we concentrate on very few. We only cover a time range of 40 years, some more than 20 years into the past and some less than 20 years into the future. We use overall population only i.e. we do not distinguish male-female, ethnicity, religion, education, region and type of residence etc. Within the population we only distinguish three age groups (Young age, Working age, Old age). To characterize the supply of health care we leave all material assets such as hospitals, practices, radiation units etc. and all consumed supply (pharmaceuticals, walking aids...) away. We rather concentrate on those resources that are hardest to multiply or to replace: physicians and nurses. Within the profession of physicians we do not distinguish specialties and we do not address part-time work at all.

2.2.2 Criteria to Select Nations

Health, diseases, suffering, and health care are universal phenomena. Qualitative aspects of disease and cure such as evolving threats (e.g. multiresistant bacteriae, the obesity epidemic, an increase in stress induced incidence of mental health problems) or evolving opportunities (e.g. minimally invasive surgery, genomic profiling, patient initiated enrollment in clinical trials) are universal but will not be addressed explicitly. However, while many other industries (traffic and transportation, finance, communication etc.) behave globally organization of health care is markedly different across countries. Therefore, trying to average across countries does not make sense. The same applies to age: trying to average across dynamics of aging populations would blur characteristic developments. Therefore, we prefer not to discuss the relation between population dynamics and health care organization with reference to the population of the developed countries as a whole but rather take two representative countries and their dynamics as examples for the following arguments. We try to derive that their national economics each almost inevitably face severe shortage of human resource or – in the unlikely case of dramatic growth of the health care workforce – severe financial demand, if present population developments continue without major interventions.

Two countries have been selected to provide most of the data and arguments for a number of reasons: The United States of America and Germany both have a solid foundation of statistical data but differ somewhat in their population dynamics and differ markedly in their organization and financing of the health care system. Some detail about the difference is supplied in Sect. 17.4. Studying other health care systems goes beyond the scope of this volume.

Publicly available figures about the population development and the quantitative development of the health care industries are retrieved from various sources and finally summarized in Table 2.2.

2.2.3 Criteria to Select Information Resources

As different as the societies and their health care systems themselves are their reporting authorities. Therefore, absolute figures may not be comparable *across* countries. However, as long as reporting authorities are used consistently and consequently *within* each country, at least trends *within* such as percent increase or percent decrease per unit time should be reliable. As to Germany not even this is easy, because Germany underwent a major turnover in 1988 through 1990 when the two states of Federal Republic of Germany ("West Germany") and German Democratic Republic ("East Germany") merged (German unification). German figures from before 1990 are, therefore, based on different polling and reporting structures and should not be used here. Hence, we compare trends from past (1990/1) to present (2008/10), the most recent consolidated data in both the USA and the unified Germany throughout the fields of population, work force, and health care.

> **Take Home**
> The USA and Germany are large representatives of very different health care systems. Reliable historical data for Germany are available since after the German re-unification in 1989. Using very coarse segmentation into age cohorts and neglecting all other health care assets and all demographic distinctions we start extrapolations from publicly available figures about the future demand and supply of health care workforce.

2.2.4 Base Figures and Derived Indicators of Health Care Demand and Supply

We compare the age segments below 20 ("Young age"), 20 through 64 ("Working age") and beyond ("Old age") in past and present and extrapolate to future (2025/30). The attributions of the age segments are somewhat arbitrary because some people start working before 20 and the retirement age is increasing in some societies. However, the segmentation and henceforth a certain amount of false attribution is done equally in the USA and Germany. Therefore, the type and amount of imprecision should be similar in both countries.

We use "workforce" for the share of a population that has or actively seeks paid work. If the age limits of 20 to 65 as "Working age" were sharp the work force figures would have to be smaller than the Working age figures. The actual limits are not sharp and especially the retirement age is moving upward, possibly leading to a larger work force than Working age population. The work force in the USA and Germany has, however, been and presently is between 83 % and 90 % of the Working age, i.e. a certain share of the Working age population does not work or seek paid work.

From retrieved statistics we calculate

- Persons in the Working age by persons in the Old age; to demonstrate the shift of the base population groups

2.2 Methodological Considerations

- Person in the Workforce by persons in the Old age; to modify for the actual participation rate of the Working age population in the Workforce
- Physicians per thousand Working age persons; to demonstrate what share of the productivity of a society is devoted to delivering health related services
- Physicians per thousand Workforce; equally modifying for the actual participation rate

and respectively for nurses.

While the above figures map a society in all its facets we now purposefully and suggestively focus on ratios that overemphasize the effects set through the aging of populations with their expected large share of high utilizers. As base figures (2008–2010) we take

- the present number of Old agers served by one physician resp. one nurse
- the present share of the Working age that serves as physicians or nurses.

We then elaborate on the following two reciprocal scenarios which reflect two opposing possible courses of future action:

- Positive formulation, the "Growth scenario": A proportionally larger health care workforce will be employed to serve a growing share of Old age high utilizers. This will allow to maintain the present quality and coverage. To substantiate the growth formulation we calculate

$$|present\ Old\ agers\ served\ by\ one\ physician| \times |future\ Old\ agers|$$

resp. for $|present\ nurses|$ where $|expression|$ denotes number of individuals identified by "expression".

- Negative formulation, the "Dilution scenario": The proportion of health care within the overall Working age will remain constant. As a consequence each health care professional will have to care for more Old age high utilizers. To substantiate the dilution formulation we calculate

$$\frac{|future\ Old\ agers| \times |present\ Working\ agers|}{|future\ Working\ agers| \times |present\ physicians|}$$

and respectively for nurses.

With a smaller share of the Working age and a larger share of the Old age it can be expected that either the proportion of health care professionals of the Working age has to be increased (Growth scenario) or the Old-age clients to be served by one health care professional increases (Dilution scenario).

> **Take Home**
>
> By calculating ratios between figures characterizing the demand (mainly Old agers) and the supply (mainly health care workforce) we extrapolate the future demand to supply prognosis under two opposite assumptions:
>
> **Growth scenario** assumes that the dependency ratios remains as today and predicts the required increase in physicians and nurses
>
> **Dilution scenario** assumes that the share of physicians and nurses of the Working age remains as today and predicts the future increase in Old agers depending on one physician resp. nurse

2.2.5 The "Best Case" Strategy of Selection

All figures carry some degree of imprecision and obviously all predictions are at best as reliable as their assumptions materialize. Therefore, we will over again be in the situation to choose between several figures within the likely range. In all such situation we will assume *best case* scenarios concerning expected shortages. For number of physicians and nurses we will adopt the largest figures projected. If population models vary in their assumption about number of yearly immigrants we will adopt the model with the largest immigration rate, because immigrants mostly are in the Working age and therefore increase the workforce pool. Proceeding like this will lead to projections that characterize the best possible future situation: in the Growth scenario the least required growth and in the Dilution scenario the least extent of dilution. In other words: it can only get worse than the projected figures suggest.

One could argue that *worst case* scenarios should rather be presented. Of course everybody is free to do so and the methods of data collection and modeling subsequently applied are equally suited for worst cases. However, the best case will already turn out so dire that its figures together with the knowledge that it can only get worse are absolutely alarming.

In an investigation for the Association of American Medical Colleges (AAMC) Atul Grover has collected a number of arguments relating to the physician workforce why we indeed have to anticipate that it will get worse [7]. They address both the supply and demand side. On the supply side they include the following arguments which leads to lower supply of physician work:

1. The physician age pyramid itself is not a pyramid but rather has largest numbers in age groups that approach retirement
2. The willingness to retire early is large
3. The enrollment to medical schools has kept declining
4. The percentage of female physicians is continually rising which makes the likelihood of periods of maternal leave and the choice for part-time work also rise

5. Only a minority would wish to work more for more money while the majority would like to reduce working hours.

Without going into detail the above effects numbered 1, 4, and to a lesser extent 3 hold for Germany as well.

These arguments about internal mechanisms that reduce actual supply of physician work hours superimposing the raw numbers of trained physicians are complemented by arguments of likely increased demand that has other causes than aging of the population. For the United States the largest potential of increased demand depends on the development of health insurance for those who are presently not insured.

> **Take Home**
> The raw figures achieved in the model 2.2.4 most likely underestimate the immanent problems because the estimated physician head counts excludes the effects of
> - the aging physician population
> - an increasing share of female physicians with their likely consequences of maternal leave and part-time work
> - reduced working hours in general
> - declining enrollment to medical schools

2.3 Sources and Results

2.3.1 The USA

2.3.1.1 Sources

US population data mostly are from Censusscope, a university institute for demographics and population studies which also makes animated population pyramids through several decades available at http://www.censusscope.org/us/chart_age.html. US work force data are taken from the report [11] available from the Bureau of Labor Statistics at http://www.bls.gov/emp/ep_pub_labor_force.htm. US physician historical data have been taken from the AMA site at http://www.ama-assn.org/resources/doc/clrpd/2008-trends.pdf [2], while for the future development reports and projections provided by the Association of American Medical Colleges (AAMC) appear like a well researched resource although it obviously is AAMC's role to lobby for an increase in physician workforce (https://members.aamc.org/eweb/upload/The%20Complexities%20of%20Physician%20Supply.pdf, [3]). Nurse supply and projections have recently been reported in a scholarly article by Auerbach and coworkers [1]. A crisp assessment of the upcoming problems can also be found in [10].

2.3.1.2 Results and Projections

For the United States population growth is expected to persist until 2030, with an overall increase from 248.6 to 365.7 million people. This roughly 47 % increase is unequally distributed through the age groups: Young agers and Working agers increase by one third while Old agers more than double from 31.2 to 71.6 million. The predicted development of workforce nearly equals the predicted growth of the Working age segment of the population. Health care professions growth outperforms the workforce growth. For physicians the expected increase over 40 years is 41 % and for nurses 254 %.

From these base figures we can derive that the Workforce to Old age ratio declines by nearly 41 %. While in 1990/91 4.09 individuals were there for one Old ager, it will be as few as 2.42 in 2030. The physician share of the work force increases by approximately 5 % while the nurse share of the workforce nearly doubles (11.70 in 1990 vs. 21.88 in 2030 of 1000 workforce).

Coming to figures that point out demand and supply of the most needy – the population of Old agers – we find that in 1990/91 one physician worked for 50.7 Old agers while according to figures from the above sources and straight projections he will be working for 82.3 Old agers in 2025. Under the dilution scenario assumptions where we assume that the share of the physicians in the workforce remains constant while the workforce itself declines one physician will have to work for 97.5 Old agers, that is nearly twice as many as 40 years earlier. Official figures from nurses are less alarming: indeed does the number of Old agers served by one nurse decrease moderately from 20.9 to 18.9, while in our Dilution scenario it increases to 25.6. Our Growth scenario requests 1226.4 thousand physicians while AMA predicts 869.9 thousand. This discrepancy goes into the same direction as a shortage predicted by AMA at http://www.ama-assn.org/ama/pub/news/news/strengthen-physician-workforce.page of 124,000–159,000 physicians by 2025. For nurses our Growth scenario requests exactly the same figure required for 2030, namely 3785 thousand.

2.3.2 Germany

2.3.2.1 Sources

Germany has had a comprehensive and all encompassing population registration and intermittent censuses introduced through the Prussian emperors in 1876 which continued into both post World War II Germanies and the unified Germany and provides highly reliable data except for the often overlooked effect of individuals moving to an abroad where they need not register as "immigrants" and hence do not notify local authorities about their emigrations. This often applies to guest workers from European Union states when they retire and return to their home countries. The primary national resource to collect and present such data is the Statistische Bundesamt with its web resource destatis, comparable to the US Census Bureau

2.3 Sources and Results

UCB. At https://www.destatis.de/bevoelkerungspyramide/ (a resource in German where bevoelkerungspyramide stands for population pyramid) offers a configurable panel that displays the age distributions of the German population from 1960 to 2008 and extrapolates until 2060. Of course, for the extrapolations assumptions must be made. Destatis offers four variants that vary by birth rate (number of children per woman, from 1.2 to 1.6), life expectancy at birth in 2060 (male: 85.0 to 87.7, female 89.2 to 91.2) (im-)migration surplus (100,000 to 200,000). The best case is high birth rate, low life expectancy, high immigration, because birth and immigration mostly add prospective or actual Working age individuals, while low life expectancy removes Old agers from the equation.[1]

German labor statistics come from Institut für Berufs- und Arbeitsmarktforschung, a research institution affiliated with the Bundesagentur für Arbeit (similar to the US Bureau of Labor Statistics). At http://doku.iab.de/kurzber/2011/kb1611.pdf [4] they provide historical data and projections into 2030 and beyond which can be varied by a few assumptions. These include reproduction rate and immigration figures.

Statistics on individuals with the academic qualification of a physician can build on data from Federal State Medical Associations. When a student has graduated from medical school he becomes a compulsory member and is inevitably registered at his Federal State Medical Association and remains registered for the rest of his life, whether he practices or not. When he moves membership automatically transfers to the new Federal State Medical Association. Compared to the US licensing where physicians can be and often are licensed in more than one state or may lose and later regain their license this means that German figures should be highly reliable.

Statistics on actively practicing physicians draw on two sources. Physicians in private practices are contracting with a social insurance reimbursement structure (Kassenärztliche Vereinigung) that geographically mirrors the Federal State Medical Associations. With the exception of very few physician who only treat patients that pay from their own purse or have a private rather than the social health insurance, this fully maps practicing medicine outside hospitals and figures are available from the Kassenärztliche Vereinigung. Physicians working in hospitals are reported through employment data of hospitals and always have a certain delay and noise due to part time vs. full time, how physicians organize their work and hence whether they are contracting with exactly one such organization or attending to more than one hospital.[2]

In Germany the Federal Ministry of Health maintains the "Gesundheitsberichterstattung des Bundes" ("Federal Health Monitoring System",) [5] which acts as

---

[1] This should by no means be taken sarcastically; it is just to illustrate the effects of assumptions made as clearly as possible.

[2] In Germany there is no one-on-one matching structure for the US licensing and license renewal process. Physicians in own private practices are obliged to provide proof of a certain amount of CME taken per 3 year interval to preserve their contract with the social insurance system. Hospitals have QA programs part of which target at qualification of employed physicians.

an authority steered by the Robert-Koch-Institut (comparable to the US Center for Disease Control, CDC), and the German Federal Statistical Office (comparable to the US Census Bureau, UCB) and assembles figures from the above primary sources to provide comprehensive reports on health and health care delivery.

The physician statistics date back to 1990, with a sharp increase owed to German unification from 1990 to 1991. To avoid the risk of badly supported figures of the period of transition we start in 1991 and compare to 2009. For physician and nurse figures mid-range projections are not available. Therefore, we use linear extrapolations from the data available for 1990/1 and for 2008/9 as a very approximate replacement. Respective figures and others derived on their bases are in italic fonts in Table 2.2.

2.3.2.2 Results and Projections

German population peaks at 81.7 million in 2008/9 and is expected to decline to 80.2 million in 2030, almost precisely back to the figure of 1990/1. Young agers and Working agers decline by 17 % respectively 14 % from 1990 to 2030 while Old agers increase by 87 % from 11.9 to 22.3 million between 1990/1 and 2030.

Expectations about workforce differ a lot from population development figures. A decrease from 42.9 to 41.0 million over 40 years – which is only 4.5 % – contrasts to the above-mentioned 14 % decrease in the Working age. Arguments in support of this higher participation rate are that more females would seek and find paid work and that retirement ages are already increasing. The latter strictly speaking is not a participation effect but an expansion of the pool from which workforce is supplied. If the assumption that more females participate materializes it is likely to amplify another critical aspect of the population statistics. Unless sophisticated financial and organizational models of care for minors become available those females who work will mostly not be mothers and will bear no or fewer children. For a longer range perspective this first reduces the Young age cohort and 20 years later the Working age cohort.

Physician and nurse figures have developed very differently. While physician figures have increased to a similar extent as in the United States and are extrapolated to grow from 242.2 to 403.5 (32 %) in 2030, the nursing workforce will decline from 913.4 towards 844.0 (thousand FTE each). This unique strange sizing of the two major professions in the German medical industry is to some extent owed to the fact that medicine is an academic while nursing to the most part is a nonacademic profession here which lends nurses less workplace and lobbying power than physicians. On the other hand it leads to physicians being seen by patients for various purposes where nurses legally offer services in many other countries (such as medication refills, wound primary treatment, ...). Germany has an amazingly high yearly frequency of patient visits to doctors of appr. 14.

The German workforce to Old age ratio declines by dramatic 49 %. In 1990/1 it was 3.61 and official agency projections predict 1.84 in 2030. During the same time interval the share of physicians of the workforce partially compensates for the decline as it increases from 5.69 to 9.84 (per thousand workforce), while the share of nurses remains nearly constant, reaching 20.58 in 2030.

The analysis focusing on demand and supply with respect to the growing Old age populations and straight projection from public resources finds that one physician will serve 55.3 Old agers, one nurse will serve 26.4 in 2030, from 48.7 respectively 13.0 in 1990/1. Assuming the Dilution scenario one physician will serve 78.0, one nurse will serve 29.0 Old agers. In the Growth scenario Germany will require 430.0 thousand physicians and 1158.3 thousand nurses in 2013, an apparently moderate 16.5 thousand more physicians and an apparently alarming 314.3 thousand more nurses than extrapolated. The projection of both physicians and nurses are, however, badly supported by evidence. The extrapolated number of physicians is likely to overestimate the true development. The 1990/1 and 2008/9 figures from which the linear extrapolations was made, represent a 2008/9 physician workforce age pyramid with overweight in the age groups beyond 50, hence a large number of practicing physicians retiring in the interval of prediction. At the same time enrollment to medical schools is lower now than a decade ago and the political pressure to finish the curriculum in time – and hence to save teaching resources – is higher than the pressure to create more study opportunities. Furthermore, from first enrollment to licensing as a General Practitioner or medical specialist takes at least 11 years in Germany. Opening (yet to be built) new medical schools in 2015 would not help until 2026. Education of licensed nurses is much shorter. That is why politics can achieve more short-term effects when the need for more nurses becomes acknowledged.

2.3.3 US: German Differences

The most notable difference between the two economies is that the USA all in all have a solid growth situation fueled through nearly sustainable birthrates and an active immigration policy directed at skilled young people. In contrast, Germany is on the verge of decline. Even in the most growth prone variant of the population pyramid by destatis Germany will keep losing 2 million per decade after 2030. No wonder, because Germany's birthrate is far below sustainable and Germany only tolerates some random influx from poor countries and some asylum seekers.

Another difference which is not so remarkable in figures today is that German statistics still believe in an unrealistically high participation rate of their Working age in the workforce as a welcome measurable productivity indicator of the national economy. While the US prediction holds a hidden reserve of more than 25 % (173 million of 199.2 million working) and therefore maintain a social fabric of continuously available individuals for family work and volunteer assistance in local or national situations of immediate need Germans believe to see more than 95 % barred in work contracts with foreseeable frictions when children want to be brought up or emergencies hit.

Table 2.1 Summary of figures from growth and dilution scenarios

	Physicians (1000)	Nurses	1 ...	Physician per ... Old agers	Nurse
USA					
Baseline ~2010	678.3	2578.8		58.4	15.4
Growth scen.	1226.4	3785.0			
Dilution scen.				97.5	25.6
Germany					
Baseline ~2010	325.9	877.4		51.9	19.3
Growth scen.	430.0	1158.3			
Dilution scen				78.0	29.0

The third notable difference between the two economies is the difference between the medical and nursing contributions to health care. While in the USA the medical contribution grows so slowly that future physicians become responsible for an unsurmountable number of elderly patients, the US nursing contribution grows much faster, but when comparing the 2009/10 figure of 15.4 versus the Dilution scenario predicted 25.6 elderly being taken care of by one nurse is still alarming. This reduction of care provision by 40 % is similar to the German one of 34 %, and precisely the same figures of reduction hold for physicians. The details are presented in Table 2.2.

> **Take Home**
> Even in best case scenarios, i.e. with all necessary assumptions made so as to overestimate future supply and to underestimate future demand, health care faces severe shortage or requires a dramatic increase in workforce, as summarized in Table 2.1.

2.3.4 Challenging the Assumptions

One can of course challenge the assumptions made as actually being best case. One challenge is to argue that a higher percentage of the Working age can actually be available as workforce because reproduction rates are declining and hence fewer Working age individuals will take parental leave. This may be correct, however, it delays the problem by 20 years rather solving it, as already outlined in Sect. 2.3.2.2.

Another challenge to the modeling assumptions is that the increased need of care towards the older end of the population is compensated for by a lower need of the Young age and Working age segments of the population because these segments get smaller. This is true to some extent. However, the absolute figures in the Young age population are already now smaller than the Old age figures. Altogether, both,

2.3 Sources and Results

Table 2.2 Development of population and health care workforce: prediction of future shortage in the USA and Germany

	Population (mio.)				Workforce (1000)			Work to retired ratio		Health care sizing (per thousand)				Inverse dependency ratio	
	Overall	Young age	Working age	Old age	Overall	Physicians (Proj: 2025)	Nurses (Proj: 2030)	Working age by Old age	Work force by Old age	Physicians by Workforce	Physicians by Working age	Nurses by Workforce	Nurses by Working age	Old agers by 1 physicians	1 nurse
USA															
1990/1	248.6	71.3	146.1	31.2	127,500	615.4	1491.6	4.68	4.09	4.83	4.21	11.70	10.21	50.7	20.9
2009/10	307.0	33.4	184.0	39.6	154,000	678.3	2578.8	4.65	3.89	4.40	3.69	16.75	14.02	58.4	15.4
2025/2030 projection	365.7	34.9	199.2	71.6	173,000	869.9	3785.0	2.78	2.42	5.03	4.37	21.88	19.00	82.3	18.9
Growth scenario						1226.4								97.5	25.6
Dilution scenario							3785.0								
Germany															
1990/1	79.8	17.3	50.5	11.9	42,900	244.2	913.4	4.24	3.61	5.69	4.84	21.29	18.09	48.7	13.0
2008/9	81.7	15.3	49.6	16.9	44,500	325.9	877.8	2.93	2.63	7.32	6.57	19.73	17.70	51.9	19.3
2030 projection	80.2	14.4	43.5	22.3	41,000	403.5	844.0	1.95	1.84	9.84	9.28	20.58	19.40	55.3	26.4
Growth scenario						430.0	1158.3							78.0	29.0
Dilution scenario															

Young agers and Working agers utilize health care less than Old agers. Therefore, the potential reduction is likely to be overcompensated by the increase requested by the Old agers.

It can also be argued that the Working age segment becomes larger because retirement ages are becoming higher. This is actually already the case. However, we are talking about a couple of months, maybe 2 or 3 years of increased retirement age at most. Therefore, even if we assume that these higher ages fully materialize in the sense that workers indeed sustain their individual workforce for three more years while staying as healthy as the rest of the Working age population we add a segment of 3 years to the Working age which in the model is 45 years, which is 7 %. Compared to that the increase required according to Table 2.2, Growth scenario, is between 32 % (German physicians) and 80 % (German nurses), with US figures in between, i.e. by far too large to be outweighed by higher retirement age. Other observations for Germany further invalidate the argument.

The following argument is double edged: More Working agers may be involved in caring for elderly family because of the shortage of qualified professionals and increasing fees. The undeniable moral responsibility to care for family may withdraw additional qualified workforce hence thus adding to the problem in a self reinforcing loop. The reverse may also be the case: With professional care for the elderly readily available qualified individuals may seek or maintain professional employment hence further reducing the size of the problem. It is up to us to make a choice.

> **Take Home**
> Developments that come to mind as being able to ease the dire prognosis either delay the problems or have side effects that aggravate them.

2.4 Options to Match Supply and Demand

From the analysis above it should be clear that health care delivery faces severe shortages in less than one generation in the future when no action is taken. Believing today that an unchanged health care system will provide equal or better treatment than we have it today for equal or longer duration than today is wishful thinking. The opposite is the likely case. We therefore introduce several paths of action that the health care systems can take and briefly evaluate their prognosis. When it comes to finance more detail can be found in Chap. 16. For all the following consideration the caveat should be in the readers mind that health care is not an open market. Increasing demand will not entail increased supply naturally for at least two reasons. First, the purchasing power of those in need is often insufficient to pay the prices that would cover the providers' cost. Therefore, not until insurance coverage is (nearly) all encompassing is there a business model for growth of the health care industry. Second, the lag time between increasing demand and increased supply is at least three plus seven years: three for building and staffing new medical schools and seven for short university and specialty training curricula. And like the financial markets – where we should have taken action before major actors collapsed – we should initiate fundamental changes early enough. We should have them in place before scores of health care professionals retire early or are burnt out, overwhelmed by continuously growing demand.

2.4.1 Rationing

Principally available services can be offered to some and denied to others. Criteria about whom to serve and whom not to serve can be diverse. The most clear-cut criterion is age: upper age limits are defined for services in general or varying by service. Harder to pinpoint criteria are merit and need. Persons can be eligible in their order of merit for the society which now pays back. Persons can be eligible in their order of need, that is a society acknowledges the severity of a problem without premises. Services can also be attributed to those who can pay as long as they can pay. This criterion can be modified as to servicing those who have sufficient insurance coverage. Whether such criteria satisfy the moral principle of distributive justice (cf. Sect. 17.11.7) may also be doubted and even if they would, determining a strict order of merits, needs etc. requires additional time and effort that we do not really want to invest.

None of these criteria are fully satisfactory and hence rationing is not something desirable but rather a backdoor when resources are just not there. In the above ways criteria are made explicit and transparent and can be subject of democratic decision-making. They become law and when the situation is there a health care professional can deliver or deny services by referring to that law rather than being seen personally responsible for a denial. Rationing can also be called reduced allocation of resources. It happens on all levels of the health care system by decisions of building or closing hospitals, by hiring or not hiring staff, and by offering or denying services. It already silently happens whenever a patient seeks hospital service and is turned away because the hospital is fully occupied. This is a rationing that just happens, accidentally, unregulated, and which only reaches the attention of jurisdiction when life-threatening situations are not handled properly. With numbers of clients continuously rising and numbers of professionals not rising it will just happen more and more often as time passes.

Criteria can be experimented with in a democratic process. However, pressure group interests can force whole societies into criteria that hurt other pressure groups' interests. Regarding the ever-increasing number of elderly age rationing may be opted out although it is the easiest to apply criterion, requiring and allowing the least deliberation.

> **Take Home**
> Rationing is a euphemistic expression for denying services to some in need. It is neither desirable nor easy, because criteria and processes for rationing are anything but easy to formulate and to implement.

2.4.2 Volume Increase at Equal Cost, with Quality at Risk

Volume increase without increasing resources is also called rationalizing. Its underlying assumption is that the same effect can be achieved with less effort. Since most medical interventions include care provider – patient encounters and care provider time cannot be split or multiplied rationalizing likely means shorter care provider – patient sessions. There is certainly potential through more structured processes, better preparation and presentation of patient data, and leaving away all communication that is not related to the medical case. It is a less humane service but when having to choose one would probably prefer some service to no service at all. The more severe risk of the rationalizing approaches is that it can be done once or twice or maybe three times and with every step the service runs thinner. But unless we take the human fully out of the equation there is a lower limit of a meaningful care provider – patient encounter. Operating in the vicinity of this lower limit increases the risks of overlooking critical signs or identifying favorable therapy options. In other words: quality of the service is at stake.

> **Take Home**
> Rationalization is an euphemistic expression for reducing effort while hoping to maintain quality. The largest proportion of health care effort is provider – patient contact times. If this is continually reduced errors are a likely consequence.

2.4.3 Reduced Effort per Case Through Quality Improvement

David Bates and his coworkers at Brigham and Women's Hospital in Boston have provided conclusive evidence of astounding reduction of efforts by consequently applying CPOE[3] in a system that backed up by comprehensive decision support and alerting functionality [9]. Over 10 years they showed that for an investment of $

---

[3]Computerized Physician Order Entry, also Computerized Provider Order Entry: ordering medications or diagnostic or therapeutic procedures online; in advanced implementations combined with

11.8 million they could collect a return of $ 26.2 million. Among the largest savings were decreased length of stay through renal function adapted dosing, nurse time in providing medication administration records, fewer ADE's etc. These three of the top four dollar savers are directly related to reduced human resource utilization. Although not explicitly stated a decrease in ADE's also means a reduction in work effort. In other words: the savings they can make due to quality improvements to a large extent are reduced workloads. The amount of savings reported here is in the order of magnitude of the shortage predicted above. So is this the solution to all our problems?

It certainly is an important step into the right direction. At Brigham and Women's they avoid many medical errors and save many lives. Most likely they still have some ADE's, and they keep trying to reduce them. But when there are no more ADE's, there are still patients to treat. Quality improvement approaches reduce efforts but this effect reaches a saturation. When saturation is reached the problem of increasing demand is still there, meeting a better prepared supply, though.

> **Take Home**
> Structures and processes to warn of errors before they happen are a worthwhile endeavor to achieve better outcomes for patients and at the same time to reduce effort. This should be a permanent undercurrent but it does not solve the problem of shortage to its full extent.

2.4.4 Growth

Growth is certainly an option. In Sect. 2.3 the required amount of growth has been outlined. It has been pointed to the fact that investment cycles to increase the medical workforce are extremely long. But after all investing into the medical industry to a major part means investing into local jobs rather than jobs abroad as they often materialize when investing into technology or less demanding or less personal services. Growth necessitates a larger amount of the GDP flowing into the medical industry. This is a likely roadblock regarding all the public uproar about the necessity to curb health care cost. Some scholars, however, go against the tides: Hall and Jones [8] use arguments of perceived marginal value of spending for health care and of spending for non-health goods and services in the USA to predict an increase of 33 % by 2050; not too far from what we find in Sect. 2.3.3 especially when regarding a widely expected slower growth of the population.

---

an electronic record system where contraindications or interactions of new orders with the present patient medication or condition can be checked and alerts can be issued.

> **Take Home**
> Although politically unthinkable to some, allowing the health care system to grow is not primarily a cost factor for an economy: It rather boosts a high end mostly *domestic* labour market rather than exporting jobs.

2.4.5 Diversification of Delivery

Three directions of delivery diversification will be presented:

- Employing less qualified or differently qualified personnel or machines
- Intensely using data in preparation and execution of patient – professional encounters
- Automated diagnosis and treatment

We already see for instance in Great Britain that nurses take far ranging responsibility in medication refills. In Germany psychologists with additional elements of clinical education can fully responsibly treat psychiatric patients. So why not give dietitians, physiotherapists, optometrists and other paramedical professions full responsibility for their diagnosis and treatment? We also already face and maybe enjoy that hotel services in hospitals are provided through hotel personnel rather than nurses. We see robots transporting all kinds of material in hospitals and other places. Why not let them transport patients within the hospital.

The more complicated a case the more important are comprehensive data and their presentation in well intelligible form. It starts with making them available for asynchronous assessment allowing the physician to take a look at not so busy hours. E-mail as means of communication has already found a place in many physician-patient relations. Furthermore, information management and processing like summarizing of patient data before a patient visit could help the physician to concentrate on the essentials. Of course signs may be overlooked because they do not fit the criteria of the summarizing software. We also see telemedicine in operation allowing the best specialized individual to offer his service through the distance rather than relying on local capacities that are not able to find the right diagnosis or therapy or need too much time and effort. We see various ways to let the health care professional – mostly the physician – act more efficiently but he is still personally actively involved case by case.

When searching the Internet we can enter symptoms, diseases, drug and treatment names, names of hospitals or physicians and will most likely find some, maybe an overwhelming amount of information. If we correctly describe our problem, select an appropriate information source and understand the information we may know how to proceed: wait, treat ourselves, maybe purchase pharmaceuticals online, see the right specialist. We also already see depression, obesity, and other questionnaires on the internet allowing us to get an idea how severe our problem is.

Without immediate involvement of the medical professional we can undergo triage and screening to help us decide whether we should seek professional advice. For various conditions we already find full-fledged treatment programs on the internet or other communications media. We receive treatment without a human being being a step-by-step provider. We may receive alerts to seek professional help when our problem escalates. This takes the health care professional almost entirely out of the operational loop and assigns him a role of developer or back-end service provider "behind" an online service. This diversification requires an investment in health care professional and other resources up front. When gone life it takes off workload because many encounters between professional and client are replaced by advice available online. From the perspective of managing their personal workload physicians should therefore be enthusiastic about investing into Consumer Health Informatics services. Of course, various other aspects play a role here, many of which will be addressed in the rest of this volume. But in the sense of taking preventive action before being overwhelmed by a continuously rising number of patients Consumer Health Informatics should be regarded as an option.

This also diversifies among the prospective clients: it can be the better educated who benefit most because they better understand provided guidance. It can as well be under-served populations in remote places, uninsured persons, who would not have access to medical services at all unless they are openly available through communications media. And we should not leave Old agers out of consideration. The Old agers we are preparing for are the mid-fifties of today, many of them computer savvy. Empirical evidence mainly in Chap. 11 demonstrate that many affected Old agers of today not only manage but appreciate being supported and safeguarded through technical means. Other evidence in sections such as Sect. 3.2 exists as well, though, which indicates that respective patient behaviors are not always rational.

Take Home

Diversification comes through

- giving paramedical professions more responsibility
- involving non-medical professions for mundane services
- employing ICT to enable the patient to become active

The latter is the call for Consumer Health Informatics. Health care professionals can see it as a preventive measure to build good Consumer Health Informatics services before the whole industry is overwhelmed with ever more patients per provider.

2.5 Benefits from Growth in Other Industries and Segments

Needless to say that all such concepts and developments benefit massively from information and communication technology that develops fast all around us. Be it the masses of data available on servers and in clouds which are ubiquitously available through fast Internet or mobile communication services. Be it the methods to make communication in open nets safe against intruders. We may think of ever more broadly available smaller and smaller high-quality devices such as smartphones or tablets. Many of us already use sensors attached to the body to track sports activities and GPS to localize ourselves. We are surrounded by surveillance cameras, motion detectors, acceleration detectors etc. This is all happening and sustained through business models of micro-payment, lifestyle and entertainment triggered purchasing power, support of business processes etc. Most of the devices we carry and the services we use are idle most of the time. Unless we need very specialized sensors, extraordinarily high resolution of images, extremely high availability, we can transport medical "payload" through an infrastructure that is already in place.

These considerations gain further attraction through the fact that – although presently they are still behind – developing countries and under-served populations catch up fast in terms of availability and command of up to date information and communication technology. Messages circulate which bemoan that there are now more working cell phones than working toilets on planet Earth and proclaim better sanitation as a major development goal (http://newsfeed.time.com/2013/03/25/more-people-have-cell-phones-than-toilets-u-n-study-shows/). It goes without saying that hygienic sanitation is an urgent need. But these same messages also support that technological and infrastructure barriers for the underprivileged to benefit from available services are dwindling.

> **Take Home**
> Many technical enablers for Consumer Health Informatics are developing fast. ICT infrastructures and ubiquitous devices are being used for lifestyle and entertainment purpose, mostly not exploiting bandwidth and processing power. They are right there as a bandwagon waiting for medical services to be added. Patients can make choices, including otherwise under-served populations who are getting access at considerable pace.

References

1. Auerbach DI, Buerhaus PI, Staiger DO. Registered nurse supply grows faster than projected amid surge in new entrants ages 23–6. Health Aff. 2011;30(12):2286–92. doi: 10.1377/hlthaff.2011.0588
2. AMA. Health care trends 2008. http://www.ama-assn.org/resources/doc/clrpd/2008-trends.pdf, 2008. 121p.
3. Dill MJ, Salsberg ES. The complexities of physician supply and demand. https://members.aamc.org/eweb/upload/TheComplexitiesofPhysicianSupply.pdf, Nov 2008. 90p.
4. Fuchs J, Söhnlein D, Weber B. Projektion des Arbeitskräfteangebots bis 2050, (in German). http://doku.iab.de/kurzber/2011/kb1611.pdf, Aug 2011.

References

5. Federal Health Monitoring System GBE. http://www.gbe-bund.de/. Accessed 20 May 2011: search string: "employment 2006".
6. Gulley SP, Rasch EK, Chan L. It we build it, who will come? Working-age adults with chronic health care needs and the medical home. Med Care. 2011;49(2).
7. Grover A. Physician workforce issues. http://michigan.gov/documents/healthcareworkforcecenter/WayneStatePresentationGROVER_192782_7.pdf, Mar 2007.
8. Hall RE, Jones CI. The value of life and the rise in health spending. Q J Econ. 2007;122(1):39–72. doi: 10.1162/qjec.122.1.39.
9. Kaushal R, Jha AK, Franz C, Glaser J, Shetty KD, Jaggi T, Middleton B, Kuperman GJ, Khorasani R, Tanasijevic M, Bates DW. Return on investment for a computerized physician order entry system. JAMIA. 2006;13(3):261–6. doi: 10.1197/jamia.M1984.
10. Sade RM. The graying of America: challenges and controversies. J Law Med Ethics. 2012;2012(Spring):6–9.
11. Toossi M. Projections of the labor force to 2050: a visual essay. http://www.bls.gov/emp/ep_pub_labor_force.htm, 2012. 14p.

Chapter 3
Level 0: Searching – Finding – Trusting – Acting – Risking One's Life?

3.1 Introduction

Health is among the strongest concerns of human living. Health and disease, and in that context risk, treatment, prognosis, prevention etc. are an extremely wide field. Health information is abundant and the search for health related information is a driver of utilization of the Internet as well as of mobile communication such as smart phone apps.

Abundance of information is an asset if it enables everybody to find appropriate quality information for his problem. However, not everybody has access as can be seen at http://www.internetworldstats.com/stats.htm.

Those, who have access may not be able to find the right search terms, and those who master the search terms problem may still be overwhelmed with a myriad of search results or trapped with faulty or even treacherous information. This chapter goes into the details of these problems and presents approaches to master them.

3.2 Facts and Behaviors

The space of information available through Internet or mobile networks is so large and grows and changes so fast that figures retrieved today would be outdated before this volume is printed. We therefore do not even try and move on to more lasting qualitative aspects.

3.2.1 Trends of Utilization of the Internet and Other Media

Impressive as the absolute figures of searchers and search results may be, better medical knowledge or healthier behavior do not emerge naturally. Two recent investigations published as Tracking Reports [21, 22] draw a detailed picture of US Americans' use and appreciation of health information from the Internet versus other resources. Drawing on telephone (2001 and 2007) and telephone and cell phone (2010) interviews with representative samples of US residents they demonstrate a strong increase in health information seeking behavior between the first and second surveys and what at first sight appears to be a plateau between the second and the third survey. The investigations differentiate in various ways between subpopulations, such as age groups, educational levels, sex, and ethnicity. Among the expected though discomforting observations is that utilization of all types of resources (print media, friends/family, TV/radio or Internet) increases with education; roughly two third of graduates but only roughly one third of no high school diploma interviewees seek for themselves or for friends or family. Women seek moderately more than men, white and African-Americans moderately more than Hispanics, patients with chronic conditions moderately more than others – as one would expect.

One would probably not expect that while first increasing from 38.3 % to 55.5 % the search for health information from any source then declines to 50.0 %. Does this mean that Consumer Health Informatics has reached its peak and is declining again? We need to look closer.

First, the percentage of information seekers that use the Internet has been continually increasing, from 15.9 %, to 31.1 %, to 32.6 %. An unremarkable increase was found from 2007 to 2010, but we will return later. The decline happened in a different place. It appears related to an economic downturn the strongest effect of which in the behaviors covered through the interviews was that the elderly dramatically reduced their purchasing of print media (from 35 % to 18 %) which had been (and still was in 2010) *that generation's* primary resource of health information. At the same time the percentage of the elderly seeking health information declined from 50 % to 42 %, while their access to Internet increased from 17 % to 24 %. Putting these pieces together they actually used the Internet more in 2010 than 2007.

3.2.2 *Increasing Compliance Meets Declining Comprehension*

Still the overall increase in Internet search is surprisingly low. The authors of the two reports provide several possible explanations. We concentrate on personal subjective assessments of those who did seek and use health information as to whether they changed behavior or understood better how to treat their medical problem. While 2007 50 % said that in response to found information they changed their approach towards maintaining their health and 80 % said that they understood their therapies better, the 2010 figures were 56 % and as low as *60 %*. There appears to be a certain disenchantment about the Internet as a source of wisdom. Truly alarming is the distinction between poorly educated and well-educated. For those with no high school diploma the percentage of believers in behavior change *increased* from 43.6 % to 44.7 % while their belief that they understood their condition better *declined* from 73.8 % to 47.4 % in not more than 3 years. At the same time the percentage of those reporting behavior change increased from 54.6 % to 60.2 % among graduates but confidence in their ability to comprehend declined from 82.2 % to 67.2 %. One third of the best educated admit that they did search but at the end of the day they did not increase their understanding. Ironically one could say that quite a few behave according to a Christian maxim, as reported in John 20:29: "Then Jesus told him, 'Because you have seen me, you have believed; blessed are those who have not seen and yet have believed."

> **Take Home**
> - The percentage of the population that searches the Internet for health information has increased only moderately (31.1 % to 32.6 %) from 2007 to 2010. Among the elderly the percentage was smaller but increased faster, from 17 % to 24 %.
> - The informational divide was disenchanting: throughout all print and digital media two thirds of college graduates but only one third of those without high school diploma searched for health information. Similar inequalities hold between well served and underserved ethnic groups.
> - Behavior modification in response to found information increased while comprehension of information declined, even in well educated subpopulations.

The authors of the two reports consider an opting out caused by "information overload, anxiety and confusion by some consumers" [22, page 4]. They appraise public resources becoming available to help clients to navigate and select, among them those by the NLM at MedlinePlus. Their value will be assessed in Sect. 3.5.1.

This was USA only. Problems on both provider and client side multiply when we think of appr. 185 countries, two handful of major languages, and countless living local languages which, small as they may be, are a lifeline for those who only speak their local language.

3.3 Effects, Risks, and Adverse Effects

3.3.1 Searching: Finding?

Often, when people start searching the Internet, it is due to a health concern or perceived medical problem. Searching cannot start without verbalizing the perceived problem. Some searches may stem from situations where presumably healthy persons are justly positively screened for a disease and get verbally precise information about the condition. In all other situations finding the right terms – or being trapped by apparently innocent yet false terms, as outlined in Sect. 3.3.2.1 – takes him who searches to good or bad places. This problem is as wide as medicine, lay language for medical terms and the Internet.

In 2006 Recupero and Rainey [19] report a spotlight of searches for psychotherapeutic counseling through the internet. Their search in Google™ and Yahoo!™ for `online counseling OR online therapy OR e-therapy` in May to September 2005 returned 55 services. The results were analyzed for various criteria of structural quality such as description of the service itself, providers' qualifications, and eligibility criteria of patients/clients. In the description of the service the term "therapy" appears frequently. This suggests that medicine is being practiced online, especially if providers indicate that they possess the necessary medical or therapist credentials. Online-only treatment is illegal but there are subtle distinctions from the non-binding provision of information which are analyzed in Sect. 17.6.2.3.

The investigation by Recupero and Rainey is detailed and to the point and a good read in the methodology of formally analyzing health websites. But at the same time and in retrospect it demonstrates how fast the field evolves and how ephemeral any such survey approach is (see also Sect. 15.7): 8 years later, in July 2013, the same queries in Google™ alone produce 113,000,000 (`online counseling`), 350,000,000 (`online therapy`) and 411,000,000 (`e-therapy`) hits. Furthermore, one of the most successful and sustained online services for depressive adolescents which has continually operated since 2000 ([24], cf. Sect. 5.2.2.4) was not even found in the 2005 search.

A fully systematic account of searching is obviously not possible. We subsequently report a longitudinal impression on the erratic nature of searching for health information on the Internet.

3.3.1.1 Thirst and Exhaustion: Phenomenology

First we report on 7 years of continuously running the same search for early indicators of diabetes – thirst and exhaustion – against the same most widely used search engine, Google™, concretely: Google.com. It should be noted that diabetes is only one explanation for thirst and exhaustion. Many of the other explanations showing in the next sections may apply as well but diabetes is by far the most widely distributed one. The number of Google.com hits for `thirst exhaustion` increased from 328,000 in February 2006, to 2.1 million in March 2011, to 6.5 million in June 2013. Google's top hits through the three samples were a computer game in 2006, vitamin B6 deficiency coming with diet recommendations that could harm diabetics in 2011, and the WebMD symptom checker suggesting dehydration as first diagnosis, next iron poisoning, then diabetes in 2013.

The computer game, top in 2006, is not the problem; the seeker would move on to the second hit which is a substance abuse self-report. All seekers not affected

3.3 Effects, Risks, and Adverse Effects   65

by addictive drugs would move on but drug addicts may feel pampered by not interpreting the new signs as a new disease but as a side effect of their known problem. Those who move on find the next two hits related to heat exhaustion or heat disorders. We identify a high risk of diabetes going unnoticed through distracting findings whereas without the Internet the client might have seen his doctor.

March 2011 is somewhat better. If seekers are not trapped by the vitamin D6 top hit they will skip the second (computer game) and then find numbers 3 and 4 pointing to diabetes.

July 2013 is more mixed and directs our attention to a new phenomenon. The top hit is medical and lists diabetes below dehydration and iron poisoning, above gastroenteritis and medication side effects, i.e. on par with very alarming and very common conditions with the incurred risk that "easy" concrete explanations such as gastroenteritis or medication side effects are preferred over the severe and abstract distant one of diabetes. Hits number 2 and 3 introduce patient blogs as a type of service that was not yet so common the years before. Hit 2 reports a discussion thread which swings back and forth between diabetes, drug side effects, malaria and bilharzia, drinking Gatorade, and vitamins, a notorious result of health related searches. Seekers who want good news will discontinue a medication they suspect to be the culprit – at their peril if the medication controls a life threatening problem –, drink Gatorade – at their peril if they are diabetics – or take vitamins. Hypochondriacs will visit a department of tropical infections, and maybe call an ambulance. Some will dig deeper into the diabetes option. Hit 3 goes into the same direction but is more intricate. The thread is labeled "resolved" and the "best answer chosen by voters" starts "Geez buddy, stress and diet can do some wicked things to our bodies if we let it." It continues with diet recommendations that are not at all suited for diabetics. Another answer in hit 3 – not chosen by voters – is a high school diploma reading level explanation of the pathomechanisms of diabetes and why they explain the symptoms. Blessed are those who keep going until hit 4. It has dehydration on top, marks it as a medical emergency and has different forms of diabetes on the next three ranks. So seekers who notice that they survive a few hours may turn down the dehydration hypothesis and take diabetes seriously. Hit 5 overwhelms with pop-ups and invitations to register as a new member but the seeker who gets through to information learns that he may have gluten intolerance.

Hit 6, at last, is MedlinePlus and has diabetes visible on the page retrieved by Google.com.[1] We will come back to MedlinePlus in Sect. 3.5.1.

3.3.1.2 Thirst and Exhaustion: Incurred Objective and Subjective Risks

This outline may appear lengthy and unsystematic. However, in its authenticity it allows so many observations that are worth pursuing in the rest of this volume that we will stick with it for another short while.

---

[1]Google is a trademark of Google Inc.

One observation is the indeterminacy. Independent of all processes of selection and interpretation the search result which necessarily is the starting point for all subsequent assessment and arbitration is beyond the control of the searcher.

Another observation is natural medicine or other evangelism, as outlined in Sect. 17.4.1.1 on the example of anti-vaccination campaigns.

Several observations relate to the contents and how it is interpreted. Truisms such as to take your vitamins and to drink enough always rank high. They are not bad as such. They are true and everybody understands. But when there is a real medical problem they are mostly not sufficient. When there is an urgent medical problem relying on a truism can be dangerous.

Among the search results containing clinical explanations of the problem, we observe the disproportion of very common and harmless diagnoses and very rare or life-threatening diagnoses next to each other as though they were equivalent.[2] Just imagine a patient in New York City who never traveled outside the US and seriously considers whether he has vitamin B6 deficiency or bilharzia.

We also observe that majority votes can have detrimental effects. In Chap. 6 we will show that crowds can know more than individual specialists. Here, however, we find a compelling example of a phenomenon that has been brought to the attention of a broad audience in "Science" [13] in 2013: crowds become impressed by communicational (mis-) conduct of self appointed opinion leaders. This has already been studied before the advent of the Internet: in Sect. 6.3.2 studies are presented where "group think" is dominated by few. In our concrete situation of the 2013 hit 2 above, the blogger whose suggestion is favored wins through a mixture of rhetoric, some facts, and bullying against others' contributions, claiming competence for himself and denying others' competence. The loser is the other blogger with a concise self-contained explanation from which the symptoms of diabetes emerge naturally for those who accept the challenge to work through the arguments. To benefit from those results the reader has to untangle rhetoric and facts and then to attempt to comprehend nearly scholarly writing. This brings up another observation: depending on their own communication patterns and education some may be impressed by the bullying and swallow the advice that it conveys. Others may feel disgusted, skip the bullying and find themselves with a challenging though nice read. The former – if they comply – will reduce stress and abandon their diet, while the latter will try to find out more about diabetes. Not only here is education the criterion that does or does not grant access to valuable information. The risks of unfair rhetoric have been systematically investigated in the medically challenging field of autism and development disorders, cf. [16].

---

[2]Some of the found websites highlight urgent diagnoses but others just list them.

3.3 Effects, Risks, and Adverse Effects

> **Take Home**
> - Systematic search with commonly used search engines does not guarantee valid or reproducible results.
> - Search results vary fast over time. Therefore, the value of a metanalysis built on search results decays fast, too.
> - Highly valuable pertinent results appear next to apparently pertinent but hazardous or inappropriate results.
> - Valuable results may not be retrieved at all.
> - Crowd votings may mislead the seeker.
>
> To summarize: The outcome of naïve search is unpredictable in each and every aspect.

We notice that high quality sources may escape the attention. We will see later that initiatives are underway to move MedlinePlus up in the search ranks. But there is no guarantee that the seeker assigns the highest trust to information that is helpful rather than dangerous for his condition. Mostly, there is an option for everyone. Everybody can find arguments in support of his hypothesis. This has been called confirmation bias of which two subphenomena, biased search and biased interpretation play a role. Consequently a person who searches may feel assured in what he already believed was his best choice, whether it was to seek or not to seek professional help.

3.3.1.3 Drugs Search: Phenomenology

An investigation by Law and coworkers [12] analyzes risks of searching the Internet on a broader scale. In one part of their investigation they show that the most commonly dispensed drugs are not necessarily the most sought after; the rank correlation between doses dispensed and number of searches is as low as 0.45. Search favorites rather are medications that call for privacy (opiates, antidepressants) followed by blockbusters such as antibiotics. In a second major part they concentrate on commonly used drugs and investigate which sites will most likely be found and the quality of the content within those sites.

For the top 198 brand names and their 278 generic ingredients (where hormones and dietary supplements have been excluded) they searched through Google™.com, Google.ca, Bing®, and Yahoo!™.[3] Google.com plays a special role because through an agreement between the US government and Google, brand name searches for pharmaceuticals originating from the USA are assigned high rankings for NLM sources. Since this is not the case for Google.ca it can be used for

---
[3]Google is a trademark of Google Inc., also in combinations google.com, google.ca. Yahoo! is a trademark of Yahoo! Inc. Bing is a registered trademark of Microsoft. For better readability the ™ and ® signs are not attached to every occurrence of the trademarked symbols in this section.

comparison. For searches only the first hits are subsequently evaluated by type of provider. The authors distinguish industry, government, merchant, user-created (including Wikipedia), independent, and unknown. Searches are equally run for brand and generic names.

Google.com fulfills the new promise: 75 % of generic name searches and 72 % of brand name searches hit NLM first. For brand names there is a clear second, http://www.drugs.com^{TM}, an independent New Zealand-based provider, while for generic names most of the rest goes to Wikipedia. The three other search engines by and large behave similarly. For generic names about 85 % first hits are Wikipedia, while for brand name searches industry is the clear winner: upper 60 % in Bing and Google.ca, nearly 80 % at Yahoo!. Correspondingly, independent providers collect upper 20 % in Bing and Google.ca while Yahoo! only directs 18 % there.

3.3.1.4 Drugs Search: Objective and Subjective Risks

One could argue that this is a nice distribution of hits among various more or less qualified providers. However, in the first place the seeker cannot predict where he will be taken. Indeterminacy is here to stay, on a much larger scale now. This would not matter so much if the pages were equally good. But they are not. The NLM plays a special role discussed in Sect. 3.5.1. Those labeled independent are a totally amorphous collection that escapes a comprehensive quality assessment. They can be brilliant or life-threatening. When visiting pharmaceutical industry sites the informed and critical reader will be watchful concerning the fair account of intended effects and adverse effects. Actually investigations have shown that some industry sites intentionally omit information about potentially harmful side effects [6]. This demonstrates an anchor point kind of problem of information logistics: even if a seeker intends to search for side effects in the material that the company offers, his search will go void although the provider knows about side effects. Finally, Wikipedia remains as the last big player emerging from Law and coworkers' investigation. Since Wikipedia does not list brand names its role is marginal there. For generic names, however, Wikipedia collects appr. 20 % of Google.com and 85 % of the other three engines' first hits.

Wikipedia is often publicly perceived as a high-quality resource because it is presumably maintained by well-meaning well-informed individuals who are themselves permanently controlled by a large community of equal do-gooders. A more scrutinized look at Wikipedia reveals other facts. [8] and [4] have shown on a very specific and on a large scale that Wikipedia information is not so high-quality as is commonly believed and is not immune against manipulation such as edits being made from IP addresses that can be traced to the pharmaceutical industry. Not until June 16, 2014 has Wikipedia reacted by changing its "Terms of Use" requesting disclosure of their source of payment for individuals who are paid for their editing (http://blog.wikimedia.org/2014/06/16/change-terms-of-use-requirements-for-disclosure/). Concerning correctness and coverage of contents only 40 % on average of what clinical pharmacology specialists regard as necessary information is present in the Wikipedia articles. Conversely, some of the presented information can be life-threatening.

What does that mean for the seeker? In the first place the qualitative observations imply that it matters whether the search takes him to a good or a bad place. And unless he uses Google.com™ and lives in the United States, there are more doubtful than truly good places. We now know what the odds are that we will reach a good site with high quality content. However, knowing the likelihood to reach a good place is not individually predictable information i.e. the analysis is as good – or as bad – for individual prognosis to find the right information as epidemiological or biostatistical data are for individual prognosis of outcome of a disease.

Take Home

- Drug search results and their quality differ whether brand names or generic ingredients are used as search terms and from which location the search is launched.
- The pharmaceutical industry and Wikipedia are likely first hits, plus NLM for seekers in the USA.
- Pharmaceutical industry sites tend to underreport side effects.
- Wikipedia is by far incomplete and not independent from the pharmaceutical industry.

The most deceptive conclusion here is that the provider that enjoys the highest trust (Wikipedia) has far lower than expected quality. This is one of those rare situation where the better educated who strive for information that is not industry biased and hence use generic rather than brand names can be trapped in two ways: information may be just insufficient or it may even covertly be manipulated by industry.

3.3.1.5 Self-Diagnosing: Error Statistics and Causes

From these observations and results we can conclude that statistically, when proceeding straightforward, the seeker has a considerable risk of not finding pertinent information but instead finding misleading information. On the other hand seekers do not just seek for curiosity and entertainment. According to the Tracking Reports referred to in Sect. 3.2 roughly one half – varying with demographic variables – of those seeking health information in various media self-report behavior changes. There is clear evidence that scores of seekers indeed act according to the insights they believe to gain. Kuehn [10] reports for AMA about a Pew[4] survey of 3000 US

---

[4] Pew Research Center is a Washington DC based "nonpartisan fact tank...trends shaping America and the World."

adults that excludes other media and interviews only on Internet search for health information. Pew probes a bit deeper into actual behaviors of interviewees once they have sought information about a health condition. Their nearly two thirds estimate of going online for health information is far more than in the Tracking Reports and the question has to be raised whether times have changed so much between 2010 and 2013, whether Pew asked differently or whether they had a different selection bias of interviewees. Kuehn's one third quoted as using the Internet "to diagnose health problems" comes much closer to the Tracking Reports in order of magnitude. About one half of the "online diagnosers" (46 %) self-assessed their findings as to requiring medical attention, 38 % believed in cure at home. Ultimately, 53 % consulted a physician. Of those, 41 % got their self diagnosis confirmed by their physician. Not too bad, one might say, but actually it means that 59 % had erred in their self diagnosis. Sarcastically, but with reason: 59 % of those who were still alive had erred. Pew could not interview those who had meanwhile died from a diagnosis where either the found information itself or the comprehension of the information did not fit their dire medical reality.

How did they search and what did they find? 75 % started with a search engine such as Google™, 13 % with a specialty site such as WebMD®, 2 % with a general information platform such as Wikipedia and 1 % with social networks. These shares have been similar the years before. If Google™ behaves for medical problems like Google.ca™, Bing® and Yahoo!™ did for pharmaceuticals, the most likely top finds would be Wikipedia and industry-sponsored, the latter maybe depending on how much sales a company associates with a search term. We have seen the risks of insufficient coverage and occasional errors in Wikipedia and the biases in industry provided information. Being aware that there are so many sources of error in the material itself let alone errors of comprehension the 41 % correct may appear amazingly good to the reader.

Take Home

- The Internet is used for self diagnosis by one third of the US population.
- Less than half of the self diagnoses are confirmed by physicians.
- It is unknown to what extent false self diagnosis is owed to deficient quality of the found information or to miscomprehension on the part of the seeker.

So the question is whether we can equip the seeker with methods, filters, and sophistication to enable him to find and correctly interpret his personally required information. Among some more arguments that Kuehn picks up from the Pew investigation we would like to point to payment for health information. Empirically, 26 % of the interviewed hit a pay wall but only 2 % paid. Most others tried workarounds, some gave up. US Americans are not alone in doing so. An investigation from Switzerland [1] shows the same effect at a lesser magnitude. If

3.3 Effects, Risks, and Adverse Effects

the Pew argument is right that quality health information has its price some may have tried to save money in the wrong place. But the proof is still due that providers who charge fees are better than those who do not, see also Chap. 16.

3.3.2 True Risks

Regarding the large number of indeterminacies in the search itself, the known quality deficiencies of resources and errors that users may make when interpreting found results, it is amazing how few reports exist that adverse events materialized as a consequence of utilization of information from the Internet.

3.3.2.1 Hidden Agendas

Some providers have hidden agendas, some of which have already been addressed (cf. Sect. 3.3.1.4) and some will be addressed (cf. Sect. 7.4). Altogether they overlay business interests or personal convictions with material that appears as information but is carefully mixed with rhetoric serving the underlying agenda. Mitchell and Read [14] and Phillips et al. [15] unmask such patterns for ADHD and for smoking cessation. No wonder that clients who have hard times anyway to comprehend the right information right are further charged to untangle rhetoric and facts.

3.3.2.2 Temptation to Overutilize

Lovett and coworkers [11] analyze the results of the search for `cancer lab testing cost` to analyze the market of direct-to-consumer (DTC) cancer screening lab tests. According to their inclusion criteria they analyze eight tests ranging in price from $44.99 to $899 which can all be ordered without consulting one's family physician. All services offer screening, some include diagnoses and monitoring. Only one offers follow-up service in form of a telephone interview, with a nurse.

Lovett's group criticizes that clients are coerced into ordering by subtly creating fears and implied obligations to early detect and treat. Providers falsely create an atmosphere of trust by pointing to FDA approval of the individual tests. The uninformed reader may therefore conclude that the tests are recommended. However, FDA only confirms that the tests measure what they claim to measure. In contrast, clinical practice guidelines advise against general population screening of many of these tests.

The real material problems, however, come with handling the consequences of a positive finding. Having done the first step of running the test the client will feel inclined to follow up on a positive finding although the specificity or positive predictive value of the test is only moderate. Following up means seeing a physician – depending on insurance policies at the cost of the general public – and then to undergo physical, x-ray, pathological or other such diagnostic tests which all have their own implied risks. Here, finally, the individual client increases his individual risk of being hit by an adverse effect of the diagnostic procedures triggered by the test he has let himself talk into and that may have been unnecessary from the start.

> **Take Home**
> Following up upon positive findings of medical tests purchased without indication entails several risks:
> - Intrusive investigations as follow up may harm the client.
> - The general public may have to carry the cost.

It should be mentioned that the described process of being coerced into taking genetic tests without indication and then having to face the consequences is not directly related to the Internet. In principle, it can be just another over-the-counter business. However, the convenience and perceived privacy of ordering on the Internet and the opportunities for the provider to use Internet and animation technology for making the case that the client needs the test magnify the business potential of such kind of an offering.

3.3.2.3 Immediate True Harm

Regarding the size of the phenomenon and the abundance of risks reported above it is amazing how little actual harm caused through Consumer Health Informatics services is publicly reported. A 15 year old survey [5] finds incidents in three out of 1512 screened article, two describing emotional distress, one veterinary medicine problems and one truly serious, fatal incidence caused through extended inappropriate medication ordered online (more on the practices of online pharmacies cf. Sect. 5.2.4). A last minute search in March 2015 did not add new insights. A likely cause for the blank sheet is that a causal trace between exposure to information and harm is hard to detect.

> **Take Home**
> The amount of harm caused through quality deficiencies of Internet health information and miscomprehension on the part of the seeker is unknown.

3.4 Trust

3.4.1 Trust as a Basic Human Notion

Trust is an essential notion of living beings existing together. It has been defined as "an expectancy held by an individual or group that the word, promise, verbal or written statement of another individual or group can be relied upon" (cf. [18]). The sense of basic trust develops among a baby or newborn animal and (mostly) his parents and enables the individual to develop trust later in life towards other individuals. Family and kin are an arena where under favorable circumstances a differentiated pattern of trusted individuals emerges. In the family we can feel safe and give and receive attention and care without which life would be tremendously more complicated. Later teachers and peers and even later bankers, travel agents, auto dealers and also physicians become trusted agents. Trauma can develop as consequence of trust being abused.

3.4.2 Innate Instincts and Their Reincarnation in the Digital Age

Basic trust cannot develop but through sensory impressions. Investigations of newborns have shown that they can already distinguish the voices of Mom and Dad from other unknown voices, as they heard their voices repeatedly throughout the pregnancy. Later, known faces provoke other reactions than unknown faces. Nobel laureate Konrad Lorenz' experiments with geese that inevitably follow the first living being that they see when they hatch are world-famous.

3.4.2.1 Applying Innate Instincts to Web Resources

These innate instincts are not invalidated by the digital age. Robertson-Lang and coworkers [17] have recently provided a detailed analysis among Canadian citizens as to how health information is being searched and when trust develops. After providing basic utilization figures for Canada like the ones by [22] for the US they first report various pertinent findings from the literature, mostly pertaining to citizens 55 or above or 65 or above. Citizens who use Internet search for health information present themselves as more active and empowered; this may, however, be confounded through the preferred socio-economic status of those who use Internet. In various investigations [17] comparisons have been found between objective quality criteria versus subjective judgments of credibility. The latter include the graphical and interaction design (color, graphics, ease-of-use), good craftsmanship (no dead links, fast download) and the existence of references. While the first group of criteria is related to comprehension and also sensual – like faces – the second is common sense ("they know how to do the job") while the third is culturally trained ("that's how science works"). Interestingly, according to [17], scientific jargon of a site cannot outweigh insufficient or incomprehensible content when it comes to credibility. Aside from references nothing really pertains to quality of the contents in an objective sense. References are indeed one of seven criteria that the authors distill from various publications and later apply to assess the quality of websites that the users in their experiment identify as their best found sources. Other distilled criteria are that authors, their credentials and contact information and the last update date should be given and that the site should not include advertisement and should not be of commercial origin.

In their own investigation, Robertson-Lang and coworkers let individuals 55+ search for health topics, let them identify their favorite source and provide argument for their choice. The results are alarmingly naïve. Ninety-six percent believe that the source was credible. However, less than one third reported that they had checked the origin of their favorite and only 17 % correctly recalled the origin. So why did they believe in the credibility? One third based on previous knowledge, one quarter because the site had good information – with whatever means they may have come to these conclusions – one fifth because they were familiar with the source, etc. When asked for the origin of a site the participants in the study also mostly erred: only 15 % correctly classified whether the source belonged to a public institution or self-help group (63 % believers), a commercial institution (24 %) etc. Actually, 42 % of the favorites were commercial and 25 % nonprofit. This distorted perception of attribution and judgment is even more surprising since participants said they used domains (.com, .gov, ...) for assessment. To summarize: as a generation for which the Internet, with all its opportunities and intricacies, comes to the end of their active period, they still have no clear strategies to identify quality and build trust. Part of this lack of orientation is that many participants, in that case younger of age, in a study by Wogalter and Mayhorn [25] cannot distinguish true health related trust marks such as HON (Health on the Net) (cf. Sect. 3.4.3) from trust pretending related or unrelated eye catchers such as "secured" or "authorize.net".

[7] provide a more formal account of credibility of Internet resources, whose established factors have also been used in other domains such as e-commerce already. Their sample (N = 561 seekers of medical information, 72 % female) is younger (18 % 55+) and more Internet savvy (98 % 3 or more years of Internet use) which leads to a more rational approach with one innate element still lurking.

They elicit subjects' attitudes towards what fosters trust and readiness to act through questionnaires which represent four academically motivated established factors (24 questions for quality information, personalization, perceived impartiality, credible design) and two new medically motivated factors which capture a being personally involved (2 questions for corroboration and 8 for perceived threat/coping). The model finds satisfactory statistical support. Many correlations among the factors and between the factors and trust and readiness to act are significant. Some observations stand out. Highest correlations are within information quality and all three other established factors. Therefore, objective quality is well represented through the three other established factors. However, the correlation of both corroboration and perceived threat/coping with trust and with readiness

3.4 Trust

to act is two to three times higher than between established factors and trust. Corroboration means "better double check than trust just one source" and indicates a mature common sense. The prominent role of perceived threat and empowerment to cope indicates innate emotions: that which inevitably affects me outperforms more remote academic indicators of quality. And remarkably: while conveying bad news is at odds with trust, conveying bad news in a way that opens doors for action is not.

> **Take Home**
>
> Trust is a vital human notion.
>
> - Innate mechanisms of building trust – partially built on sensory information – still exist in spite of the digital age.
> - It is mainly elderly seekers who do not command criteria and procedures to check trustworthiness of digital media.
> - In the absence of innate mechanisms and trained criteria and procedures to allocate trust to or withdraw it from Internet resources, seekers apply a strange portfolio of sensory, common sense, and culturally imposed heuristics for quality assessment.
> - Features of web sites used for quality assessment are poorly recalled and respective heuristics often fail.
> - Appeal to the seeker's situation and empowerment for action are perceived as trust building.
>
> Malevolent providers can easily abuse such deficiencies of human judgment and build trust gaining websites to "sell" evil services, products, or convictions.

3.4.3 Trustmarks

As early as 1995 HON[5] was founded in Geneva in Switzerland, as a non-for-profit organisation targeting at transparency of quality of health information on the Internet. Others followed suit, such as URAC, MedCertain, Discern, but HON achieved the widest though still disenchanting coverage. The aspiration was that health websites were rewarded one of these trustmarks when their quality had been examined. Citizens were supposed to learn the meaning of the trustmarks and consequently trust so designated sites and not trust others.

HON and URAC still exists, URAC with a scope much broader than Consumer Health Informatics but very few Consumer Health Informatics services are URAC trustmarked. HON is also rarely seen, even at high quality resources. So what happened?

The still valid highest standard of unbiased assessment of quality of contents, peer review, was not realistic for websites, regarding the close to eternity turnover

---

[5] Health On the Net Foundation, http://www.hon.ch

times that scientific journals achieve with the much lower volume of articles submitted. We just do not have enough reviewers for the plethora of writers on the web. So, HON was wise enough and not even tried peer review. What they rather set up was a face validity approach: self-declaration of providers about their qualifications, scientific rationale and transparency of contents provided, sources of funding etc. (cf. http://www.hon.ch/Conduct.html as entry panel to the application process to become a HON trustmarked provider). Few providers, however, actually applied. Keselman and coauthors [9] on behalf of the AMIA WG Consumer Health Informatics[6] investigated the situation a decade later and provide some arguments for an explanation of the phenomenon. One is competition of trustmarks. Keselman and coauthors found nearly 100 different initiatives to determine and demonstrate medical quality of websites. To the author's knowledge the following has not been investigated systematically but the multiplicity may have irritated providers who did not want the effort to apply manifold and had no clear idea about the future reference trustmark. As a consequence not a single trustmark achieved wide positive public recognition. Consequently, again, clients did not develop the habit to seek trustmarked sites and to avoid others, hence there was no incentive for providers to seek the seal. A negative feedback loop. Additionally, we learn from [9] that the face validity approach of HON and equally its competitors, badly correlated with quality. So discouraging news was all around.

HON has meanwhile also started to trustmark mobile apps [2]. The need is immense, as Sects. 7.3 and 7.4 demonstrate. Maybe an opportunity for a rebound for the HON foundation.

> **Take Home**
> Trustmarks such as HON, URAC never achieved the sweeping recognition that had been hoped for to establish them as a safe and versatile instrument for the citizen to check trustworthiness of information in the Internet and in mobile networks.

3.5 Trustworthy Providers: More or Less

3.5.1 NIH and Its Organisations

Regarding the outstanding and lasting role of the NLM in providing quality information for health professionals its patient directed service is a natural candidate for the trustworthiness award.

---

[6]Meanwhile merged to form the WG Consumer and Pervasive Health Informatics.

3.5.1.1 MedlinePlus as a Collection of Resources

http://www.MedlinePlus.gov has an alphabetical directory of conditions and a search function (which makes it a Level 0 service) but transfers to various kinds of Level 2 online counseling, mostly information broker and logistics support services (cf. Sects. 5.2.5.1 resp. 5.2.5.2). It has featured topics by target groups, i.e. a minimal amount of personalization, (seniors, men, ...) and some amount of static (e.g. on vaccinations) and context dependent (e.g. winter health hazards) public health outreach messages. Through a "Popular searches" panel it includes minimal Level 3 functionality (for Levels cf. Chaps. 4, 5 and 6). When a client chooses an entry point and then dives in he hits an enormous variety of material. If e.g. selecting the tab men, then `Health Checkup`, then `Journal articles`, he has a selection between diverse educational material, diverse information brokered, and dead links to the AHRQ and to Medline articles about "School sports preparticipation" and "Kenya's Report Card on the Physical Activity". Remember? He was seeking for Men's Health Checkup. It makes an impression of lost in cyberspace reinvented.[7]

3.5.1.2 MedlinePlus's Search Engine

So quantity is sufficient, if not more than that. Quality is hard to judge, regarding the huge amount. Few systematic investigations have been reported in the past years but at least did Chumber and coworkers [3] compare the MedlinePlus search engine medical quality with that of Google™, Yahoo!™ and Bing® through applying criteria by JAMA [20] and HON (cf. Sect. 3.4.3). Knowing that these criteria are of face validity type and knowing that face validity is not strongly correlated with correctness these results are of limited value only, but still a surprise. Google™ comes out first, and MedlinePlus at similar ranks as the large general purpose search engines. How come, knowing the highly erratic nature of Google™ search outlined in Sect. 3.3.1.1? Chumber and coworkers' query was `diabetic nerve pain`: much better targeted than `thirst exhaustion` used in Sect. 3.3.1.1. So this need not amaze the reader but it should concern him: Those who already know a lot about their condition, such as the specialty language term diabetic nerve pain, find out more. Those who do not know to describe their condition precisely may find themselves arbitrarily taken into diverging directions.

3.5.1.3 PubMed Health

For seekers who want to look behind the scences http://www.ncbi.nlm.nih.gov/pubmedhealth/ by the National Institutes of Health touches upon the scientific

---

[7]These observations were collected on March 14, 2015, and things may be different on March 15. However, the general impression of NLM's policy of "Let's show all the related stuff we have" has been the same throughout visits in the past.

background of citizens' health concerns. Those clients to whom all the concerns raised in Sects. 8.4.3 and 12.4 about cognition and comprehension do not apply can dive right into a collection of selected abstracts and articles from scholarly journals with titles such as "Antibiotics for meconium stained amniotic fluid in labour for preventing maternal and neonatal infections".

3.5.2 Wikipedia's and MedlinePlus's Contents

In Sect. 3.3.1.4 we find Wikipedia®'s presumable independence at risk. Here we ignore that threat and report results of an impartial investigation of the quality of Wikipedia articles, in comparison with MedlinePlus and emedicine (http://emedicine.medscape.com/)(and various others not so widely used which will not be followed up upon). Regarding the queries and the material studied the investigation by Volsky and coworkers [23] is not core Consumer Health Informatics. It can be regarded Consumer Health Informatics because the general purpose search engine Google™ is used to search sources the quality of which is subsequently analyzed. It turns out to be some Consumer Health Informatics because of the three resources that cover the searches best two are meant for the general public (MedlinePlus and Wikipedia) while one is meant for professionals (emedicine). It is professional information seeking rather than Consumer Health Informatics through the terms for which Google™ searches: Acute otitis media, ..., cervical lymphadenopathy, ..., epistaxis . Given this coerced focus on professional material it is no wonder that the service meant for professionals performs nearly twice as well (84 % correct contents) as the two services for lay citizens (MedlinePlus 49 %, Wikipedia 46 %).

Some further investigations address the user satisfaction with health resources and their search, reading level of presented material, etc. However, none of these investigations answers the question: Which resource delivers the highest quality information for the lay citizen who asks a question in lay language?

Take Home

MedlinePlus cannot demonstrate the excellence hoped for as a reference where the lay citizen can conveniently find correct health information.

Repository for the lay person As a resource it offers an enormous amount of information. This gives the seeker hard times to not lose orientation.

Repository for the professional It could not compete with resources built for the professional.

Maintenance The contents has formal deficiencies. Regarding its sheer size it is hard to maintain.

Search engine It could not compete with Google™.

Some of the mediocre performance can be attributed to research designs that penalize MedlinePlus' aims.

> **Take Home**
> When queries are medical specialty terms neither lay citizen search engine (MedlinePlus, Wikipedia) can compete in quality of found resources with professional search engines.

3.6 A Short Note on apps

Apps for smartphones or tablet computers are a fast-growing segment of consumer communication technology. A short summary of its present importance and limitations for Consumer Health Informatics in general follows in Chap. 7. This section deals with those aspects that are specific for Level 0: searching and eventually finding.

In the open space of the Internet, content is harvested and made available through search engines which boast themselves as registering and making searchable each and every quote in a website. A search for "thirst" retrieves all sites in the depth of which thirst occurs, be they medical and pertinent or totally off the mark. On the contrary, the space of apps is regulated and made accessible through major platform providers such as Apple for the iOS^{TM} and Google^{TM} for the Android ^{TM} architectures (and some others with a smaller market share). They tag their respective registered items by major descriptors such as "medical" or "diabetes" only, which are, therefore, not found when searching for "thirst". The Internet normally has extremely high – in the millions – recall at the price of low precision while the opposite holds for the app market.

Registration with the providers and henceforth distribution through their portals ("stores") requires compliance with their technical specifications rather than with standards of (medical) content quality. Consequently, authors of apps often provide technical credentials – as opaque and doubtful as they may be –, sometimes a legal notice and a street address of the responsible person or company, and even more rarely credentials as a health professional. Paradoxically the client has to use the Internet as a parallel source of information to assess the standing of an author of an app he is about to purchase, and there is no guarantee that something be found. In the "fun" and "convenience" place of apps, legal accountability seems to be an out of place notion. Waivers of liability are normally present in marginally or truly medical services but the client often searches in vain for the entity that he might take to court.

It appears that the app stores are not the best place for searching in the Level 0 sense. Only when the client knows the right descriptors will he find apps. The number of apps when searching for medicine, diabetes, blood pressure, smoking (cessation) is impressive (several thousand) but by far smaller than the number of hits on the Internet. In Sect. 5.3 we will analyze some apps which broker and locate other apps by exploiting health terms that the client uses.

> **Take Home**
>
> Search and quality assurance is even harder and more fragmented for apps than it is for Internet resources.
>
> - Names of requested services must be known or guessed very precisely.
> - Providers' medical credentials – if any – and terms of use are often hard to find.

References

1. Brockes MC, Neuhaus Bühler RP, Schulz E, Neumann CL, Schmidt-Weitmann S. Medizinische Online-Beratung im Universitätsspital Zürich vor und nach Einführung einer Bearbeitungsgebühr (in German). Dtsch Med Wochenschr. 2010;135:231–5. doi: 10.1055/s-0029-1244838.
2. Boyer C. e-mail Feb 8, 2015. Personal communication. C. Boyer is Executive Director of Health On the Net Foundation.
3. Chumber S, Huber J, Ghezzi P. A methodology to analyze the quality of health information on the internet. Diabetes Educ. 2015;41(1):95–105. doi: 10.1177/0145721714560772.
4. Clauson KA, Polen HH, Boulos MNK, Dzenowagis H. Scope, completeness, and accuracy of drug information in wikipedia. Ann Pharmacother. 2008;42:1814–21. doi: 10.1345/aph.1L474.
5. Crocco AG, Villasis-Keever M, Jadad AR. Analysis of cases of harm associated with use of health information on the internet. JAMA. 2002;287(21):2869–72. doi: 10.1001/jama.287.21.2869.
6. Davis JJ, Cross E, Crowley J. Pharmaceutical websites and the communication of risk information. J Health Commun. 2007;12:29–39. doi: 10.1080/10810730601091326.
7. Harris PR, Sillence E, Briggs P. Perceived threat and corroboration: key factors that improve a predictive model of trust in internet-based health information and advice. JMIR. 2011;13(3):e51. doi: 10.2196/jmir.1821.
8. Jank S, Bertsche T, Herzog W, Haefeli WE. Patient knowledge on oral anticoagulants: results of a questionnaire survey in Germany and comparison with the literature. Int J Clin Pharmacol Ther. 2008;46:280–8.
9. Keselman A, Logan R, Smith CA, Leroy G, Zeng-Treitler Q. Developing informatics tools and strategies for consumer-centered health communication. JAMIA. 2008;15(4):473–83. doi: 10.1197/jamia.M2744; http://jamia.bmj.com/content/15/4/473.short.
10. Kuehn BM. More than one-third of US individuals use the internet to self-diagnose. JAMA. 2013;309(8):756–7. doi: 10.1001/jama.2013.629.
11. Lovett KM, Liang BA, Mackey TK. Risks of online direct-to-consumer tumor markers for cancer screening. J Clin Oncol. 2012;30(13):1411–4. doi: 10.1200/JCO.2011.37.8984.
12. Law MR, Mintzes B, Morgan G. The sources and popularity of online drug information: an analysis of top search engine results and web page views. Ann Pharmacother. 2011;45:350–6. doi: 10.1345/aph.1P572.
13. Muchnik L, Aral S, Taylor SJ. Social influence bias: a randomized experiment. Science. 2013;341:647–50. doi: 10.1126/science.1240466.
14. Mitchell J, Read J. Attention-deficit hyperactivity disorder, drug companies and the internet. Clin Child Psychol Psychiatry. 2012;17(1):121–39. doi: 10.1177/1359104510396432.
15. Phillips CV, Wang C, Guenzel B. You might as well smoke; the misleading and harmful public message about smokeless tobacco. Biomed Cent Public Health. 2005;5(31). doi: 10.1186/1471-2458-5-31.

16. Di Pietro NC, Whiteley L, Mizgalewicz A, Illes J. Treatment for neurodevelopmental disorders: evidence, advocacy and the internet. J Autism Dev Disord. 2013;43(1):122–33. doi: 10.1007/s10803-012-1551-7.
17. Robertson-Lang L, Major S, Hemming H. An exploration of search patterns and credibility issues among older adults seeking online health information. Can J Aging. 2011;30(4):630–45. doi: 10.1017/S071498081100050X.
18. Rotter JB. A new scale for the measurement of interpersonal trust. J Pers. 1967;35(4):651–65.
19. Recupero PR, Rainey SE. Characteristics of E-therapy web sites. J Clin Psychiatry. 2006;67:1435–40.
20. Silberg WM, Lundberg GD, Musacchio RA. Assessing, controlling, and assuring the quality of medical information on the internet: caveant lector et viewor – Let the reader and viewer beware. JAMA. 1997;15(277):1244–5.
21. Tu HT, Cohen GR. Striking jump in consumers seeking health information. http://www.amcp.org/WorkArea/DownloadAsset.aspx?id=12579, 2008. Tracking Report 20, Accessed 21 Sept 2013.
22. Tu HT. Surprising decline in consumers seeking health information. http://www.hschange.org/CONTENT/1260/1260.pdf, 2011. Tracking Report 26, Accessed 21 Sept 2013.
23. Volsky PG, Baldassari CM, Mushti S, Derkay CS. Quality of internet information in pediatric otolaryngology: a comparison of three most referenced websites. Int J Pediatr Otorhinolaryngol. 2012;76(9):1312–6. doi: 10.1016/j.ijporl.2012.05.026.
24. van Voorhees BW, Hsiung RC, Marko-Holguin M, Houston TK, Fogel J, Lee R, Ford DE. Internal versus external motivation in referral of primary care patients with depression to an internet support group: randomized controlled trial. JMIR. 2013;15(3):e42. doi: 10.2196/jmir.2197.
25. Wogalter MS, Mayhorn CB. Trusting the internet: cues affecting perceived credibility. Int J Technol Hum Interact. 2008;4(1):75–93. doi: 10.4018/jthi.2008010105.

Chapter 4
Level 1: Enhancing the Provider – Client Relation Through IT

4.1 Introduction

Today, most physicians answer patients' telephone calls. Some call themselves when lab or other results have arrived or examinations are due. Hospitals, public health authorities and others call whole target groups of medical or preventive programs or to advertise new treatment options. In a way they all apply `telemedicine` as the NLM defines it as a MeSH keyword (1993): "Delivery of health services via remote telecommunications. This includes interactive consultative and diagnostic services." Telemedicine has the sub concepts `teleradiology` and `telepathology` which point into a different direction but also `remote consultation`. While the two former deal with specimens or images taken from the patient that are viewed and diagnosed by a specialist in a different place the third involves the patient personally: "Consultation via remote telecommunications, generally for the purpose of diagnosis or treatment of a patient at a site remote from the patient or primary physician."(MeSH 1996) However, the patient still is the object of physician's activity while in Consumer Health Informatics we emphasize that he be an agent, a person who actively contributes or takes the initiative. A patient who calls his doctor takes initiative. Or a patient who sends his doctor an e-mail. This takes us right into Level 1: physician and patient enhancing their face-to-face visits through intermittent synchronous and asynchronous exchange of information.

4.2 Level 1 Consumer Health Informatics Versus Telemedicine

While telemedicine sees the patient in a passive role we find a good definition of telemanagement that includes the Consumer Health Informatics typical client activity in [4, p. 236]: "In this review, telemanagement will be defined as an interactive and proactive management approach consisting of an ongoing partnership of patients and professionals supported by ICT and focused on clinical outcomes and patient goals in the individual."

> **Take Home**
> Telemedicine and Consumer Health Informatics share the property that health information and data are exchanged through the distance. Consumer Health Informatics differs from telemedicine through the client's active responsible role.

4.3 Incorporating New Media into Patient-Physician Communication

Physicians have used the telephone for ages to communicate with patients. This started to become an accepted practice in times, when awareness for risks was much lower than enthusiasm for technology. Telephone still plays an essential role today but subsequently we concentrate on more recent digital media and their role for health.

4.3.1 E-Mail

E-mail is the first means of electronic communication that entered the field after telephone. Like telephone e-mail is one-to-one or one-to-few: The sender selects the recipient(s) and relies on secure delivery according to the criteria in Sect. 13.3.

An analysis of its advantages and risks that have to be controlled has already been provided in 2003 by Bovi and the Council on Ethical and Judicial Affairs (CEJA) of AMA [1]. It also forms the basis of Derse's (2008) outline about the legal nature of different electronic communication means provided in Sect. 17.5. In the respective chapter the distinction has also been made between so far illegal use of electronic means of communication to *establish a new* patient physician relationships while it can be legal – if done properly – to *enhance an existing* patient physician relationship. Level 1 means enhancement of existing relationships which we will now look at.

Bovi establishes an analogy between a surface letter and e-mail. She rightly states that the written character of the message avoids the busy setting of the face-to-face visit with its time pressure. It rather allows thorough consideration and structured writing, plus a feeling of anonymity, compared to a face-to-face setting, to easier voice sensitive or personal issues. She leaves out of consideration whether conversely the lack of a sensory impression the provider would collect in a face-to-face meeting compromises the quality of his decisions. She also does not address whether the need to write widens or narrows the gap between more or less literate subpopulations.

Basically, e-mail is an asynchronous form of communication. However, in case of need of the client and opportunity of the provider turnover times can be minutes. Of course, this bears risks. Expectations of clients for expedited response to urgent requests may be in conflict with physicians' routines and scheduled time slices when to work through their e-mails. Since physicians have lots of other obligations which do not go away when e-mail enters the scene such schedules and respective delays in replying to e-mails are fully legitimate. Therefore, a necessary precondition for mutual trust with the medium is that rules about response times and other rules have been agreed upon before including e-mail as a means of communication. A further legal analysis for the USA is in Sect. 17.4.1.2 while the respective German Professional Code only covers telemedical activities (Sect. 17.4.2.2).

We address some other aspects here, some of which are just practical and some others that also call for legislation. The asynchronous nature has many blessings. Both, client and provider, can smoothly integrate the communication in their personal chores. Although financial compensation for e-mail is not yet a sure thing physicians may like to gain control over the sequence of addressing their patients' requests. E-mailing also is – or should be incorporated to be – self-documenting. An e-mail correspondence entered into an electronic health record is an authentic trace of advice sought and given.

Authentic at least if the identities of writers and readers can be doubtlessly asserted. However, this is not the case with conventional e-mail. The client cannot normally confirm the credentials of a writing entity that claims to be a physician. Actually, automatically generated message will in some projects pass like ones written by a human, cf. Sects. 5.2.2.2 or 17.6.2.3.

The provider cannot normally be sure whether an individual he writes to is the patient he knows, whether the client's e-mail account is under the client's exclusive control, or whether he shares it with family or friends. A highly effective but also resource demanding approach to guarantee authenticity of writers and readers of e-mail – as well as for other communication media – is presented in Chap. 13. Assuming that with these or other methods authenticity can be made sufficiently secure e-mail as part of provider-client communication has various advantages. With present bandwidths it can even be used conveniently for bulky attachments such as images or biosignal recordings.

> **Take Home**
>
> E-Mail as an enhancement of an existent patient physician relation is a convenient upgrade of face-to-face, telephone, and written communication.
>
> - E-Mail combines the advantages of considerate written communication with speed, availability, and authentic dump into an electronic record.
> - Exaggerated expectations must be managed through clear and agreed upon rules.
> - Identity, authentication, and privacy bear certain risks and must be managed thoroughly.

4.3.2 Social Networks

While e-mail still is a major and apparently stable factor of online communication new media are gaining ground that are different in one essential aspect: Blogs, feeds, and social network communications lack the one-to-one or one-to-few character of e-mail; they rather broadcast. They are perceived by many, not only younger generation, as a convenient way of sharing and exchanging contents and way of life. According to Hawn [5] they may be experienced as "simpler, more elegant, and more fulfilling experience for physicians and for patients". This raises the question whether a more elegant, more fulfilling experience is central to, unrelated to, or in conflict with the necessary clinical core of a good treatment. In Chap. 15 we address such question as how "good treatment" can be operationalized and how a client's positive perception of his therapist can appear like a therapy effect that does not exist. Here we concentrate on facts and side effects of the communication method as such, irrespective of the meaningfulness and effectiveness of contents conveyed.

The social network way of showcasing and peeking is perceived as normal and natural by many who consequently expect their doctors to also join the medium of their choice. We do not yet have a mature cultural feeling or professional rules for this phenomenon although a gut feeling of professional discomfort about being Facebook "friends" with their patients can be read from letters to journal editors such as [6].

In the first place the basic principles of growth and spread in social networks have as consequence that newly created information reaches ever-growing circles ever faster irrespective of whether the information is good or bad. For medicine this means approved and unapproved, curative and harmful, caring and advertising information all travel equally fast and equally far. The search problem of Chap. 3 turns into a filter problem when all our friends place contradictory and variably relevant posts on a topic.

Besides this problem of quality and reliability we face several problems of confidentiality and privacy that are typical for social media. The underlying structural cause is that with growing membership "communication channels grow exponentially more diffuse" [5]. There are privacy settings to delimit the circle of spread. But privacy may be breached through intruders or insiders. Even if principles are implemented securely by providers they may be undermined by member behavior. For some setting privacy appropriately is so complicated that they give up while others draw a narcistic gratification from the unlimited spread of what they post and what is posted about them and do not want privacy. Whatever the reasons, such members become seed nodes in the network from which information spreads to other members where it was not meant to spread.

Respective risks have been analyzed by Guseh and coworkers [3]. The risks hit both ways. For the first information from the private sphere may intrude the patient physician relationship. The physician may self-disclose about his personality, such as sexual orientation, which for some patients may jeopardize their trust into their provider. Conversely, the physician may "see" patient behaviors (such as smoking) not meant for him and henceforth is in doubt and has no legal guidance whether he must, may, or must not use such information in his therapist role, as well as whether the information must, may, or must not be part of the medical record. Consequences for all parties can be dire: for the physician if a court holds violation of confidentiality, for the client when an insurer refuses coverage of treatment cost.

For the second information from the patient physician relationship may be disclosed and become publicly known through "private" "friends" who get access to information exclusively meant for the therapeutic context. Patient problems become publicly known, with larger risks for the patient's family and social and professional circles. In conclusion, social media "friendship" between physician and patient may lead into attitudes and behaviors other than the therapeutic best.

Patients may not be aware of all these consequences and may therefore feel rejected if the physician refuses an invitation to be a "friend". This is taken into account in [3] where four guidelines for physicians concerning their participation in social networks are suggested. Apart from under no circumstance initiating "friending" with a patient himself the physician should

1. Avoid social network dual relationship; if patient may feel hurt, discuss risks face-to-face; maybe get ethics or risk management consultation
2. Carefully manage info inadvertently received through social sites
3. Exercise restraint in what to disclose as profile; concentrate on administrative info (specialty, contact info, address, office hours, ...)
4. Read and *understand* (emphasis by author) the privacy settings; use language and style that fits a physician's role and perception; be aware that conservative privacy settings do not safely prevent breaches

Regarding the complexity of managing one's privacy settings at providers that continually change the privacy options as such and the methods to check and adapt individual settings, the request to *understand* seems like wishful thinking.

> **Take Home**
>
> Social networks foster unintentional broadcast of information often not meant for many of the recipients.
>
> - Physicians may unintentionally self disclose information that undermines their patients' trust.
> - Patients may find medical or behavioral information widely disclosed that they meant designated for the clinical relation alone or for their private circles alone.
>
> Social networks should, therefore, be used with great caution and very restrictively for client physician communication.

4.3.3 Electronic Health Records

Health Records are the collections of data that health care providers or patients gather about the diagnosis, treatment and other relevant information. In earlier times they were on paper and each provider had its own collection but here we concentrate on electronic media which opens the doors for merging data from different providers and the patient himself.

The topic is so wide that it deserves a book of its own. Rather do we provide an entry level description and comparison with e-mail and social networks here. Chapter 14 provides much more detail from history through function, contents, quality, to role in the Meaningful Use campaign.

A major distinction to be made pertains to the center of gravity. In Chap. 14 we distinguish between provider controlled Electronic Patient Portals (EPPs) and patient controlled Personal Health Records (PHRs). An advanced notion of the latter client centered approach are self tracking services, combined with quantified self devices, where patient-provided data originate from vital sign sensors.

All these variants of electronic resources for the provision of medical data have different communication properties than both e-mail and social networks. Primarily they are passive resources from which information is retrieved upon need. Like e-mail they may include messaging to the patient or a selected caregiver such as alerts when tests or treatments are due or monitored vital signs deteriorate. But these are advanced functions on top of the repository. EPPs and PHRs definitely do not broadcast. Information is accessible to a clearly designated and limited set of clinically qualified and authorized individuals plus the client, plus family or friends that he may involve and who must be given an authentication and who cannot pass authentication on to friends of friends of friends. This assumes of course that the infrastructure that hosts the resource and manages access is equipped with a highly secure concept and implementation for privacy and confidentiality. In Chap. 13 we demonstrate that this can be done.

For the sharing of health information between providers and clients in an Electronic Resource (ER) of either of the above types or any intermediates to be meaningful a variety of aspects have to be dealt with. They include:

Unique identification It must be secured that all information collected in one ER actually relates to the same client and that all information available about one client gathers in the same ER.

Integration of past data When the present problem suggests that past data may help to interpret and make right decisions it must be possible to access them from within the present ER without prohibitive effort.

Comprehension While in Chap. 14 the challenges of technically managing ones data are addressed we point to the challenge of intellectual comprehension of difficult to read material. Specialties such as medicine have specialty languages for good reason; they are instrumental to concise and unambiguous communication among those who are in command of the specialty language. On the other hand clients report about their problems in lay language and need information and explanations in lay language unless they can be taught some medical literacy. In any case it is not sufficient to grant logistic access as a straightforward interpretation of the term EPP might suggest; rather must the bridging of the different sociolects be constructively addressed. More on comprehension and the risks of non-comprehension can be found in Chaps. 8 and 12.

Quality of client provided "data" The more actively the patient contributes or assumes the role of the owner of the ER the more does the helpfulness of the overall resource depend on the trustworthiness of the client's observations and measurements. Although a cooperative attitude can normally be assumed it may be absent in some psychiatric conditions and it does not guarantee professionalism in taking data and reporting symptoms. Therefore, policies have to be defined and services implemented accordingly that allow the provider to incorporate client provided data into his decisions and set him free of accountability when he relies on inaccurate data.

Data "patchwork" When clients in their role of providers of PHR's selectively grant and deny access to parts of the data the provider cannot know whether he sees the whole story. He may for instance see three medications that would not interact with one he plans to add but does not see a critically interacting fourth one. Therefore, policies have to be defined and services implemented in such a way that fairly assign accountability between provider and client for harm caused through data that the client made invisible .

Besides these subtle ingredients of functionality we must also have the considerable additional cost for sustained operation in the absence of an immediately visible ROI in mind. EPP's may pay through an intensified "customer relationship" or more effective processes through better scheduling, reduced readmissions etc. The Mayo Clinic and the St. Johannes-Hospital apps discussed in Sect. 4.5.1 are examples. Still providers are in a situation to justify the investment to their shareholders. PHR's have even harder times to come up with business models. With the exception of high prevalence chronic conditions such as diabetes clients typically are not sufficiently organized among themselves and by no means legal entities that could assume the role of provider organizations for sustained provision of PHR's. Health plans may step in but this interferes with the patient centered idea and may raise concerns as to what information leaks out to the health plan. These and other funding models are discussed in Chap. 16. Other core aspects are outlined in Chap. 14.

> **Take Home**
> Different forms of electronic resources (ERs) dedicated to health content and shared between physician and client offer various opportunities to enhance care and pose specific challenges.
>
> - ERs have the potential to develop into a full account of a client's health history including physician and client provided data.
> - When made available with great care and through a well designed set of services with up to date privacy safeguards they enable to grant access exclusively to precisely designated qualified individuals.
> - Safe and secure logistics to provide data are by far not sufficient for beneficial use. Solutions must be found for safe medical practice when clients hide data or report findings in lay language, or when clients are confronted with data they do not understand or which sound intimidating.
>
> Technical solutions are by far not sufficient. Trusted and efficient communication must be established on top.

4.4 Condition Specific Services

4.4.1 Discharge Management and Follow-Up Care

Patient discharge and follow-up after surgery is a process that requires high attention. True complications and patient perceived threats both have a certain likelihood to happen, the more likely the sooner after surgery patients are discharged to their home environment. The distinction between true complications and harmless perceived threats is a matter of information processing and communication. Some of the true complications can also be managed at home through appropriate bidirectional flow of information. When a complication or perceived threat is not appropriately managed the frequent cause of action is readmission into inpatient care. This is a considerable burden on the patient, on hospital staff and also financially. Therefore, Consumer Health Informatics support of the discharge and follow-up home care process suggests itself. However, few services exist as yet. This may be due to the high criticality and vulnerability of the patient right after intrusive treatment. Very high safety standards have to be met before postoperative homecare services can be established. We briefly describe a very densely knit service to allow safe discharge of selected patients 1 day after carotid endarterectomy.

4.4 Condition Specific Services

In an experiment in Genoa, Italy between October 2005 and June 2006 Palombo and coworkers [8] showed that a carefully selected one seventh of the patients where certain risks were not present can be safely released home at 12 noon on the day after the surgery when the subsequently described support structure and monitoring scheme is in place and stays in place for 48 hours. Discharge after 24 hours was an ambitious goal knowing that the typical length of stay after this surgery still is several days.

The conditions under which patients became eligible to the 24 hours regime included that surgery could be done minimally invasively, that a certain standard policy for the surgery itself and the material used could be applied, that patients did not show postoperative complications such as fever, cervical hematoma or abnormal tests and that their personal home equipment and regional coverage allowed UMTS communication and less than 30 km transport distance to an appropriately equipped emergency care hospital. Those patients received detailed information about the experiment and about complications they might be aware of, as well as hands-on training with the video equipment. They were equipped with a bag holding an electronic blood pressure meter, a smart phone with video function and calcium antagonist medication.

A complete monitoring videoconference was scheduled every 4 hours at daytime, each checking the optical appearance of the surgical wound, blood pressure, heart rate, and general conditions as communicated by the patient. All communication was logged and monitored at the study center. Patients also had to fill a four item questionnaire at the time of discharge, at every videoconference and before and after a control examination on the eighth day.

For 21 of the 36 primarily eligible patients there were no complications in the 24 hours after surgery such that the 1-day discharge schedule could be initiated. Medically, the 1-day discharge patients fared well. Compared to 126 patients undergoing the same surgery during the same time period but for some reason were not eligible for the 1-day discharge regime (the control) no medical prior risk or outcome variables differed notably. Since the assignment of patients to one-day discharge or control could not be random for medical reasons the assumptions underlying the statistical test theory do not apply, but if they would, no difference would be significant. Three hypertensive crises could be handled in the home environment through video communicated advice to administer the calcium antagonist medication.

From the perspective of Consumer Health Informatics the time course of questionnaire filled values is equally interesting. From beginning to end the 1-day discharge patients were asked ten times (including at every videoconference) whether they felt insecure, skeptic, enthusiastic, or satisfied, yes or no. The control patients were equally asked at discharge and before and after a control visit after 8 days. Overall, the control arm had seven questionnaire presentations, i.e. four in the days between discharge and final control visit.

At discharge about 60 % of the control felt insecure compared to nearly 90 % of the 1-day discharge patients. Conversely, none in the 1-day discharge arm felt satisfied at the time of discharge while at their individual times of discharge (i.e. individually varying some days later) the control arm had more than 20 % satisfied patients. On the first videoconference the 1-day discharge arm even finds all their members insecure. These perceptions later turn out as deceptions. In the cause of time perceptions reverse. While the percentage insecure in the 1-day discharge arm falls continually, videoconference by videoconference, to 60 %, then 30 %, ending at nearly zero after the 8 day control visit, insecurity remains high in the control, at around 40 % and boosts to 95 % after the control examination on the eighth day. It appears that the sequence of videoconferences step-by-step builds trust in the 1-day discharge arm about the signs of their postoperative state and how to handle them while the control arm remains ignorant. After the control examination on the eighth day control arm patients are fully hit in the face by the expectation that they are now alone with their fate. No wonder that the enthusiasm and satisfaction scores remain at a moderate level in the control arm while they keep growing in the 1-day discharge arm and satisfaction reaches 100 % on the eighth day. As a side effect of an information flow regime primarily meant to curb actual medical risks patients were emotionally and cognitively empowered.

Caveats should be raised whether the medical non-inferiority and emotional superiority of 1-day discharge reflects that the 1-day discharge cohort was the lower risk cohort, whether we see a dose effect that the 1-day discharge patients were exposed to a higher "dosis" of information flow, or whether some of the perception biases described in Sect. 15.2.3 blurred the actual results.

This notwithstanding the regime of rapid discharge and dense videoconferencing surveillance worked medically and emotionally, but at what price? Moderate, as it turns out. Videoconferencing alone, assuming that the equipment can be reused, costs 25 Euro per patient, compared to one in-patient day at 470 Euro. So with very few unnecessary readmissions avoided through careful video consultation, like hypertension treated at home with calcium antagonists, makes the service cost-effective.

4.4.2 Managing Chronic Diseases

Level 1 Consumer Health Informatics services exist for various chronic conditions including asthma, diabetes, hypertension, depression, rheumatism and pain. We subsequently analyze the *Pain Course* as a well considered recent example of wisely combining consumer health with classical elements of service and TASMINH2 as an equally well considered monitoring and management of hypertension.

4.4.2.1 Pain Course

Dear and coworkers [2] have developed the therapy concept for patients with chronic pain as an Internet delivered CBT (iCBT) service. Its standardized Internet delivered part consists of didactically designed "5 online lessons, 5 lesson summaries combined with homework assignments, and 9 written resources ... " on topics such as sleep hygiene and managing attention .... "These components are released sequentially and serially over eight weeks." [2, p. 944] Patients also receive narratives about other patients who mastered certain problems. Standardized e-mails announce the availability of new material or remind of due assignments with already available material.

For the purpose of the trial reported in [2] the authors also try to standardize the human part: one designated clinical psychologist does all the following activities with all clients, although in a naturalistic environment other clinical psychologists of about the same qualification who know the contents of *Pain Course* could equally well do the client contacts. These consist of weekly telephone calls and depending on circumstances e-mails. In the phone calls the psychologist "summarizes content, answers questions, reinforces progress and encourages skills practice" ... [2, p. 945] etc. A target of 10–15 min contact time per telephone call was set but not taken strictly when the client situation required less or more time.

Trial subjects were solicited through advertisements in various media that address pain patients in Australia. Besides chronic pain of at least 3 months diagnosed by a general practitioner or specialist clients had to present a somewhat stable situation, i.e. mainly stable medication and absence of severe psychotic or depressive disorders or life-threatening risks. To connect to classical care the authors also sent letters to their clients' physicians to invite them to contact and to report any concerns they might have about their patients participating in the treatment or the trial.

Since chronic pain after a while may impact various aspects of quality of life the authors decided to check whether their intervention is able to reduce the activity level of various problems: depression, anxieties, and disability as primary outcome measures[1]; and pain, self-efficacy concerning pain management, kinesiophobia and self statements, mainly catastrophic cognitions and coping strategies.[2]

Eligible clients were randomized to either treatment (*Pain Course*) or control (3 months waiting list, then *Pain Course*). Measurements were taken at pre-treatment, posttreatment, plus 3 month follow-up for the treatment arm. For the treatment arm telephone calls were scheduled at 6-week intervals during the follow up period.[3]

The results are impressive. Except for coping all differences between the treatment and the control arm at the end of the intervention are highly significant.

---

[1]PHQ-9: Patient Health Questionnaire 9-Item (for depression); GAD-7: Generalized Anxiety Disorder 7-Item; RMDQ: Roland Morris Disability Questionnaire, developed to identify activities endorsed or avoided due to back pain, but can also be used for other pain.

[2]WBPQ: Wisconsin Brief Pain Questionnaire, subscale for average pain intensity; PSEQ: Pain Self-efficacy Questionnaire; TSK: TAMPA Scale for Kinesiophobia; PRSS: Pain Responses Self-Statements, catastrophic cognitions and coping subscales.

[3]Three month follow-up data capture could not be taken in the control arm because for them waitlist was followed by the *Pain Course* treatment.

The therapy arm maintained their achievements: 3 months after termination none of the scores had changed significantly. The effect size for all scores was at least moderate as judged by Cohen's $d > 0.5$, and large for self-efficacy ($d > 0.8$). Many effect sizes kept growing after termination of the therapy: they were large at 3 month follow-up for depression, anxiety, pain, kinesiophobia, and catastrophic cognitions, and remained large for self-efficacy. One patient each had a deterioration of more than 30 % for depression resp. anxieties at the termination and four for anxiety at 3 month follow-up. Clients attested that *Pain Course* had not contributed to these deteriorations.

All these apparent improvements have to be seen in the light of subject reflection effects as discussed in Sect. 15.2.3.3.2. However, the size of the changes, the number of changes going into the same direction and the standardized instruments used to assess activity of symptoms clearly suggest that *Pain Course* is effective. The authors regret that they cannot measure the influence of the factor iCBT versus the factor therapist. They also report that therapist time varied a lot from client to client, with no visible impact of the time spent with a client on the outcome the client achieved. What may appear as a weakness of the experimental design may as well point to the true strength of this Level 1 service: the fact that the human therapist was right there (per telephone or e-mail) when he was needed and to the extent he was needed; that he was available for the unforeseeable, the deeply human, without counting and without extra billing, ready to reconfirm those in need and to let the others alone. On an average *Pain Course* still saves a lot of therapist time and effort. Without insisting on a precise estimate on the size of the savings the authors report that the average time devoted to one client within the trial was approximately 80 min (standard deviation 30 min) while offering the same CBT concept in a face-to-face group setting would take approximately 8 therapist hours per client. Furthermore, the presented combined approach allows the therapist to fully concentrate on what he is really needed for and to relieve him from the routine of over again teaching the same class. At the same time the majority of the clients is truly empowered: they keep improving after the end of the therapy and they trust their own power, as visible from the large effect size of the self efficacy score at post treatment and at 3-month follow up.

4.4.2.2 Hypertension Management

In a mid sized RCT McManus and coworkers ([7], project TASMINH2) demonstrate how a sophisticated scheme with Consumer Health Informatics and face-to-face elements reduces blood pressure more than usual care. Patients under regular in-person treatment could enroll.

Intervention arm participants ($N = 234$) received equipment for convenient automatic RR measurement and to transmit values daily for every one in 4 weeks. Easy individualized traffic light coding of the measured values let the clients know how they were faring daily. Four or more red days a month was classified as above target. Family doctors were involved in corresponding medication changes or increments when a months was above target. They were on no a specific algorithm for such changes but had received and been encouraged to use the NICE (National Institute for Health and Clinical Excellence) guidelines. Two subsequent changes could be initiated through the distance while for a third change a visit was requested. For deeper insight into the treatment effect and control the involved family doctors received monthly summary reports. Patients with internet access could view their readings themselves.

Control and intervention arms improved on the main outcome variable systolic blood pressure at 6 and 12 months by noteworthy 9.2 (6 months) resp. 12.2 (12 months) in the control and 12.9 resp. 17.6 (all readings in mmHg) in the intervention arm. Noteworthy, because positive effects kept increasing i.e. the intervention was tailored intense enough to have an effect and low key enough to avoid fatigue (cf. a lessons learnt in various interventions for the metabolic syndrome, 9.5.3 and 9.6.1.2). Noteworthy also because the control arm improved by an enormous decade. This seems to call for checking biases discussed in Chap. 15. However, we may have a very simple reason here, kind of a functional underpinning for what appears like a Hawthorne effect: Participating physicians all received the encouragement to apply the NICE guidelines. Assuming they are good physicians on an average they likely treated everybody more consciously with the onset of the trial, so on the average everybody benefited.

To conclude with an appraisal of the tested Consumer Health Informatics service: Intervention arm participants benefited so much and highly statistically significantly more than control arm participants that an Consumer Health Informatics effect on top of more conscious physician performance can safely be claimed. Active patient participation and better timely transparency about the effectiveness of the past medication likely are its effective agents.

Take Home

Condition specific services can achieve good care by purposeful use of technology and communication:

Rapid discharge Videoconferencing and automated blood pressure measurement.
Pain management Online courses and telephone reenforcement.
Hypertension Intertwined partially automated, partially visit based dose control based on automatically transmitted data.

4.5 A Short Note on apps

4.5.1 Customer Relationship apps

Organizations that have started offering apps for their clients are insurance/health maintenance organizations and providers such as hospitals. Health care providers primarily present more or less personalized logistics information, logistics transactions such as making an appointment, medical education etc. To some extent and when the client so wishes and agrees with disclaimers concerning the risk of both data exposure and unforeseen clinical events will medical records data and advice be shared between the client's smartphone and the provider's server.

The Mayo Clinics are a major US example. A client who knows that institution and its reputation will search for `Mayo clinic` and find it immediately. Others who seek `patient` may as well come across the Mayo Clinic apps but equally well hit other apps that are not that quality. When searching for `hospital` (2180 hits) Mayo clinic is not among the first 150, however, a somewhat informed seeker will notice that a large share of the findings are infotainment and may change his search term. `clinic` (1143 hits) has Mayo Clinic as 30th,[4] among other health providers from around the world, but as well computer games, `Debt clinic` .... When finding Mayo Clinic from Google play and App Store, he is informed that he may gain access to various medical (labs, pathology reports, medications, ...) and logistics (appointments, directions, ...) information and is invited to sign in. With an ongoing treatment at one of the Mayo Clinics the service is Level 1. The Mayo Clinic also has a small suite of Level 2 apps (cf. Chap. 5). They provide access to a considerable amount of quality information such as `Mayo Clinic ...Meditation, Diet, on Pregnancy` etc. Search in the Apple App Store is highly sensitive to small variation in search terms, though. `Mayo clinic pregnancy` returns 0 apps, while `Mayo clinic o` delivers Mayo Clinic on Pregnancy from Google play and App Store. Another point of confusion is that about half the apps found with `Mayo clinic` are for health care professionals. A Level 3 (cf. Chap. 6) service `Mayo Clinic Health Community` which was available in June 2013, had been withdrawn by December 2014. Apparently, also best hospitals still have to learn lessons in Consumer Health Informatics.

JoHo Dortmund Innere Medizin I from Google play and App Store by St.-Johannes-Hospital Dortmund, (found through `Krankenhaus`, the German translation of hospital) is a German service offered by St. John's Hospital Dortmund which shares many of the traits described for Mayo Clinic. In addition it offers two kinds of support for emergencies: relevant phone numbers (including space for the client to add personal ones) and which are dialed right through after one tap of confirmation, and GPS localization to guide the dispatching of an ambulance. It offers patient maintained profiles and diaries. It does, however, not offer an internal

---

[4]Figures about apps are from December 2014.

4.5 A Short Note on apps

social network function, i.e. communication between users of the app. The hospital also offers an app to guide parents through pregnancy with a combination of advice and diary function. There they can upload content into some of the existing social networks.

`Kaiser Permanente` with its dual nature of a provider and a health maintenance organization is slightly different in character: for nonmembers it mainly is the invitation to become members. For members it offers all kinds of personalized medical and account information. Kaiser Permanente explicitly excludes emergencies, although for emergencies and the possibility to report an emergency with automatic transmission of GPS coordinates is a specific opportunity of mobile Consumer Health Informatics services. Here as in many cases medical software concerns may be the reason.

> **Take Home**
> Large providers and health plans enhance their customer relationships through patient portals, partially exploiting the convenience and ease of use of smart phones.

4.5.2 Condition Specific apps

Although it suggests itself to have app support after a clinical encounter (surgery, chemo, etc.) or chronic conditions (diabetes, asthma, COPD, etc.) hardly any apps exist for the post inpatient situation, while most of the apps for the second type of situation are Level 2 and will be discussed in Sect. 5.3.4.

While most Level 1 apps that are presently available in the stores deliver some data sharing and more or less personalized information provision purposes a recent development AERIAL from the Netherlands tries to reach farther: in its present version it offers decision support about seeking or not seeking professional help. In the foreseeable future it may include recommendations for adapting pharmaceutical treatment.

The development reported in [9] addresses COPD. Patients with medium to severe COPD and frequent exacerbations are equipped with a smart phone app AERIAL that interprets recent signs and distinguishes between "stable COPD" and "active exacerbation". It is then up to the client to seek professional help. The app normally reminds one time per week to checkmark eight symptoms (present/not present), to take a FEV_1 (Forced Expiratory Volume 1 second) test and a pulse oximetry measurement. Reminder frequency is automatically increased to maximally one per day when there is an apparent risk of a beginning exacerbation. Measurement values are both transmitted to the smart phone through a specialized medical Bluetooth® interface. The set of 10 parameters feeds a momentary Bayesian network that has been trained to discriminate with high precision between a stable and a deteriorating situation. The Bayesian discriminator is implemented on the smart phone such that the client has his decision support at his disposal anytime anyplace, independent of net coverage and availability. However, recorded data are also transmitted at the earliest convenience to a server where nurses, general practitioners and respiratory medicine specialists who are treating patients that are using AERIAL can also double check and take action when they deem it necessary.

In tests with some patients van der Heijden and coworkers found that when well instructed and being provided with text and images about how to handle the app the patients felt confident that they could use it. In a test on data sets from patient records the discriminatory power of the Bayesian network could be proved. Therefore, prerequisites have been accomplished for AERIAL to become a serious Level 1 smart phone app. However, since it actively impacts patient behavior it is a medical device according to European legislation. Before bringing it into use, i.e. placing it into one of the app stores, it has been filed for release as a medical device.

Future planned developments require even more scrutiny to get approval as a medical device. They include to use the temporal development of signs in order to predict a forthcoming exacerbation and to recommend adaptation of dosage of drugs already used or of adding antibiotics if a beginning infection is diagnosed by the future algorithm. While in the present version the scope of the app "only" is to equip the client with a better decision bases to seek or not to seek professional help – which he would do anyway when the exacerbation comes, but maybe so late that it takes an unfavorable course – the future one would actively change the therapy. The legal implications of such an expansion of functionality are analyzed in Chap. 17.

References

1. Bovi AM. Ethical guidelines for use of electronic mail between patients and physicians. Am J Bioeth. 2003;3(3):W43–7. For the council on ethical and judicial affairs of the American medical association. doi: 10.1162/152651603322874771.
2. Dear BF, Titov N, Perry KN, Johnston L, Wootton BM, Terides MD, Rapee RM, Hudson JF. The *Pain Course*: a randomised controlled trial of a clinician-guided internet-delivered cognitive behaviour therapy program for managing chronic pain and emotional well-being. Pain. 2013;154:942–50. doi: 10.1016/j.pain.2013.03.005.
3. Guseh JS, Brendel RW, Brendel DH. Medical professionalism in the age of online social networking. J Med Ethics. 2009;35:584–6. doi: 10.1136/jme.2009.029231.
4. Van Gaalen JL, Hashimoto S, Sont SK. Telemanagement in asthma: an innovative and effective approach. Curr Opin Allergy Clin Immunol. 2012;12(3):235–40. doi: 10.1097/ACI.0b013e3283533700.
5. Hawn C. Take two aspirin and tweet me in the morning: how twitter, facebook, and other social media are reshaping health care. Health Aff. 2011;28(2):361–8. doi: 10.1377/hlthaff.28.2.361.
6. Lacson SM, Bradley C, Arkfeld DG. Facebook medicine. J Rheumatol. 2009;36(1):211. doi: 10.3899/jrheum.080750.
7. McManus RJ, Mant J, Bray EP, Holder R, Jones MJ, Greenfield S, Kaambwa B, Banting M, Bryan S, Little P, Williams B, Hobbs FDR. Telemonitoring and self-management in the control of hypertension (TASMINH2: a randomized controlled trial. Lancet. 2010;376:162–72. doi: 10.1016/S0140-6736(10)60964-6.

8. Palombo D, Mugnai D, Mambrini S, Robaldo A, Rousas N, Mazzei R, Bianca P, Spinella G. Role of interactive home telemedicine for early and protected discharge 1 day after carotid endarterectomy. Ann Vasc Surg. 2009;23:76–80. doi: 10.1016/j.avsg.2008.06.013.
9. van der Heijden M, Lucas PJF, Lijnse B, Heijdra YF, Schermer TRJ. An autonomous mobile system for the management of COPD. J Biomed Inform. 2013;46:458–69. doi: 10.1016/j.jbi.2013.03.003.

Chapter 5
Level 2: Services Without In-Person Contact Between Provider and Client

5.1 Introduction

Services and business transactions that used to be conveyed face-to-face two decades ago are now normally expected to be offered online. Cooking recipes, language classes, training programs, navigation aids, investment counseling come through the Internet, as smart phone apps or on kiosks in public places. The knowledge and advice included in such digital services may be provided through some knowledgeable authority – or at least claiming to be such – or may be the common shared knowledge of the community. For the latter "wiki" has established itself as a term and a movement that draws more and more attention. For the purpose of this textbook we want to make the conceptual distinction between the two – professional provided or community provided – although in practice the borders may be blurred. The necessity to distinguish the two in the arena of medical advice and treatment derives from the fact that the legal character and ethical obligations differ fundamentally when a provider acts in his capacity of a health professional as opposed to a member of the community sharing his personal experience and observations. Wiki i.e. community-based knowledge sharing will be handled in Chap. 6. This chapter rather introduces services provided by professionals i.e. Level 2 services through various examples. A legal assessment of such online only professional services follows in Chap. 17.

> **Take Home**
> Much alike other domains such as retail, travel, etc. health information and services are conveyed through the distance through businesses and volunteering community members. In the medical domain legislation and ethics differ fundamentally whether lay persons or professionals publish.

5.2 Examples

5.2.1 Health Awareness

Awareness of health hazards and opportunities to prevent hazards empowers clients to improve on their personal medical prognosis. The problem with health and awareness services is that there is no problem, at least not a perceived problem on the part of the prospective client. Therefore, health awareness services need to get into the way of unsuspecting clients, draw their attention or spot patterns of hazardous behavior to start intervening. The subsequently offered contents typically consists of education and chunks of knowledge. Some of the following examples demonstrate that because unawareness often coincides with low education level and literacy contents must be packaged for related target groups.

5.2.1.1 Child Health Promotion

Limited awareness of child health prevention programs is a public health concern. Thompson and coworkers [24] address this concern through a service implemented on touchscreen kiosks placed in a McDonald's restaurant, a Department of Motor Vehicles and a public library. The kiosks advertise themselves through labels "Child health information" visible on the sides and also on the idle screen. The information conveyed has been tested and found appropriate in a clinic-based study. It covers incidental risks such as frequently occurring injuries, smoking and television overuse, sudden infant death syndrome prevention. Three information packages address screening for common developmental or health problems and one assists in interpreting breathing problems that may be related to asthma. Clients get the advice based on the age of the child. Clients can register and continue former sessions upon revisit. The whole menu structure is totally user driven. Contents has been provided at eighth grade reading level.

Thompson and coworkers report a variety of results concerning utilization of the service. They achieved at least two noteworthy tangible clinical or behavioral improvements. Eighty-seven percent of the information requests concerning asthma led to better controlled management of the disease. Forty percent of the ADHD sessions initiated clinical follow-up of a respective risk. The authors also found out from optional exit surveys that users with high (above high school graduation) and low educational level rated information equally as easy to use. On the contrary, users without any Internet experience found the information hard to use. This indicates that the child health promotion kiosks are an example to analyze whether Consumer Health Informatics reduces or increases the digital divide, as briefly addressed in Sect. 1.9.2.

5.2.1.2 Sexually Transmitted Infection Prevention

Prevalence of STI is outstandingly high in a subpopulation of young adults, gay males and female sex workers. This population uses the Internet over proportionally and to some extent to seek sex partners. Curioso and coworkers [6] set up the service that tried to identify web sessions meant to find sex partners and to inject risk alerting and preventive information into such sessions. Their initial setting is public Internet access booths (cabinas públicas) in Lima/Peru, a kind of Internet café with a bit more of privacy, i.e. no other visitors being able to watch a visitor. Other investigations had shown that such cabinas are actually used for sexual contacts.

The technical background of the service is to parse blogs for words or phrases typically used when seeking sexual contacts. Whenever such a pattern is identified the blogger is provided with information about safe sex practices. Major advantage of this approach is to be highly specific: it addresses precisely those presumably in need of the respective information and spares all others. It can easily also be offered on a much wider scale, maybe nationwide while still only filtering individuals by their blogging contents. This is briefly addressed in Sect. 1.9.1. Filters have to be adapted for other countries and updates may be required as the sociolect evolves. Of course, privacy concerns are imminent: it certainly feels as a major intrusion when such a blog is monitored and leads to a third-party intervening. This serious subjective concern of the to-be-client contrasts with the objective usefulness of his authentic behavior in a virtual environment for diagnostic purposes. In Chap. 13 a technical ground will provided for tracing clients' behaviors in virtual social networks while maintaining anonymity. Section 17.11 investigates whether such intrusion into the patient's autonomy is in acceptable balance with potential health benefits.

> **Take Home**
> Early on low intensity – low commitment services achieved improved health awareness by injecting their message into normal "work"-flows of prospective clients: shopping, reading, driver license renewal, Internet surfing.

5.2.2 Mental Health Coaching

Mental disorders suggest themselves as another field for Level 2 services. For many conditions both, diagnosis and therapy are based on communication. Physical encounters required for functional diagnosis, lab tests, or physical examinations play a minor if any role. For those diagnoses that can be established through standardized questionnaires and interviews and where appropriate communicative setting and exchange of contents is the core part of therapy, delivery through the Internet or other medium of communication is an obvious option.

In the following we will analyze one example of panic disorder, of addictive behavior, and of mild depression. As we will see this is conceptually from easiest to hardest which is not meant as a ranking of the severity of the diseases.

5.2.2.1 Anxiety and Panic

Panic disorder, if untreated, is a debilitating condition that decreases life expectancy in general and may even lead to suicide. Besides pharmacological treatments Psychodynamic Therapy and Cognitive Behaviour Therapy (CBT) have been successfully applied. However, access to face-to-face therapy is limited by the number of therapists available. Group CBT reduces the impact of such shortage at the price of more complicated scheduling and patients having to comply with provider schedules rather than taking an active role.

Bergström and coworkers [3] present a service where CBT for panic disorder with or without agoraphobia is conveyed through the Internet. Ten modules are offered that are composed according to CBT principles (1: psychoeducation, 2–3: cognitive restructuring, 4: interoceptive exposure etc.). Each ends with an assignment for the client. Approval of an assignment through a therapist enables access to the next module. One module can be finished per week. Therapists answer e-mails within 24 hours during weekdays and react to delivered assignments when need be. Clients can join un-moderated discussion forums with other clients.

Generally, enrollment to the service can be client initiated online only. For the purpose of their clinical trial [3], however, started with a face-to-face session. All patients, i.e. referrals from GPs or outpatient clinics as well as clients that had come spontaneously were seen by a psychiatrist to verify the diagnosis and to check inclusion criteria for a randomized trial. The trial compared the new Internet CBT with the standard group CBT. For the purpose of that trial therapists assessed outcome in a blinded setting, coming to the conclusion that internet CBT and group CBT did not differ a lot in the percentage cured (reduction of the diagnostic instrument Panic Disorder Severity Scale (PDSS) value by 40 %) at the end of the therapy and at 6 month follow up.

A more differentiated outline of the trial is in Sect. 15.4.2. There we also follow up upon the authors' claim of reduced therapist hours per client in the Internet CBT arm claimed to lead to improved cost-effectiveness as the major new outcome.

Face-to-face interactions can be cut down further in this service if client assessment can be achieved through the internet or other communication media. For the PDSS where therapists stage patients face-to-face it would mean that they can reliably stage a client after a phone or video call. Client self report measures also exist (cf. [21]). With their application we would fully abstain from human "gatekeeper" involvement. Risks and limitations of client self assessment as outlined in Chap. 8 must then be considered.

Since exposure can be an element of therapy and virtual reality offers unprecedented opportunities to create nearly real exposure without physical risk respective approaches may attract more interest soon. An impression can be gained through www.virtuallybetter.com. Some of the providers of those services have also written an early review article including some ethical issues [1].

5.2.2.2 Addiction

Addiction can have different targets, including alcohol, substance, hallucinogens, and smoking, but also internet and gaming and behavioral patterns such as in eating disorders. Examples of Level 2 services exist for all except obviously Internet and gaming. We present an example of Internet mediated smoking cessation therapy here. An example of therapy of uncontrolled drinking is further analyzed in Sect. 15.4.1.1. Bauer and Moessner provide an up to date survey on Consumer Health Informatics services for eating disorders [4].

Strecher and coworkers are pioneers in the field of Internet mediated smoking cessation. In [22] they report about a tailored program where depth of tailoring of the components is varied experimentally between randomized arms. Generally, the service is based on "cognitive-behavioral methods of smoking cessation and relapse prevention, including an appeal to motives for quitting, stimulus control, self-efficacy enhancement, and suggestions for coping with tempting situations and emotions." [22, p. 375]. Clients receive advice to increase their self efficacy and hence to increase their odds to overcome barriers. This advice can be general or personalized to the client's known most recent barriers. Clients are offered success stories of individuals who are their age and gender and can be further matched by ethnicity, marital and family status, their individual motivation and other environmental and personal variables. They receive the material as a whole bunch or cut into individual pieces. The service provider introduces itself as an institution only or with personal reference (photographs, personal messages) including signature of the therapists. Therefore, the various mechanisms above to personalize on the side of the client find a complement in personal reference on the side of the provider. Among the latter, signature as a cultural token of creating a trusted personalized setting plays a special role that will be outlined in Sect. 17.5.1.

In a sample of 1866 subjects each receives one combination of more or less personalized treatment elements. The material is available or is made available in pieces over a period of 5 weeks and remains available. Therapy effect is measured through 7-day abstinence according to subject responses in telephone interviews 6 months after termination of the therapy. Smoking cessation rates are not impressive, between 23.1 % and 39.1 %, but they never are [14], even in face-to-face intensive classical treatment settings. Reported smoking behavior may even be biased due to the subject expectancy effect described in Sect. 15.2.3.3.2, see also [9]. This notwithstanding, we find interesting differences between the effectiveness of personalization of parts of the service. The difference between marginal and in-depth personalization is highest for success stories (p = 0.018), also significant for the other more personalized variants but unsignificantly inverse for packaging: getting the whole material in one bunch is superior to provision piece by piece. It is interesting to note that the highest single combination of factors is individualized success stories for clients without high school graduation. Unless we have the highest subject expectancy effect here this points to the necessity to be concrete and detailed for those who cannot get the message from abstract specifications.

5.2.2.3 Depression

Depression is a widespread condition through all ages. Approved behavioral therapy forms do not essentially require physical presence, i.e. lend themselves for being offered as Consumer Health Informatics services. Depression is sometimes associated with anxiety or panic disorders which makes combined treatment offers also appear worthwhile (for a review that also covers conventional therapies cf. [8]). Depressive patients may have suicidal ideations which may take them as far as successfully committing suicide. Therefore, dealing with such ideations, either through exclusion of respective subjects from services or through thoroughly detecting respective cues is a must. That it can be done has been shown for a Level 1 Internet CBT therapy [27]: In a sample of patients where their GPs had first excluded "people who were 'actively suicidal'" in the remaining patients suicidal ideations were common (54 %) before and dropped to 30 % after the therapy.

On the other hand, persons with mild depression may not even think they have a disease and need treatment while those with major depression may no longer be active enough to seek any form of help. Therefore, getting the right persons to subscribe as clients to Consumer Health Informatics services for depression is a problem in its own right.

Spek and coworkers report about an Internet-based CBT service for mildly depressed elderly. For the purpose of the investigation [23] they snail mail to all inhabitants of the target age group (50 to 75) in the city of the investigation (Eindhoven, The Netherlands) and do a primary screening for inclusion by a paper-based depression scale EDS. Subjects exceeding the EDS threshold of 12 are telephone interviewed to exclude too severe or suicidally inclined cases.

Apart from this safeguarded enrollment procedure the service operates virtual only, it does not include any patient – provider contact. For those eligible the service consists of a thoughtfully remodeled course of eight modules each consisting of text, exercises, videos and figures. In contents and spirit it corresponds to a classical therapy approach that has already proved effective in face-to-face group settings (CWD) and that has been adapted to Dutch, and makes use of the additional illustration and animation opportunities of the new medium. The included instructions encourage clients to complete one session per week.

The authors present the service as part of an RCT. Besides the waiting list control condition which will not be addressed further here there is the classical CWD in 10 group sessions. For this and for the Internet based interventions the proportional completion rates of the course and posttreatment outcome assessment are reported. Turnout for posttreatment outcome measures to be taken was 65 % in the Internet versus 55 % in the course condition. Average completion of the presented material was 78.1 % versus 98.3 %. 48.3 % finished the Internet course, 94.5 % the group course. Therefore, in terms of dose effect considerations the Internet course was unpurposefully under dosed. Nevertheless, the Internet course reduced the primary outcome variable, an indicator of clinical activity of depression (BDI II), by about the same amount as the face-to-face course (Internet: 19.17 to 11.97, group setting 17.89 to 11.43). Possible limitations of the design of the trial notwithstanding we see the positive effect that while saving workload on the side of the provider and offering the client the opportunity to take the course according to his personal time management rather than being constrained through the schedule of his therapeutic group the Internet treatment achieves about the same therapeutic effectiveness.

For the purpose of the investigation the clients were thoroughly selected using telephone interviews and other psychometric instruments. Therefore, the setting is not truly Level 2. It contains elements of face-to-face or at least "voice-to-voice". We now consider options to make it fully Level 2.

Instruments to diagnose and severity stage depression typically are questionnaires from the paper ages which technically can be transformed and have been transformed into similar looking online questionnaires. If their sensitivity and specificity for depression itself is sufficient and if they reveal serious suicidal ideations with sufficient sensitivity they suggest themselves as methods to control enrollment to Consumer Health Informatics depression services.

Even for the psychometrically approved paper-based instruments, however, results are controversial about the use in routine health care settings such as primary care. An AHRQ report comes to the conclusion of "the need for more detailed follow-up by a clinician to determine ... diagnostic criteria ... other possible causes ... coexisting psychiatric disorders" [18, p. 5]. Furthermore, base psychometric validity has not been shown in a convincing way for internet versions of classical instruments. Existing investigations appear too optimistic regarding the response rate of only about one third among those invited as volunteers to help calibrate the Internet versions of psychometric instruments [7].

> **Take Home**
>
> Mental conditions principally lend themselves for Level 2 services because compared to somatic diseases the amount of instrumentation and physical presence in centers of care plays a smaller role. Inasmuch as risks outlined in Chap. 8 are carefully attended the following are examples of successful services:
>
> **Anxiety, depression, panic** Internet adapted CBT performs equally well as group CBT for anxiety and depression. Virtual reality exposure therapies are under development.
>
> **Addiction** In a smoking cessation service differential effectiveness of different personalization strategies can be shown although the overall success rate is as disenchanting as in face-to-face therapies.
>
> Results are based on standard paper questionnaires where some concern still exist whether they are valid and equally calibrated when presented online.

5.2.2.4 C-Referral

What might help to legalize services meant as purely virtual, Level 2, is what we suggest to call c-referral. It means that a prospective client of a Consumer Health Informatics service for a condition two is a patient in the classical sense for some other condition one and enrollment is initiated or safeguarded through the health professional who treats condition one.

Depression along with some other disease is an example. A care provider for the other disease who believes to see signs of depression can mention the opportunity to his patient. He can take some precautions for clients not to enroll to virtual only services if they hold some of the typical risks of depression that can escalate. For those eligible he can encourage and approve; this corresponds to a referral if it were between classical care providers. Van Voorhees and coworkers [26] present a well considered example how this can be made work. In a RCT they identify patients visiting primary care physicians and compare different means of motivating those patients eligible for treatment of depression to first visit to an information portal and in case of interest to join a well established Interactive Support Group (Psycho-Babble, http://www.dr-bob.org/babble, cf. [12]). A major result of that trial is that appealing to patients' internal motivation is most effective to get them enrolled with Psycho-Babble. To establish this and other results the process of the RCT was split into nine major steps which include different stages of patient consenting and being randomized to a study group. More important for the concept of c-referral is that selected steps of the RCT can be collapsed into not more than extending one routine in-person primary care encounter. When the primary care physician gets the impression that the patient should receive depression treatment and can confirm the impression by presenting a depression staging questionnaire whose application does not require the specialty qualification of a psychiatrist (PHQ-9, [15]) he can motivate and approve enrollment to a Level 2 Consumer Health Informatics depression service. Another positive result in [26], which may to some extent be confounded through a selection bias of those consenting to participate in the trial, is that 87 % of those who visit the information portal subsequently join Psycho-Babble. That means that the collateral impulse provided by the primary care physician does not only address the legal problem of the only virtually conveyed Interactive Support Group treatment but is also very effective in helping patients accept that treatment offer.

Van Bastelaar and coworkers report about another approach with minimal attachment to classical care. Originating from a pre-existing Coping With Depression Consumer Health Informatics service they develop a variant for diabetics. Heavily drawing on early user participation they replace or modify general topics to enhance diabetes related coping targets. For a prospective client to get enrolled he must have been referred through his treating physician or agree that he be informed, thereby safeguarding against potentially hazardous provider client relations. Once enrolled clients take the online lessons, submit their exercise results, get e-mail reminders when overdue, and receive minimal guidance through human coaches checking the exercise results. Van Bastelaar's group could show high user satisfaction mainly caused through the tailoring to the specific stress factors and concerns that diabetics face. Their cohort, though, mainly was well educated, young, and had diabetes mellitus 1 over-proportionally represented. A positive pre-selection of individuals who want to manage their health related issues anyway and found the right means here may be the explanation [25].

Other diseases for which c-referral may be productive include asthma, COPD, arthritis, congestive heart disease. The question remains whether a physician licensed for one specialty may legally make patient related decisions or transactions pertaining to a different specialty. We address this question in Sect. 17.7.2.

> **Take Home**
> Presently medical Level 2 Consumer Health Informatics treatments are illegal (cf. Sect. 17.6.2.3). C-referral suggests itself as procedure that allows to legalize them without laws having to be changed.

5.2.2.5 Concluding Remarks

Clearly, the above examples demonstrate limitations of the purely virtual approach. In Chap. 8 we analyze how respective risks can be detected and curbed. These risks and limitations should, however, be traded off for the advantages of Level 2 services being conveniently available 24/7 at equal quality any place. At the end of this chapter we also address to what extent they are scalable (Sect. 5.5).

5.2.3 Somatic Diseases

Virtual only management of diseases that affect the human body is much harder to achieve than of diseases that affect the mind. Mostly, it requires some kind of physical examination and the application of a certain physical, be it pharmaceutical treatment regime which normally can only be provided through the presence of a professional. On the borderline we find equipment such as blood oxygen or blood glucose meters or peak flow meters for residual breathing capacity which the client can use by himself after being instructed. Nevertheless, the Level 2 examples presented below are less pervasive and by the same token less persuasive as the examples above. We still want to explore the opportunities but also want to point to the fact that in Chap. 9 the large field of the metabolic syndrome is covered much more widely and elements of all levels will become apparent there.

5.2.3.1 Urinary Continence

Urinary incontinence is an embarrassing problem the prevalence of which increases with age and which hits women more than men. Although being physical in nature it can be modified if not avoided through appropriate behavior changes. Because the problem as such is not a topic of choice in face-to-face communication anonymous online advice seems to be a preferred alternative.

An online portal to advise elderly women at risk has already been built as early as 2003. Its contents draws on a large body of knowledge which relates specific forms and situational variants of the problem to concrete behavioral preventive measures which also still help at a moderate level of clinically manifest urinary incontinence. The measures include pelvic muscle exercise, fluid management techniques, avoidance of caffeine etc. which can all be applied without physical presence of a care provider. An expert system has been developed and implemented as a web portal where clients checkmark their specific problems and the rule base infers their suggested measures for them. In this sense the selection of recommendations is personalized but advice in canned text form adds to just naming behavior modifications.

The system has been built with all knowledge engineering and usability methodology of that time being applied and received very favorable feedback from prospective users. There seem to be no experimental evaluations of the effect. Indeed they would be hard to achieve because the anonymous one-stop shop nature of the portal where the client collects her advice without uncovering her identity is part of the success that such a system might achieve but adverse to the researcher's interest to provide proof [5].

5.2.3.2 Asthma

Asthma is a widespread disease the prevalence of which is paramount in highly polluted urban areas. It affects all ages with children being at special risk because asthma may go unnoticed and at the same time can be fatal if not attended and treated appropriately. In Sect. 5.2.1.1 we have described a combined public health – Consumer Health Informatics effort to help identify children that need to be tested for asthma. In Sect. 12.2.1.1 we analyze the risks of impaired perception of the level of activity of one's asthma. Here, we concentrate on a compact concise service for adults developed for use on smart phones in the city of Taipei/Taiwan.

The problem with asthma is that as long as you keep it under control by appropriately dosed corticosteroid aerosols, systemic corticosteroids or antileukotrienes it will not progress and its inflammatory side effects will not materialize. However, such appropriately dosed base anti-inflammatory medications will let the patient feel healthy and will let him believe that he can reduce or even terminate the treatment. He may then encounter a relapse and find himself in a worse shape than before his last start of a treatment episode. Therefore, feeding back to the patient as accurately and as timely as can be the presently required dosis is a key for long-term successful management. This is explained nicely in [2], see also Sect. 12.2.1.1. There we learn that relying on clients' perceptions alone is not enough. Objective readings are taken from a peak flow meter. The Peak Expiratory Flow Rate (PEFR) reading indicates the present capacity to exhale, which is the most sensitive short term indicator of the asthma activity. The client subjectively reports symptoms such as sleep quality, severity of coughing, difficulty in breathing and use of relief medications (symptomatic treatments such as β_2-agonists when the corticosteroid base medication is felt to be insufficient). Liu and coworkers [16] have developed a system that has a smart phone front end for clients and a backbone rule engine on a server which together provide the following information flow and service: The client enters his observations including the PEFR and for the subjectively reported complaints and behaviors specifies how severe they were (on a scale from 0 to 3). From this cross-section of observations and from the variation of the PEFR recordings of the past 7 days the client is assigned a severity score which draws on a Global Initiative on Asthma (GINA) 2006 guideline. The score value is classified as "controlled" or "partially controlled" or "uncontrolled" given the GINA threshold values. Based on that classification the client receives the advice instantaneously as to dose adaptation if required, plus general recommendations to attend and possibly to control environmental factors and stress, and how to apply concomitant medications re upper airway diseases.

In the setting of the trial about which Liu and coworkers report here, the automatic recommendations were cross checked by professionals at short intervals. But if the effectiveness and safety of the service can be proven in various aspects (see Sects. 15.4.1 or 15.5 and 15.8) and if additional safeguards would be built in that in the case of doubt, i.e. a set of readings that is not in accordance with common knowledge about asthma or the individual patient history, a professional would automatically be called in, the system can be considered as a Level 2 virtual only service.

In the trial measurements were taken at monthly intervals starting after 3 month. We report the 6 month endpoint data here. Compared to a randomly assigned control arm (n = 60) which received a passive asthma symptom diary booklet and was asked to record the same variables daily as did the smart phone arm (n = 60) the adherence of the experimental arm (smart phone) with the protocol was about the same (77 % control, 72 % smart phone still reporting after 6 months). The main physical target variables PEFR and FEV_1 and the SF12® physical for physical facets of health related quality of life came out significantly better in the smart phone arm, e.g. PEFR 383 $Lmin^{-1}$ smart phone vs. 343 $Lmin^{-1}$ control. The most important behavioral change, however, is that the smart phone arm increased their dosage of corticosteroid base medications significantly and continually throughout the 6 month interval while the control stayed the same. Unscheduled visits to the emergency department were 2 (smart phone) versus 12 (control). This clearly indicates that the increase in dosage in the smart phone arm was reasonably sized on average and not, as could be assumed, an indicator of oversupply. Rather were the lower doses that the patients in the control chose to apply undersupply with unfavorable consequences as to individual health and utilization of resources.

5.2.3.3 Cancer Survivors

Having survived cancer and mostly having undergone extended intrusive treatment finds clients in the strange role of being healthy and, therefore, not qualifying for receiving financially covered medical care and on the other hand being objectively at higher risk for future cancer and subjectively highly insecure about one's prognosis and potential to curb risks. An overwhelming amount of information exists about life expectancy, beneficial and detrimental factors, new signs to attend, late side effects to be aware of etc. Therefore, offering the individual survivor just that selection of information that pertains to his case and sparing all the rest may be instrumental to more empowered behavior.

This has already been requested in a 2005 Institute of Medicine report "From Cancer Patient to Cancer Survivor: Lost in Transition" and has led to an initiative of the University of Pennsylvania Abramson Cancer Center to provide a respective Consumer Health Informatics service OncoLife. At http://www.oncolink.com/oncolife/ clients are informed about the fully anonymous and transient nature of the subsequent service and are then encouraged to provide a detailed account of their past cancer case. This includes lists to be checkmarked about type and location of cancer, treatment modalities and targets, names of chemotherapeutic agents, and various demographic and behavioral information. Having finished clients can request their individualized cancer survivorship plan as a PDF file.

The cancer survivorship care plan has a major logistics support and a major knowledge and behavior component. The logistics part consists of forms for various types of information that typically gather in the course of a cancer treatment but may be spread across various locations and care providers (treatment schedule, treatment summary, blood count reports, family history, insurance information etc). Knowing

5.2 Examples

what to search for allows the client to pull together a comprehensive retrospective record of his treatment. The knowledge and behavior component consists of chunks of text (typically a fraction of a page long, some hyperlinking to more in-depth further reading) that address risks, signs, preventive measures etc. carefully selected to cover the individual situation of the client and not to overwhelm with non-pertinent information. For instance, if there was no radiation therapy, the client will not be offered texts about late effects of radiation.

All information is conveyed very empathetically. The service takes the attitude that it is the client who chooses and the web portal that holds underpinning information in support of well-informed choices. It makes very clear, though, that the information provided is "not a substitute for professional care". This is also clearly stated in a report about utilization of the service in 2007 through 2008 [10]. The authors point to the fact that in the present implementation all medical facts are being supplied by the client and are not and can presently not be validated against electronic records. Linking to electronic records is mentioned as a possible future development which would, however, trade validity of the information for the anonymous nature of the service.

The analysis of 3647 surveys delivered by clients draws an interesting picture about who does and who does not use such information and how well or not so well cancer survivors are being taken care of. The majority of the users were female, Caucasian, college educated and with 51 the median age was much younger than the typical cancer survivor part of the US population. Breast cancer survivors make up 22 % of cancer survivors in the US but 45 % of OncoLife users. The reverse is the case with prostate cancer survivors (17 % versus 6 %). About one half of the whole population (1869) did receive some follow-up care but only a small percentage of these had been given concise survivorship information (235). Most users were highly satisfied with both the data that the system requested and information that it provided. Obviously, those that used OncoLife were well enough informed about their past treatment that they felt confident to precisely name the medications they had received. OncoLife had mostly been used by survivors or family/friends. Professionals, though, also appreciated the service.

Besides the core functionality of offering selected survivor information the following additional services are worth mentioning. In some aspects OncoLife is really personalized. Clients can for instance request a cancer survivor care provider within their ZIP Code neighborhood. They can even recommend one, giving the service a Level 3 flavor. The information, though is taken as provided and not quality checked. In another population of clients characterized through not having had cancer yet and trying to figure the individual risks and behavioral modifiers, users are taken through a similar in style dialogue as survivors – just concentrating on biography and other diseases rather than on cancer – and receive textual advice and graphical display of individual risks. Finally, persons diagnosed with cancer and seeking treatment options can request clinical trials that they might be eligible for. This, however, is not anonymous; clients have to enroll and register personally for good reason. Since, when seeking this kind of referral we are clearly entering the stage of medical treatment or medical research which is a service provided by professionals to contracting patients who have to identify themselves.

OncoLife has millions of potential users worldwide. Thousands have voiced their satisfaction in the survey presented after the consultation. It is likely that those who were satisfied also felt better with their survivor role and took a more active stance in following up on healthy behaviors, interpretation of new signs and handling late side effects. If it is true that the more active initiative taking patient has better odds to manage his disease it is likely as well that OncoLife improves outcomes. However, with the present instantaneous anonymous consultation and no chance to follow up on client careers without risking the atmosphere of privacy and trust that OncoLife presently creates, it seems impossible to prove that outcomes change. Therefore, rather than trying to prove direct effects the authors suggest to consider as a major indicator for success that considerable workload can be taken off the health care system. They report that a personally prepared cancer survivorship plan takes a professional 20 min. With OncoLife it happens fully automated. The creation of the individual plan does not consume a single second of a professional's worktime. Maintenance of the knowledge built into OncoLife of course requires permanent professional attendance and intellectual as well as logistic effort. A well-maintained service, however, fully scales up to virtually unlimited numbers of users in virtually unlimited regions. Presently, it is still underutilized by generally under-served populations, but the Spanish version is a first step into the direction to make it a service that also helps to reduce disparities.

> ## Take Home
> Level 2 services exist for a host of somatic conditions and types of service:
>
> **Behavioral advice** Against early stage urinary incontinence behavior modifications can sufficiently help and be commu-nicated without embarrassment and noteworthy risk.
>
> **Treatment** Precise medication dosage in diseases such a asthma defines treatment quality. Automated dosage adaptation proves superior to constant dosage in trials but cannot legally be brought into routine use.
>
> **Case management** For complex long lasting treatments with many care providers the patient is the natural protagonist to assemble his treatment history and to follow up where necessary. Regard-ing the complexity of the task a portal for cancer survivors has been a welcome support for a decade.

5.2.4 Online Pharmacies

While all examples above each are dedicated to a circumscribed medical problem and tailor the general character, the contents, admission and inclusion, allocation of initiative, liberalism or directiveness of the service to the requirements of clients who have that medical problem, the following two areas claim to cover medical care across all specialties and all target populations. They are Online pharmacies and general Online counseling.

With online pharmacies we enter the world of shopping carts, discount coupons, express delivery, return policies and disclaimers. Clients are encouraged to behave like when ordering electronics, apparel etc. Since pharmacological treatment is big business, online pharmacies can be big business and the services that clients hit when searching for `<drug name> no prescription` look like big business. And since big business means sales the common client expectation that his order will be served without asking painful questions meets the common provider interest to maximize sales.

Pharmaceuticals can be as life-saving as they can be life-threatening. They can lead into addiction and society wise, in the case of overuse of antibiotics, they can enhance the spread of resistant germs. Fake pharmaceuticals that include the active substance at too high or too low concentration or do not include it all can kill. Therefore, pharmacy is a health care profession with high requirements on education, licensing, quality assurance, and not just another industry. In another sections we analyze legal principles underlying online pharmacy services (cf. Sect. 17.11). In yet another section we investigate extra legal challenges in an international market in the absence of international legislation and licensing (Sect. 17.8). Present mostly national regulations are rather conservative and prefer client safety over client autonomy. Still, the volume of drugs shipped at lower prices from Canada to the USA, partially paid by US insurers, has already aroused political turmoil and called the FDA, the regulatory agency in charge for the USA, into place years ago. In this section here we concentrate on the processes for clients to get drugs that they feel certain they need.

The client has a safe yet convenient choice of presenting a regular prescription from a classical or Level 1 Consumer Health Informatics service to a mail order pharmacy registered through health authorities in his country of residence. He may benefit from free shipping of over-the-counter extra purchases. Some mail order pharmacies offer additional convenience for the client to scan and upload a prescription for immediate processing. The client will, however, also find service providers that advertise as "prescription free" or "no prescription". There he goes the direct way by providing the drug name, selecting a dosage and quantity, as well as delivery and payment terms, finalizes the shopping cart and moves on to payment and thereby closes a deal that the provider typically confirms. Before confirming, the provider will insist that the client accepts the terms of service which almost inevitably include that the delivery cannot be stopped and the merchandise cannot be returned under any circumstances and that the client is fully responsible in any conceivable way for all kinds of effects that the merchandise may have, now or in the future. Some providers request that the client declares that he has a valid prescription from a physician licensed where the client lives and that he takes responsibility to discuss the application of the drug with a respective physician.

There are some variants of this common pattern. An obvious one is that the client subscribes with one online pharmacy and has all the convenience of using the same logistics information over again and at the same time normally receiving discounts from the provider.

An interesting variant in terms of suggesting that the service is medically safe is a British one, cf. http://www.euroclinix.de for the German presentation. Being located in the UK with street address in London and referring to all kinds of British credentials for legal licensing and quality it confirms that "registered physicians check your medical data and then prescribe". Actually, the client can answer several medical questions favorably, declare that he agrees to the terms and conditions without ever having been there and reaches the payment and delivery part of the transaction without anybody apparently checking medically.

www.euroclinix.de's declaration of patient's obligations are marked as such and are reached through one click from the bottom of their homepage. The header of that part of their service reads "Patient obligations and declaration of consent" but does not request a consent giving transaction here. As seen above, clients can order without taking notice. Implicitly, then, they concede that they are responsible for taking all kinds of actions to avoid foreseeable risks and indemnify www.euroclinix.de from all consequences of adverse events.

A legal assessment of such transaction designs of Consumer Health Informatics services is provided in Sect. 17.5, coming to the conclusion that transactions that qualify as practice of medicine and do so without any in person provider-client encounter, are illegal. One condition listed there clearly renders delivery of prescription drugs without regular prescription illegal: the condition of a closed deal. Other conditions need a closer look.

Generally, online pharmacies implement lean processes for mass shipping according to clients' orders. They request some data concerning the indication and contraindications of the requested drug to be filled into structured forms, for instance blood pressure history when the client tries to order beta blockers, but it is not apparent what consequence the check marking of potentially harmful signs will have. Some online pharmacies have Q&A features. Optically these are far less prominent than ads for all kinds of over-the-counter well-being products and Viagra. The client self-assessment is not validated in any way; it is the client who solemnly declares that what he wrote is true. Validating clients' data by linking to electronic records would increase the complexity of the online pharmacy business and likely also reduce the volume because a certain amount of the attempted purchases would have to be blocked for medical reasons. Therefore, there is no interest on the part of a provider to deny client requests. One provider (http://www.acmeds.com/) even boasts of a "99 % approval guarantee".[1] No wonder that Orizio and coworkers [17] show in an investigation about 57 online pharmacies that the diligence in

---

[1]This was the case in April 2013. In a final check of resources in February 2015 the service no longer exists, at least not evident through any referencing information when using the above link. No wonder, somewhat.

checking clients' condition, comorbidities, other medications, situations of life such as pregnancy or breastfeeding is far from the medically necessary on average. Not even known drug allergies are asked by all (55 of 57). This is clearly negligent and not attending to foreseeable risk might be regarded reckless. Definitely criminal, as outlined by Jena and coworkers is the Internet delivery of controlled substances without valid prescription [13].

Orizio's and coworkers' assessment dimension can also be regarded in the context of client assessment in Sect. 8.4. Their scheme is, however, limited in coverage and reliability. First it is meant for the restricted purpose of safeguarding the dispensing of pharmaceuticals. Second it was generated bottom up through systematic exploration ("Content Analysis", [20]) of the assessment dimension that happened to be covered in 57 online pharmacy providers investigated. Dimensions that none of 57 addressed necessarily lack in [17] as well. Third it assumes face validity of the answers clients give for directly asked questions such as alcohol use or whether a doctor made the diagnosis the drug is requested for. Obviously a client who really feels an urge for a drug may fake answers to avoid denial of the purchase according to the pharmacy's criteria.

What else do we know about the client himself? Few systematic investigations about online pharmacies and their effects on clients and the health care system have so far been published. But there is one that makes hope with respect to a responsible client role despite all temptations to consume. Hou and coworkers [11] found out in an investigation in spring 2009 through spring 2011 that 3560 users of online pharmacies behaved more rationally and consequently than 3560 matched non users (control), i.e. a cohort that matches the user cohort in terms of age, gender, chronic condition score, copay rank, household income and urban versus non urban address. For both cohorts eight drug agent subgroups (such as antidepressants, beta blockers, ulcer drugs) were traced as to ordered quantities, anticipated consumptions and due dates of refills. The proportion of days covered (PDC) is the number of days for which the client presumably has the drugs he needs at his disposal, divided by 365. PDC was 73.19 % in the user vs. 61.64 % in the control group. This, as well as the by agent differences for all agents except beta blockers were significant. These and other statistical results suggest that those making use of online pharmacies at least take better care of the logistics of their drugs. Doubts are nevertheless in place whether more consequential drug logistics implies better drug compliance in the central meaning of drugs being taken as prescribed. For the first, despite all attempts to match users and controls we may have a selection bias; users may differ in their personality from controls in traits which influence drug logistics behavior but escape quantification. For the second numerous investigations have shown that getting the drug and actually taking it are two pairs of shoes. So proof is still due whether superior stock of drugs translates into superior use of drugs.

> **Take Home**
>
> Online pharmacy is big business with all advantages of convenience but also ramifications of opaque non-traceable practices.
>
> - Authorities in the national medical industries have defined procedures that legally map the over the counter process into a remote one based on valid prescriptions (mail-order pharmacy). Lists of approved pharmacies are available.
> - Other pharmacies use the fragmented legislation between national states to conveniently deliver prescription and other drugs without checking a prescription. Their terms typically transfer all incurred risks to the buyer.
> - A survey of the safeguards that online pharmacies apply before clearing a customer for shipping shows grave deficits.

5.2.5 Online Counseling

Clients may be interested for numerous reasons to seek medical advice and treatment through services other than their GP or local specialist. Besides not being satisfied with the services they receive locally clients may seek convenience such as avoiding waiting times and traveling. They may wish to conceal embarrassing conditions from their home environment. Searching for terms such as "internet physician" makes them find something. It actually makes them find much more than they want: appr. 180,000 hits, a problem addressed in Chap. 3. So it needs some sophistication to find out which of the hits hits the mark of ones personal quest.

> **Take Home**
>
> Four major models of online counseling can be distinguished, subsequently ordered from least to most personal and pervasive:
>
> **Information broker** Client readable educational material on common conditions.
> **Logistics support** Referral to local physicians, pharmacies, partially enhanced through educational material and physician rating.
> **Pre-Screening** Entry point into a telephone consultation setting; internet forms help to screen requests and collect complaints and history, but the care itself is conveyed through "voice-to-voice" communication and typically leads to a prescription.
> **Virtual service** Online provision of care without compulsory "voice-to-voice" or other synchronous communication between provider and client; treatment can happen through mail delivered prescriptions.

5.2 Examples

To classify a service as one of the above may require to dive deeply into terms and conditions, disclaimers, etc.

5.2.5.1 Information Broker

The US based http://www.webMD.com and the British http://www.netdoctor.co.uk/ which has national clones in other European countries are typical examples of this type of service. We will mostly use netdoctor, one of the oldest prominent such services to demonstrate the properties of Information brokers.

http://www.netdoctor.co.uk/ is linked to the UK NHS (National Health Service). To some extent information brokers resemble the good old dictionaries: they have educational material and their contents is provided by distinguished clinicians listed by name. Names and often portrait photos of those who provide the service are an ingredient of most online counseling offerings of all types.

Information brokers use the opportunities of Internet technology to add other types or information or infotainment to the text cores. Contents can be assessed via affected body part, symptom name in plain language, questionnaire type symptom checkers, therapy names. WebMD's Symptom checker assists in seeking classical care by convenient printouts of symptoms and questions to ask your doctor summaries. In addition we find community forums for conditions (asthma, depression, etc) or situations of life such as pregnancy, advertisements for third party paid services, and stories about blockbuster topics such as ADHD, men's health, smoking cessation etc.

Information brokers declare very clearly that they cannot answer personal medical questions and instead refer to their archive of articles. However, they may request of their community members that they reveal their identify and transfer copyright of all uploaded contents to the holder of the service.

5.2.5.2 Logistics Support

Logistics support services, also called physician referral services, normally promote a search function. http://www.jameda.de is a very comprehensive German example. It includes 250,000 of the approximately 330,000 physicians in Germany. Search is by medical specialty and town or ZIP Code. Physicians are listed with address, some detail about their specialty and patient ratings on a general satisfaction score plus text. The search can be narrowed by checking male or female physicians only and which health plan or social insurance plan a physician is contracting with. This is the core function. If the client wonders why some physicians show with a portrait photo and others do not he may look into other functions offered and may discover that doctors may become premium members at a certain fee. This is one part of the business model.

Another part of the business model becomes visible when the client selects "pharmaceuticals". A certain selection is offered for mail delivery at discounted prices. They are all nonprescription drugs, i.e. well-being products and other merchandise not subject to the regulations of the health care system (cf. Sect. 17.5.2). Implicitly this underlines that the service concentrates on logistics. It does not support transactions that require a client – provider contract where the provider takes responsibility as a health professional.

Other search functions contribute to the convenience of the client. He can search for conditions and will find his search strings orthographically corrected. He can search by medical problem, drug name, and finds highlighted topics of interest, where, again men's health and sexuality are prominently displayed. So we find a different type of convenience shining through here: collecting information about embarrassing conditions without revealing one's identity. Indeed do logistics support services offer one-stop shop behavior without enrollment and provision of identifiable information; so traceability is confined to identification of IP addresses of clients. The real medical services happen in the real medical word and may go unnoticed for the provider of a logistics support service unless the client decides to return and rate a doctor that he visited. This is still an exception rather than the rule in the case of http://www.jameda.de: since the foundation in 2007 few votes have been provided. It should be mentioned that the core information of logistics support services may be available through government or boards of physicians agencies such as the Medical Board of California at http://www.mbc.ca.gov/Breeze/License_Verification.aspx or the German federal state of Baden-Württemberg based licensing board http://www.aerztekammer-bw.de/20buerger/20arztsuche/index.html. There are two major dimensions of distinction between commercial and governmental agencies: The commercial ones offer quite some more convenience while governments reflect accurate and up to date information on licensing state. The commercial ones can be nationwide, could be beyond if there were business models for referral out of country while the state authorities are confined to their state or nation by law.

5.2.5.3 Pre-screening

At first sight, pre-screening services and virtual services may not look too different from logistics support services. However, while logistics support services *refer to* classical providers region or nation wide, pre-screening services are *front ends to* self offered telephone based services and virtual services *replace* classical services. While logistics support is paid by classical providers, mostly physicians, who want premium placement, pre-screening and virtual provider services have a clear business process which takes the client from enrolling or logging into an existing account to an accomplished and paid consultation including a prescription, mailing of a lab test kit etc.

5.2 Examples

We use http://www.quickrxrefills.com as an example of what it means to "Consult with a doctor online & get your prescription now! Doctors respond within 30–60 min!" as the client reads in block letters on the home page. Pre-screening services have a streamlined convenience oriented process that leads from registration or logging into an existing account through pre-payment, filling a medical history form, being called back, have a telephone consultation, and receive pharmaceuticals from a local pharmacy. As the Q&A tells the service includes prescription drugs but excludes narcotics and controlled substances. QuickRxRefills plays its role and the risks down by its name alone but also by using the diminutive "ailments" instead of "diseases", by creating the impression of a temporary substitute of classical medical care in transient situations such as having run out of medications, changing one's office-based physician etc. But actually the services are not confined to transient situations. They are confined to a list of frequent conditions, which do, however include such serious potentially chronic and life threatening conditions as asthma and high blood pressure. QuickRxRefills declares that their service cannot replace the office based doctor but doesn't enforce that he be involved. Actually it detaches itself from the classical service by not using the medical record but rather builds its own parallel record that grows with repeated pre-screened telephone consultations. The client has to look into the Terms and Conditions to find out that QuickRxRefills makes no warranty whatsoever and that the client and his physician are solely responsible and that QuickRxRefills' service is not meant for emergencies and 911 should be called. QuickRxRefills, though, confirms that US licensed, more so, "US based physicians" provide the telephone conversations. We analyze in Chap. 17 that this actually makes a difference compared to physicians licensed or residing abroad if it comes to having to sue a provider for malpractice. To summarize: as long as the client does not look into the smallprint, QuickRxRefills maintains the impression that the right treatment can be purchased there for those able and willing to pay the price: $ 99 for a first and $ 79 for a follow up visit. Testimonials underline this impression.

Some other convenience service elements come for free alongside with the paid consultation. They include medical Q&A, educational articles, and hit lists of ailments treated, led by the notorious erectile dysfunction.

5.2.5.4 Virtual Service

Virtual services are an apparently small step farther away from classical face-to-face practicing of medicine by the fact that they do not necessarily include a "voice-to-voice" part of the consultation. That this may be a giant leap as to the legal consequences of this virtual only process is analyzed in Chap. 17. Economic opportunities of such a model are analyzed in Sect. 16.3. Here we concentrate on the properties of the service and will come to rather critical conclusions as to the conduct of providers of virtual services. It should, therefore, be noted that others have reached a positive assessment of function and contents [19].

http://www.revolutionhealth.com was an early protagonist whose fate will be addressed later in this section. We rather use http://www.dred.com, DrEd for short, for illustration of the concept because it clearly shows typical ingredients of a virtual only Consumer Health Informatics service. The home page transfers to www.dred.com/CountryCode of the client and switches to the main language of the respective country but the client can choose to see the services for other countries as well. In the respective context DrEd replicates numerous elements of the classical medical care process. They request registration, have forms to fill about the condition for which advice is being sought and build and maintain their own electronic medical record which they hold for 10 years (in compliance with legislation). Medical advice is generated from that record, potentially without any person to person contact. The record may include photos that the client is encouraged to upload, e.g. when suspecting an STI. Advice may turn into treatment by providing prescription drugs to be delivered through a pharmacy that the client chooses or one that DrEd suggest, www.apo-rot.CountryCode. DrEd offers to inform the client's office based physician if the client agrees.

DrEd is a UK based company that offers identical services to Germany, Austria, Switzerland, some northern European countries and UK. They declare British law as applicable unless compelling local laws supersede British law. A contract is being closed, i.e. a "treatment is purchased" and payment is due when the client so chooses by clicking a respective button. They have short and extended consultation. Short consultations ("one step") cost 9 €, extended ones ("two step") 29 €. Short ones definitely are virtual only, extended ones include a more detailed check of eligibility for online consultations and additional asynchronous (SMS or e-mail) elaboration of the condition. DrEd lists the specialties or domains to which it confines its services which include blockbuster topics already mentioned.

Refunding of paid fees through client's health insurance is handled differently and confusingly in different country versions. The UK version does not mention it. The German version is contradictory in itself because in one section of the Q&A it says that client should check refundability with his health insurance while in another section it says that unfortunately there is presently no contract with the German health care system and therefore no refunding. To add to the confusion the Austrian version offers the absolutely not applicable German regulations.

Payment and truthful filling of questionnaires are the only client's obligation. Then DrEd accepts to be liable but the liability may be less impressive than it sounds as outlined in Chap. 17. DrEd has a returns and refunds policy and a London street address and a UK e-mail address as contact points for any kind of legal dispute. They try to create the impression that they are liable without limits for all incurred damage. When the client reads further he sees the restriction to foreseeable and typically occurring damage and finds himself in the role of finding out what that is. If he reads thoroughly enough he notices that DrEd refers to product liability which applies to movable property *excluding* pharmaceuticals. Movable property is not what they deliver. So the declaration of liability goes void.

The client encounters more contradiction in the small print of well sounding declarations meant to create an atmosphere of trust. He reads that "we comply with the Health and Social Care Act 2008 (http://www.legislation.gov.uk/ukpga/ 2008/14/contents)" and "doctors ... regulated by the General Medical Council" and "comply with ... Good Medical Practice Guidelines". Their chief medical officers' careers sound impressing but their formal qualifications fall short of the expectations created.

The impression remains that DrEd carefully wraps its core service in a coat of declarations that sum up to the client being fully responsible. This corresponds to the caveat emptor maxim described in Sect. 17.5.2. The maxim is meant for businesses among partners who can get access to all information and freely choose. In Sect. 17.5.2 we also analyze that caveat emptor can legitimately be applied to well-being and some preventive service but not to core practice of medicine.

It should by no means be concluded that DrEd is the only Virtual service provider whose practice needs good attention. DrEd may be a fast and cheap track for those clients who are aware of the consequences and want to exert choices, in the sense of Sect. 17.11.4.

http://www.healthcaremagic.com boasts itself as a service with numerous physicians online. They offer a more personally looking interface than DrEd by allowing free text description of symptoms. Physicians will then provide advice at a price that varies whether the client wants a GP or a specialist to respond. Response is through e-mail, and delivers "medically correct health information ... guide ... in choosing the right course of action" or, in the case of a specialist responding a "Specialist Opinion Service". Careful reading reveals that this should not be taken as medical treatment but rather as provision of information, albeit personalized. The terms and conditions confirm that intention, by block letter emphasis in the disclaimer that "healthcaremagic ... (is) not responsible for the results of your decisions". In Sect. 17.5 we analyze whether for such a combination of apparently personal advice that is being paid for the claim can be upheld that healthcaremagic is not offering practice of medicine. The attempt to find out more about the provider failed repeatedly. We do not find any legal notice and e-mails to the only visible contact point customercare@healthcaremagic.com were not answered for months. Therefore, legally binding information about ownership, legal affiliation, board certification of their physicians etc. could not be found out.

www.justanswer.CountryCode takes a different approach to blur the highly delicate nature of medical counseling. The service used to be called justananswer and is one of two successors of what used to be called www.revolutionhealth.com, later renamed to justanswer® the other being everydayhealth.com,[2] a combination of Information broker and Logistics support services for the USA.

Justanswer® has national variants that similarly offer answers to questions about health, medicine, vehicles, computers, education, law and other fields. It is a paid service which is provided when a down payment has been made. In the Q&A section

---

[2]Everyday HEALTH is their trademarked name.

it reads that the customer chooses the amount while in the terms and conditions Justanswer® does. The terms and conditions furthermore state that in the case that a customer contracts for an answers he makes the contract with the specialist rather than with Justanswer®. Therefore, Justanswer® is not liable at all except in rare exceptions. The specialist is not liable either because the customer has agreed to the regulation that he is not expecting personalized advice and that he should seek advice from professionals directly.

Justanswer® does not distinguish in its terms and conditions between medical and not medical. Therefore, the client is fully turned into a customer who buys nonbinding information about a topic of his interest.

5.3 A Short Note on apps

5.3.1 Information Broker apps

Some apps assemble health information across wide domains, somewhat like a dictionary, just smaller and available wherever there is cell coverage. Information brokering alone is not really a stronghold of the medium because the small screen limits reading convenience. A good Austrian example, though, is Medizin populär, the online version of a monthly journal provided by the Austrian Association of Physicians for the lay population.

Some apps take a dedicated position. Gesundheits-Irrtümer (Health Misapprehensions or Myths) lists 144 popular beliefs on health and why they are false. The contents is a perfect replica of a book with the same title. The author is a certain Andros Link who also authors Business quotes, Weight reduction tips and introduces himself as "Energetischer Heiler" (energetic healer), without further reference. Some more detail about him and the likes follows in Sect. 7.4.

The following two apps have some flavor of logistics support in addition to their core function of information brokering. Patient.co.uk is a nongovernmental organization that, however, refers to the UK NHS by advertising for instance that their apps include the same leaflets as doctors would hand to the patient. Additionally, the app has a search function for symptoms plus locating nearby health services.

Fitfortravel has English and German advice. Organized by world region and often broken down to country it informs what health hazards to be aware of. Access to information is easy and fast but the advice itself is lengthy flat text and does not make use of the opportunities of interactive media. Checklists about medical and other preparations for travel are convenient other functions. The app clearly declares its contents as general information only which does not replace individual counseling with a professional. Consequently it includes a locator function for tropical infection specialists which, however, is not very helpful. When

5.3 A Short Note on apps

searching for a provider to advise on infectious disease prevention in preparation of developing country traveling the client may receive the address of a local general practitioner who retired 2 years ago rather than being pointed to the regional university center of tropical hygiene at less than eight miles away.

5.3.2 Logistics Support apps

`find doctor` as search key in the app store returns more than 70 apps the majority of which actually finds doctors, often by state of the United States. `jameda` finds 250,000 of the 330,000 German doctors. All such locator services and the accuracy, timeliness and pertinence of their suggestions should undergo some systematic test. As already pointed out in section `Fitfortravel`: perfection should not be expected. `jameda` fails on the same test where fit for travel also gives inappropriate advice.

In this sense the following apps are presented to provide an idea of the scope of the type of service. They are not meant as recommendations of good Consumer Health Informatics services; nor is there any immediate evidence that they are bad services. `Catamaran` (formerly `informedRx` by SXC Health Solutions Corp) add the management and home delivery of valid prescriptions in the US to various functions of tracking ones medications, of receiving reminders for due doses, of finding nearby pharmacies etc. `rxbattle` is a best price search engine for prescribed drugs in the US. `medikamente-per-klick` is a German mail order pharmacy app certified by DIMDI (cf. Sect. 5.4).

5.3.3 Reminders

Reminders are galore in app stores. Client requirements and opportunities of services provided through ubiquitous devices cannot fit any better than for reminders. Precautions made in Sect. 7.3 hold here as well. But most clients will find something that meets their expectations and personal preferences. What they do not find is a pervasive system of medical quality trustmarking.

Presently available apps remind according to fixed schemes that the client sets according to instructions from his physician, instructions for use coming with a medication or alike. Reminder apps that adapt their scheme of reminding to the course of the disease and severity of symptoms are a totally different story because they assume a role that is normally reserved to the physician. One such app that is being tested for release as a medical software is discussed in Sect. 4.5.2.

> **Take Home**
> The diversity in function and quality reflects the bonanza type perception of the infotainment apps market that developers have. Apps work somehow and deliver some information. Through their convenience and appeal they suggest medical benefit, which the lay persons has hard times to verify. This does not mean that there are no nuggets in the heap, such as combinations of medical advice, safe delivery of prescription drugs, and reminders.

5.3.4 Condition Specific apps

Besides medical education and instruction, which often is not more than delivering known texts in electronic form, the majority of medical apps supports the client in taking notes (diary) on his condition, getting more or less personalized behavior advice, and convenience functions such as statistics, graphical display of trends, short-term reminders for daily routines as well as long-term for visits or drug refills. The examples selected here do not claim to be perfectly systematic but rather try to point to some typical aspects.

Condition specific apps typically are for prevention such as smoking cessation or weight control or for chronic conditions such as asthma, high blood pressure, diabetes, etc. Their major function is diary, i.e. personal notes, short questionnaires about symptoms or quality of life, and recorded values such as body weight, blood pressure, heart rate, venous glucose concentration, air flowmeter readings, blood oxigenation etc. measurements, and graphic displays of time courses for recorded values.

Equipments to measure glucose concentration, FEV_1, etc. of course are no off-the-shelf consumer products. Clients who hold them must have seen a physician who has established a respective diagnosis and has recommended or ordered for such equipment to be bought and used. Therefore, it may appear that apps that require clients to enter glucose or FEV_1 readings must be Level 1 because the initiation was through the classical health care system. However, most of the subsequently outlined apps enact their service detached from the classical health care system. They assist in recording readings, they provide good graphical displays of trends, they send encouraging notes etc. but they do not hook up with the client's provider.

5.3.4.1 Smoking Cessation

Smoking cessation is a cannot do harm situation. The largest risk is that smokers who use an app do not quit and get more frustrated ...but that they do anyway. Success rates in personal or group therapy settings rarely exceed one third but the societal effort and cost is by far larger than programming an app.

5.3 A Short Note on apps

Three German apps nicely demonstrate the axes of variation in the smoking cessation league: `Rauchfrei gratis`, `Rauchfrei Pro` and `Rauchfrei durchstarten` all offer some kind of goal setting, recording of smoked and not smoked cigarettes, self rewarding, financial savings made, and encouragement messages. The first two are more entertaining and stylish, with no medical credentials, while the third refers to a well validated test score for dependency (Fagerström-test) and marginally implements elements of CBT – reflection on situations of temptation and how to avoid them in the future. The first two get positive client ratings and reviews, the third gets nothing.

Some smoking cessation apps advertise hypnosis as a successful and approved method to quit smoking. They include the two English ones `Stop Smoking Self Hypnosis by Jere Parker` and `Stop Smoking Forever - Hypnosis by Glenn Harrold` and the two German ones `Get smoke-free Fleckenstein` and `Jordan Rauchfrei`. Reports by happy clients are overwhelming as are some of the abbreviations of academic qualifications and affiliations of the providers. This apparent success story in variations contrasts harshly with scientific evidence of effectiveness of hypnosis as a therapy for smoking cessation: when searching MEDLINE for "Hypnosis" [Mesh:NoExp] AND ("Smoking Cessation/methods" [Majr] AND "Smoking Cessation/statistics and numerical data" [Majr]), two articles in the past 17 years are retrieved one of which denies effectiveness of hypnosis while the other article attributes some supportive role of hypnosis in conjunction with workplace smoking ban programs. This does not necessarily mean that hypnosis – and hence self hypnosis apps – should not be used for smoking cessation. But several places in this volume allow the interpretation that it is not the hypnosis as such but the belief of a client in hypnosis that makes it individually effective (Sects. 3.2.2, 3.3.1.3, and 15.2.3.3.2). In that case the huge marketplace of therapy concepts at our fingertips lets many people find their personally appropriate approach. And, after all, MEDLINE does not retrieve any article on adverse effects of hypnosis for smoking cessation.

5.3.4.2 Overweight

Overweight is similar in character – unhealthy behavior gotten out of control – with different values and behaviors to record, feedback through graphical display of past behavior, encouragement and, depending on specific diets quite a bit of knowledge on nutrition facts, healthy recipes etc. As long as it is overweight, the advice conveyed through apps can be regarded as support of well-being, whereas apps that suggest themselves to treat obesity are entering the core medical arena where medical device regulations may apply. Therefore, it may come as a surprise that the following numbers of apps are found in the Apple Appstore: Overweight: 64; weight control: 90, obesity: 154. There is some overlap in the apps found and no clear criteria to distinguish between the three. As with smoking cessation some apps emphasize fun and appeal to the ludic drive while others explicitly refer to scientifically founded methods. Here it makes no difference as to client reviews or ratings.

> **Take Home**
> Problems such as smoking and overeating have a strong situational character where advice on the palmtop when the temptation is there is promoted as a factor. Respective apps are galore, proofs of effectiveness are in short supply.

While smoking and overeating doubtlessly have long-term negative effect on quality of life and health they hardly ever lead into life-threatening emergencies immediately. Therefore, by and large, their realm is well-being and prevention. The following conditions, in contrast, are manifest diseases where loss of control can lead into severe crisis if not death.

5.3.4.3 Asthma

As outlined in more detail in Sect. 12.2.1 asthma is a condition where the patient may have hard times to subjectively assess his breathing capacity correctly and faithfully. Therefore, here as also for COPD, flow meters and FEV_1, PEFR or alike recordings are essential.

AsthmaMD nicely puts peak flow measurement values, medications, subjective observation of symptoms and suspected triggers for an exacerbation together and offers displays of trends. Mostly the same, except triggers, holds for the German AsthmaCheck . Both are for free, both have mostly positive reviews for older versions, for both the responsible medical professionals or organizations can be identified – through www search though. For AsthmaMD Glaxo Smith Kline appears as a sponsor together with easy to read disclaimers that using the app does not replace treatment through a medical professional. Neither app hooks up with the classical health care system tightly; only standard export formats for documents can be created "to show to your doctor". Apart from this limitation these are two positive examples in the list of more than 100 apps found when searching for asthma . Some other apps have more educational material, some have fewer parameters to record, and of course the style varies. Generally, for asthma the quote of apps that are worth considering is high compared to overweight and smoking cessation. With asthma, miracle cures are harder to sell, it appears, than with the addictive patterns of behavior.

5.3.4.4 Diabetes

Among the various apps for diabetes mySugr (junior) plays a special role because it makes sophisticated use of the opportunities of mobile devices. It comes

5.3 A Short Note on apps

in two apps, one for a child diagnosed with diabetes and one for a parent. The app for the child allows him to register behaviors, meals including assistance in calculating nutrition values for unknown dishes, blood glucose readings and planned insulin shots. For each accomplished data entry the child gets reward points. Entries are immediately mirrored to the parent's app who can but need not necessarily react. Especially can a parent make suggestions about insulin dosage hence safeguarding the kids therapy.

mySugr (junior) has a medical advisory board. It appears well considered and well implemented. It still is a service that calls for in-depths investigation of various aspects dealt with in other parts of this volume. One is legal responsibility resp. guardianship, cf. Sect. 8.4.4.1. Another is an ethical weighing of risks, some foundations of which are in Sect. 17.11. For both the consequences of advice and instruction that the parent conveys solely based on data entries provided by the kid has to be raised. Also, protocols between mobile apps must be established that guarantee integrity of the communication, cf. Sect. 13.3.

5.3.4.5 Images and Vital Signs

Some apps use the smart phones as measuring or recording devices. Cardiograph measures heart rate from a short video of the fingertip. It does just that, plus recording measured values. So as long as the measurement is accurate a sequence of values is a small piece of evidence in tracing cardiovascular conditions.

Skinvision analyzes images of skin regions whether they are indicative of a melanoma developing. Registered clients can take and archive pictures, can record a skin health profile, can check for UV exposure expected in the (GPS located) neighborhood and try to identify a nearby dermatologist. The app is clearly structured and images are analyzed at the provider's server reporting a result and recommendation within seconds.

What appears to be a valuable well considered service in the first place still raises some questions. First, the provider cannot be identified. Not at all from the app and when trying on the Internet traces lead to the Netherlands and Ireland, without clear account for who is responsible for what, based on what medical credentials. The privacy policy is far from what is recommended in Chap. 13, although at least this fact is obvious from "Privacy policy" which is easy to find on the Internet. The highest risk, however, results from false positive and more so false-negative recommendations based on the automatic analysis of the picture. The provider offers a human consultation based on a recorded image, for a fee of €4.99. If the client trusts this diagnoses through the distance and its advice is right, Skinvision is the perfect shortcut for high-efficiency autonomous screening. However, if the advice is wrong, nobody can be made liable. So better not trust? In that case the false positive entails an unnecessary utilization of a dermatologist's service whereas the false negative delays a necessary visit, with potentially fatal consequences.

> **Take Home**
>
> Some specially developed apps for frequent conditions build on well considered medical models and package their functions to bring safety and convenience to managing ones condition.
>
> **Asthma** Behavioral advice, integration of flowmeter readings, graphical display of time course and other pertinent information helps the client to control the disease.
>
> **Diabetes** Among numerous apps for the individual diabetic mysugr (junior) stands out because it combines a creative concept of bonding parents' and minors' devices with a model of parent personalized advice.
>
> **Images and vitals** Built in camera, microphone, motion sensor etc. lets mobile devices successfully be used as recorders. Processes of interpretation and follow up upon recorded signals need good attention.

5.4 Variety of Service Characteristics

As the reader has certainly expected the examples demonstrate a rich choice of Consumer Health Informatics services that vary along various dimensions. Some are very narrow, focussed on one medical problem, some cover the whole health care sector. Some request contracting and encourage to reveal highly personal information, others assist sniff viewers in finding their information without revealing anything but an IP address. Some charge the client a fee, some are for free for the client. For the apparently free ones there must still be some funding or business model which raises the question of sustainability to be addressed in Chap. 16. As outlined in more detail in Chap. 3, using the typical search mechanisms produces between several thousands and several million hits. Therefore, it is hard for the client to find a service that fits his problem, has the right quality and tolerable exposure of personal information, and has a business model that the client agrees with.

Some services help the client in matching his problem with the coverage of their service. Criteria of inclusion or eligibility are checked through questionnaires. Therefore, if the client truthfully fills them he will only be encouraged to subscribe if the service fits his request.

The fees – if any – charged for the business are normally easy to check, although coverage through health insurance may be harder to find out. It is easy, too, to find out whether the service requests registration and disclosure of personally identifiable data and sensitive health information. Providers that ask such data typically declare that for them privacy matters. However, regarding the sophistication visible in Chap. 13 that is required to live up to such declarations providers and clients are challenged to establish a safely private relation. Such a relation may be regarded as a contract although without electronic signature its validity may be challenged.

To support the client in assessing quality and trustworthiness trustmarks have been introduced, such as HON (Health On the Net) and URAC. Their limited impact and respective limited help for seekers has been analyzed in Sect. 3.4.3. For none of the services described in this chapter's parts Sects. 5.2.1, 5.2.2, and 5.2.3, certification could be found although quality was moderate to good throughout. Mostly, these services are described on the basis of scholarly publications, and their portals are not reported in the articles or may meanwhile have been withdrawn or hosted by providers other than the authors.

None of the online pharmacies in Sect. 5.2.4 is HON or URAC certified. www.apo-rot.CountryCode, subcontractor of DrEd, instead has an accreditation of the German HTA authority DIMDI, which it strangely also presents for its Austrian customers. DrEd itself presents a certification through the UK Quality Care Commission (http://www.cqc.org.uk/), which is, however, only valid for practice at a London street address. DrEd also declares that its physicians are certified through the UK General Medical Council (http://www.gmc-uk.org/). This cannot be checked by the client but assuming that it is true it still does not warrant that they are entitled to offer their services virtual only, cf. Sects. 17.11 and 17.8.

The information brokers WebMd and netdoctor.co.uk and the combination of information broker and logistics support everydayhealth are HON certified, WebMd by URAC as well.

These are few examples only but they add to the picture already drawn in Sect. 3.4.3 that there is no highway to confidence in a service provider's trustworthiness.

5.5 Considerations on Scaling Up

In the previous sections we have analyzed the nature of various Level 2 virtual provider services on an as is basis. We now take a brief look into scaling up and sustainable operation. According to Chap. 2 one of the drivers behind developing and propagating Consumer Health Informatics is the need to relieve the health care industry and to reduce the workload for health care professionals while maintaining the overall standard of health care. This calls for sustainable funding models and scalability. Funding models have been comprised in a chapter of its own (Chap. 16). Scalability is fostered through a configuration of automated services wherever appropriate and human provider involvement when the automated services touch their limits. This is informally investigated in the sequel.

For a service to scale up it must be available in an n-fold increased volume with the required effort increasing less than n-fold. This typically holds for fully automated software solutions such as online banking, electronic flight tickets etc. Of course servers have to be added on the part of the provider when numbers of clients or of transactions increase. But since human workforce is much more expensive and scarcer than hardware, networking etc. capacity we do not take increase in ICT expenses into account here unless a massive investment is required.

It turns out that among the health awareness examples only the child health promotion service which has been tested at kiosks in three public places requires kiosks in many such places i.e. a major investment in hardware and probably also maintenance effort regarding the exposed nature of appropriate places. The anxiety and panic service requires psychiatrists checking assignments and answering e-mails, i.e. service effort conveyed by humans increases in proportion to the number of clients. Therapists, however, gain convenience by not having to stick to tough schedules or hold themselves available for phone calls. The addiction (smoking cessation) services scale up easily. In the smoking cessation example a feature becomes apparent that may even make online services more efficient: the wide range of opportunities to personalize according to personality, individual risks, success stories of individuals in a similar situation with a similar risk structure etc. With the generally low success rate of smoking cessation programs it makes even more sense to save human workforce. Depression CBT scales up inasmuch as service providers find ways to curb the suicidal risk.

Among the online counseling services information brokers and logistics support scale up easily. They may both, however, have adverse effects. The convenience of finding a nearby physician who has good patient ratings may invite for a visit that would be spared with more uncertainty about what to expect. A symptom checker of an information broker may make the user feel sicker than he is – aka Molière's "Imaginary Invalid" – and seek professional help that he does not actually need.

Among the services for somatic diseases the urinary continence and the cancer survivor services scale up easily, too. The asthma one does except the apparently additional small investment in peak flow meters. Apparently, because to be taken good care of the respective clients need them anyhow. So the Consumer Health Informatics service is not the cause for an investment but a service that makes an existing but not yet articulated need obvious.

Online pharmacies are a somewhat different story. Their sales volume is their major business model. When it increases they can invest in both equipment and staff. The point here rather is that, when they are successful, they contribute to an increase in health care spending. Some of this additional volume will be out of pocket, which the customer accepts more easily for matter that he purchases than for advice that he collects. That is why business models for Pre-screening and Virtual services appear more fragile. Virtual services, though, do scale up. Pre-screening service do not really scale up because every consultation involves individual attention of a health care professional, mostly physician. Some increase in efficiency may still be achievable through specialization, load balancing among doctors on duty and other improvements in convenience.

> **Take Home**
>
> An ad-hoc collection of indicators suggests that Consumer Health Informatics services scale up easily when they do not require multiplication of user access point hardware or services conveyed by humans. This mainly applies to services that convey logistic or medical advice, dosage recommendations etc. automatically.
> Services with human contribution may at least offer convenience and load balancing through asynchronous communication.
> Services such as online pharmacies follow a different model because their source of revenue is sales volume.

References

1. Anderson P, Jacobs C, Rothbaum BO. Computer-supported cognitive behavioral treatment of anxiety disorders. J Clin Psychol. 2004;60(3):253–67. doi: 10.1002/jclp.10262.
2. Anhøj J, Nielsen L. Quantitative and qualitative usage data of an internet-based asthma monitoring tool. J Med Internet Res. 2004;6(3):e33. doi: 10.2196/jmir.6.3.e23.
3. Bergström J, Andersson G, Ljótsson B, Rück C, Andréewitch S, Karlsson A, Carlbring P, Andersson E, Lindefors N. Internet-versus group-administered cognitive behaviour therapy for panic disorder in a psychiatric setting: a randomised trial. BMC Psychiatry. 2010;10(54):1471–244X. doi: 10.1186/1471-244X-10-54.
4. Bauer S, Moessner M. Harnessing the power of technology for the treatment and prevention of eating disorders. Int J Eat Disord. 2013;46:508–15. doi: 10.1002/eat.22109.
5. Boyington AR, Wildemuth BM, Dougherty MC, Hall EP. Development of a computer-based system for continence health promotion. Nurs Outlook. 2004;52:241–7. doi: 10.1016/j.outlook.2004.04.014.
6. Curioso WH, Blas MM, Nodell B, Alva IE, Kurth AE. Opportunities for providing web-based interventions to prevent sexually transmitted infections in peru. PLoS Med. 2007;4(2):e11. doi: 10.1371/journal.pmed.0040011.
7. Cuijpers P, Boluijt P, van Straten A. Screening of depression in adolescents through the internet. Eur Child Adolesc Psychiatry. 2008;17:32–8 doi: 10.1007/s00787-007-0631-2.
8. Cuijpers P, Reynolds CF, Donker T, Li J, Andersson G, Beekman A. Personalized treatment of adult depression: medication, psychotherapy, or both? A systematic review. Depress Anxiety. 2012;29:855–64. doi: 10.1002/da.21985.
9. Gorber SC, Schofield-Hurwitz S, Hardt J, Levasseur G, Tremblay M. The accuracy of self-reported smoking: a systematic review of the relationship between self-reported and cotinine-assessed smoking status. Nicotine Tob Res. 2009;11(1):12–24. doi: 10.1093/ntr/ntn010.
10. Hill-Kayser CE, Vachani C, Hampshire MK, Jacobs LA, Metz JM. An internet tool for creation of cancer survivorship care plans for survivors and health care providers: design, implementation, use and user satisfaction. J Med Internet Res. 2009;11(3):e39. doi: 10.2196/jmir.1223.
11. Hou JG, Murphy P, Tang AW, Khandelwal N, Duncan I, Pegus CL. Impact of an online prescription management account on medication adherence. Am J Manag Care. 2012;18(3):e86–90.
12. Hsiung RC. The best of both worlds: and online self-help group hosted by a mental health professional. Cyberpsychol Behav. 2000;3(6):935–50. doi: 10.1089/109493100452200.
13. Jena AB, Goldman DP, Foster SE, Califano JA. Prescription medication abuse and illegitimate internet-based pharmacies. Ann Intern Med. 2011;155:848–50. doi: 10.7326/0003-4819-155-12-201112200-00008.

14. Kirshenbaum AP, Olsen DM, Bickel WK. A quantitative review of the ubiquitous relapse curve. J Subst Abuse Treat. 2009;36(1):8–17. doi: 10.1016/j.jsat.2008.04.001.
15. Kroenke K, Spitzer RL, Williams JBW. The PHQ-9. Validity of a brief depression severity measure. J Gen Intern Med. 2001;16(9):606–13. doi: 10.1046/j.1525-1497.2001.016009606.x.
16. Liu W-T, Huang C-D, Wang C-H, Lee K-Y, Lin S-M, Kuo H-P. A mobile telephone-based interactive selfcare system improves asthma control. Eur Respir J. 2011;37:310–7. doi: 10.1183/09031936.00000810.
17. Orizio G, Schulz P, Domenighini S, Bressanelli M, Rubinelli S, Caimi L, Gelatti U. Online consultations in cyberpharmacies: completeness and patient safety. Telemed e-Health. 2009;15(10):1022–5. doi: 10.1089/tmj.2009.0069.
18. O'Connor EA, Whitlock EP, Gaynes B, Beil TL. Screening for depression in adults and older adults in primary care: an updated systematic review, volume 75 of evidence synthesis. Rockville: Agency for Healthcare Research and Quality; 2009. AHRQ Publication No. 10-05143-EF-1.
19. Cohen R, Elhadad M, Birk O. Analysis of free online physician advice services. PLoSONE. 2013;3(8):e59963. doi: 10.1371/journal.pone.0059963.
20. Riffe D, Lacy S, Fico FG. Analyzing media messages. Using quantitative content analysis in research. Mahwah: Lawrence Erlbaum; 2005.
21. Shear MK, Brown TA, Barlow DH, Money R, Sholomskas DE, Woods SW, Gorman JM, Papp LA. Multicenter collaborative panic disorder severity scale. Am J Psychiatry. 1997;154:1571–5.
22. Strecher VJ, McClure JB, Alexander GL, Chakraborty B, Nair VN, Konkel JM, Greene SM, Collins LM, Carlier CC, Wiese CJ, Little RJ, Pomerleau CS, Pomerleau OF. Web-based smoking-cessation programs. Results of a randomized trial. Am J Prev Med. 2008;34(5):373–81. doi: 10.1016/j.amepre.2007.12.024.
23. Spek V, Nykliček I, Smits N, Cuijpers P, Riper H, Keyzer J, Pop V. Internet-based cognitive behavioural therapy for subthreshold depression in people over 50 years old: a randomized controlled clinical trial. Psychol Med. 2007;37:1797–806. doi: 10.1017/S0033291707000542.
24. Thompson DA, Lorenzo P, Christakis DA. Parent use of touchscreen computer kiosks for child health promotion in community settings. Pediatrics. 2007;119(3):427–34. doi: 10.1542/peds.2006-2669.
25. van Bastelaar K, Cuijpers P, Pouwer F, Riper H, Snoek FJ. Development and reach of a web-based cognitive behavioural therapy programme to reduce symptoms of depression and diabetes-specific distress. Patient Educ Couns. 2011;84:49–55. doi: 10.1016/j.pec.2010.06.013.
26. van Voorhees BW, Hsiung RC, Marko-Holguin M, Houston TK, Fogel J, Lee R, Ford DE. Internal versus external motivation in referral of primary care patients with depression to an internet support group: randomized controlled trial. JMIR. 2013;15(3):e42. doi: 10.2196/jmir.2197.
27. Watts S, Newby JM, Mewton L, Andrews G. A clinical audit of changes in suicide ideas with internet treatment for depression. BMJ Open. 2012;2:e001558. doi: 10.1136/bmjopen-2012-001558.

Chapter 6
Level 3: Patient Power on the Web: The Multifaceted Role of Personal Health Wisdom

Andrea Hartzler and Jina Huh

6.1 Conceptualizing the Wisdom of Patients: A Unique Value Proposition

Individuals develop a wealth of expertise from managing day-to-day health experiences. For example, a cancer survivor may have valuable strategies for tracking medical bills and benefits, updating her social and professional networks about her health, scheduling chemotherapy appointments to minimize disruptions to her professional work, or dealing with the pain of hair loss and wigs. Similarly, a diabetic may develop a range of personal strategies, such as tracking diet and blood glucose levels, as he gains experience managing his personal health. Much of this personal health wisdom is experiential in nature, drawn from personal experience, rather than from professional training. Personal experiences result in unique wisdom that clinicians cannot necessarily provide. Personal health wisdom offers valuable insights for those facing a similar health situation for the first time. En masse, personal health wisdom has the potential to reveal patterns in health and uncover biomedical discoveries.

From the dawn of folk medicine, people facing new health conditions have sought the support of someone who has been there. Modern society has devised a number of peer support mechanisms to meet the need expressed by patients for experiential wisdom that other patients can provide. For example, people who share similar health situations help one another to cope with illness by sharing their personal health wisdom through patient-led support groups, self-help groups, chronic disease self-management programs [22], or through mentoring programs,

---

A. Hartzler
Group Health Research Institute, Group Health Cooperative, Seattle, WA, USA

J. Huh
Department of Biomedical Informatics, University of California, San Diego, CA, USA

such as "Reach to Recovery" [4]. Experienced patients have offered valuable information to other patients by providing illness narratives as educational resources [31] and by acting as peer navigators who provide newly diagnosed patients with assistance that busy professionals are often unable to provide [11]. Such peer support programs benefit patients through provision of informational, emotional, and instrumental support [6].

Although historically bound to face-to-face settings, technology is significantly enriching the reach of peer support mechanisms for patients. Steady evidence points to the prevalence of personal health wisdom exchanged through online forums [16, 17]. The wisdom of patients has continued to gain visibility with advancements in social media (e.g., forums, social networking tools, blogs, wikis) that help people exchange personalized health advice. Researchers mine this patient-generated health data for patterns, such as detecting adverse drug events embedded in message board posts [3]. Clinicians can also leverage patients' personal experience to support individual treatment through mechanisms such as e-mail aftercare programs. Recent developments in 'citizen science' point to the broader potential of large scale personal health sharing through social media research platforms that crowd source this data en masse and report research findings on par with clinical trials [35, 39].

This unprecedented explosion in the social use of Internet-based technology by real people to solve real problems brings personal health wisdom center stage. Treating personal health wisdom as a serious knowledge source across this spectrum of uses spawns new questions about the ways people use technology to share their experiences, including risks associated with potential misinformation or loss of privacy. Minimizing such risks (cf. Chaps. 8 and 12) could lead to substantial benefits from broad use of social media to exchange health wisdom. The reach and potential of this widespread patient power on the Web can benefit not only individuals, but also biomedicine and society at large.

6.2 Exchanging Patient Wisdom Online: An Evolving Landscape of Social Media

An increasing range of social media enables diverse interactions for exchanging personal health wisdom [32]. Many tools are condition-specific and moderated, while others are not. Social media sites provide several building blocks for expertise sharing, such as user-generated content, recommendations, and social connections, the result of which can be used as collective knowledge. In light of this evolving landscape, this section covers four specific social media platforms well-suited for supporting the exchange of patient wisdom: Internet forums, blogs, wikis, and social networking tools.

6.2.1 Interacting Through Internet Forums

An Internet forum brings people together for interaction around a shared interest through a 'birds of a feather style' of collaboration [25]. Some variations of Internet forum platforms include threaded discussion boards, mailing lists, and newsgroups. On question and answer boards, such as Yahoo! Answers (https://answers.yahoo.com), several users post responses to a question, rather than appending replies within the flow of a discussion thread. Forums can vary along a number of characteristics, including size, composition, level of moderation, nomenclature, structure, and group dynamics (e.g., lurkers vs. contributors). Forums have become a common feature offered by many health-related social networking sites, such as PatientsLikeMe (http://www.patientslikeme.com).

Obtaining support on day-to-day health issues is a common reason for participation in an Internet forum. Health-related discussion emerges through patients' use of general-purpose forums, such as Yahoo! Answers (https://answers.yahoo.com). Other forums are designed specifically to support patient discussion around a specific health topic, ranging from cancer to chronic illness to everyday well-being.

Similar to traditional face-to-face patient support groups, Internet forums provide a mechanism for psychosocial benefits of peer support, but this support system is not constrained by time or geography [37]. In parallel, Internet forums have witnessed disparities in access with the "digital divide between those with and without Internet access". Forums can be distinguished by discussion that is moderated by peer "counselors" versus professionally-moderated. Because of the large-scale interactions that Internet forums facilitate, health professionals' engagement in support groups can also differ from traditional face-to-face settings.

Compared to other social media, Internet forums have a longer history of use and are associated with a larger body of research on their usage patterns [26] and psychosocial benefits [9]. As a knowledge source for personal health wisdom, Internet forums offer free-form flexibility to capture the contextualized detail of patients' personal stories and encourage interactive dialogue. The resulting richness of this interactive medium can help individuals to share tacit knowledge while retaining the detail necessary for reuse by others [1].

6.2.2 Capturing Knowledge Through Blogs

A blog is a website created by an individual blogger to share personal opinions, views, and experiences through regular detailed commentary on sites, such as LiveJournal (http://www.livejournal.com). Other tools, such as how-to web pages, offer blog features for individual contributors to easily capture and share their knowledge with others. Broadcasting brief, real-time commentary through micro blogging has become a popular use of social media through services, such as Twitter (http://www.twitter.com). Blogs encourage an 'opinion leader model' of collaboration [25] because they showcase an individual's opinions and experiences that serve as influential examples for others to follow.

Many patients increasingly turn to blogs to share personal health wisdom within a public space. Early blogs for patients include DIPEx (http://www.dipexinternational.org), which publishes video and transcripts from patient interviews, and Experience Journal (http://experiencejournal.childrenshospital.org), which showcases personal stories contributed by patients and family members. More recently, blogs have become a common means for health advocates to reach a wide audience, such as e-Patient Dave (http://patientdave.blogspot.com). Others have quickly followed suit through micro blogging on Twitter (http://www.twitter.com) to broadcast experiences around chronic illness management or health promoting physical activity.

Compared to other social media, individuals generate blog content with the intent for mass consumption. Although this potential for wide spread reach is impressive, the lack of corroboration through collaborating authors can raise questions around quality and fit of the personal health wisdom broadcast through blogs. For example, bloggers might exclude pertinent details of their experience or highlight uncommon or negative experiences even though patients can benefit from both positive and negative as well as mundane and unusual experiences. Although many blogs allow readers to comment on content, the perception of the blogger's ownership of content makes this platform less conducive to corroboration than more collaborative platforms like wikis that enable the critical reader to directly edit content. However, blogs often carry implicit advice through the detailed narrative of personal stories [14]. This natural expression captures detailed health experiences and has been highly valued for supporting expertise sharing in other contexts, such as professional organizations [24]. Similar to Internet forums, the rich contextual detail retained in blogs can help others to assess the quality and fit of advice to their own personal situation [1].

6.2.3 Building Collective Wisdom Through Wikis

A wiki is a web page or a collection of web pages that acts as a communal document by enabling anyone who accesses it to contribute content. Unlike blogs that restrict editing to the owner, wikis harness collective wisdom through a decentralized process of collaborative consensus building among contributors. Thus wikis reflect a 'democratic model' of collaboration [25]. One of the best-known wikis, Wikipedia (http://www.wikipedia.org), is one of the most extensively used platforms for health-related use aside from historical Internet forums.

Whereas general-purpose wikis (e.g., Wikipedia) incorporate a range of health topics, health-specific wikis, such as wikiCancer http://www.wikicancer.org, pool collective wisdom to recommend personal health articles and websites. Similarly,

Weiss and Lorenzi [21] designed a community-driven tool to synthesize and share local knowledge about cancer resources. A different example is Flu Wiki [28], which pools collective knowledge to help local communities prepare for and cope with a possible. These examples are akin to collaborative recommendation systems that help users share their expertise through item evaluations and benefit from each other's views, opinions, and experiences [36]. Although wikis are thought to be a valuable channel for promoting community health [7], relatively little research has explored their health-related use [29].

Compared to other social media, wikis can synthesize a wealth of wisdom from many individuals within a single location. This integration of knowledge contrasts with Internet forums, which can scatter that wisdom among forum threads. Wikis can compliment educational materials obtained from the healthcare system by meeting patients' needs for generalized health information that embodies experiential perspectives. Although the open nature of wikis encourages collaborative self-correction of misinformation, information quality is a common concern particularly in the health domain. Even when information is accurate, conflicting information can still be problematic. Because wikis strive for collective concordance, they are not designed to easily accommodate divergent or conflicting perspectives. Compiled information on wikis often loses the detailed context of narrative experiences reported on Internet forums or blogs. This distillation of detail can make it difficult to re-contextualize the shared wisdom for re-use [1].

6.2.4 Collaborating Through Social Networking Tools

Social networking tools differ from other social media in the vast range of interactive features they offer for sharing wisdom. These tools typically incorporate a collection of traditional social media features, such as discussion forums and blogs, for use among members of an online community. A defining feature of social networking tools is the user profile through which individuals can describe their personal interests and share a range of content (e.g., pictures, web pages, videos) with community members with whom they establish "friend" connections. Popular social networking tools include the friendship-focused Facebook (http://www.facebook.com) and the professionally-focused LinkedIn (http://www.linkedin.com).

Social networking tools can be used to stay connected with one's existing network of family and friends or to extend one's personal network with new social connections. For example, cancer patients need ways to keep their personal network up-to-date about their cancer experience, but often need ways to reach beyond their existing network when it lacks sufficient support. Extending one's personal network, by establishing "weak ties", enables patients to garner expertise that can be different from the information available from family and friends [12]. Several health-related tools have been designed with these different uses in mind, such as CarePages (http://www.carepages.com) for supporting existing social networks and PatientsLikeMe (http://www.patientslikeme.com) for extending social networks.

Although general-purpose social networking tools, such as Facebook, can be used for health-related exchange [2] differences in patients' use of health-specific and general-purpose social networking tools warrant further investigation ([27], cf. also Sect. 4.3.2).

Social networking tools can also facilitate the exchange of personal health wisdom when used as 'people finders' to locate individuals with similar health situations for personalized interaction around health [5]. For example, user profiles on PatientsLikeMe form the basis for searching for users who manage the same health condition. Frost and Massagli [11], through a content analysis of profile comments on PatientsLikeMe, discovered that experienced patients who reviewed profiles of peers often picked up on potentially problematic patterns they recognized from their own similar health experiences. These 'experts' would then provide peers with feedback to alert them to the potential problem and offer advice.

Beyond facilitating individual connections, social networking tools can also pool wisdom across community members to target personalized recommendations. For example, Khan et al. [20] designed a tag-based recommendation system using community ratings of health-related content. Others have joined the Quantified Self (http://www.quantifiedself.com) movement as a popular means of sharing quantifiable information about oneself to monitor health and network with others. Aggregation of health experiences across community members is gaining credence as a community-based participatory approach to patient-reported outcomes research [35]. This collective use of crowd-sourced wisdom is part of the growing 'citizen science' revolution.

In summary, the evolving landscape of social media enables the spread of patient wisdom across the Internet. From interacting on Internet forums, to capturing knowledge through blogs, collecting wisdom through wikis, and collaborating through social networking tools, the growing use of social media illustrates its potential as a premier nexus for personal health. Not only serving as marketplaces of crowds willing to share their own knowledge, social media offer resources that can be mined to generate new knowledge across the masses. By supporting a range of personal health wisdom, from patient narratives to quantified self, social media is well positioned to facilitate multifaceted use.

6.3 Leveraging Patient Wisdom: Varied Levels of Use Among Individuals, Groups, and Crowds

The wisdom of patients can play a powerful role across a spectrum of uses. From the individual level of shared experience, to the collaborative level of the group with specialized interests, to the collective action of the masses at the crowd level, personal health wisdom is making its mark. Across this multifaceted use, this section covers benefits and challenges of leveraging personal health wisdom at three important levels: individual, group, and crowd. The three levels are illustrated in Fig. 6.1.

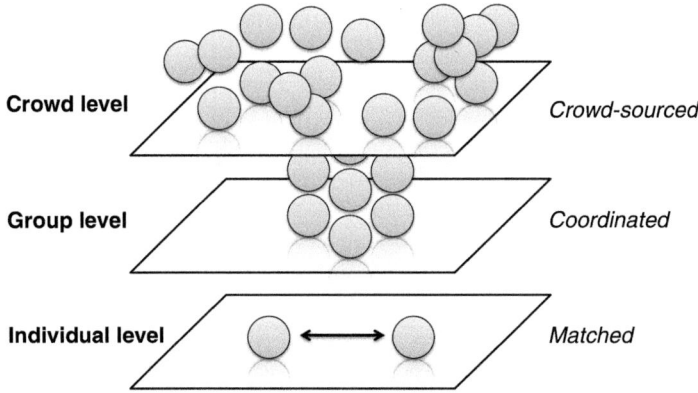

Fig. 6.1 Levels of shared personal health wisdom

6.3.1 Individual Level: From Foraging Alone to Shared Experience

At the individual level, people both seek and offer highly individualized personal experiences. For example, a breast cancer patient may seek help deciding between lumpectomy and mastectomy. She may seek the advice of another patient who faced the same diagnosis and treatment decision by posting a request for help on an Internet forum. In response, she receives advice from a 5-year cancer survivor who shares her personal experience choosing lumpectomy, considering issues such as prognosis, recovery time, and body image. As this example illustrates, sharing individual experiences can facilitate highly customized problem-solving. The value of sharing wisdom at the individual level is in learning to manage personal health from others rather than learning on one's own.

Classic peer support mechanisms, such as patient support groups, emphasize the sharing of individual experience. Some mechanisms foster a mentoring relationship between more and less experienced patients, such as the "Reach to Recovery" breast cancer program [4] or patient-led chronic disease self-management programs. As peer support mechanisms move online to social media, a strong motivator of use remains individual problem solving [18]. For example, users of PatientsLikeMe benefit from health promoting support they receive from other users in response to sharing their experience with treatments, symptoms, and outcomes. By understanding others' personal health management strategies, online communities help patients find individualized management strategies for themselves.

Beyond providing individualized solutions, a major benefit of sharing personal health wisdom at the individual level is exchanging social support. Connecting with individuals who have similar health experiences not only offers the emotional support of empathy and concern, but can also provide a wealth of informational support in the form of experiential advice. In addition to benefits of peer support

[15], sharing personal health wisdom can benefit the helper as much as the helpee through the "helper therapy principle" [30]. In particular, patients who help other patients can experience physical and emotional benefits of the "helper's high" [23] as well as arrive at a deeper understanding of their own health situation [33].

Despite these benefits, sharing personal health wisdom at the individual level can present a number of challenges, particularly to personal privacy and personalized fit. Obtaining peer support often requires disclosing sensitive personal information about one's health. Health-related social media need enhancements to facilitate tradeoffs between personal disclosure and safeguarding personal privacy. The potential for misinformation is also a common concern, although studies of peer interactions in online communities have found low levels of inaccurate medical information [8, 9]. Even when information is accurate, shared advice can have a poor fit due to misalignment between the situation of the helper and the helpee, resulting in the misapplication of sound advice that simply does not transfer from one situation to another. Work to overcome challenges surrounding privacy, misinformation, and fit of information will advance the future of social media for sharing at the individual level and beyond.

6.3.2 Group Level: From Shared Experience to Collaborative Bricolage

At the group level, individuals work together towards a common goal by taking part in a larger dialogue that extends beyond one's individual interests. Contributors bring specialized wisdom into a collaborative process of problem solving in which individual solutions are stitched together into a diverse 'bricolage'. For example, patients in a diabetes support group might exchange strategies to generate a comprehensive list of low-carb diet options. Newcomers can challenge the group's agreed on knowledge with their own experience, pushing the group's wisdom one step further by incorporating a greater diversity of opinions. Wikis are well-suited to support this type of group work to collate generalized wisdom. The value of sharing wisdom at the group level is in working together, through a common interest among group members, to develop a shared understanding, means, and ends. The combined effect of the group acting in sum can often be greater than the parts acting alone.

Collaborative bricolage involves several types of knowledge work. For example, members of online health communities often work together to enhance the quality of information they share through safeguarding strategies, such as, self-correction among watchful members [8]. Individuals often compare and contrast their health experiences with the illness trajectories of other patients. Through this collaborative "alignment work" [13], a support group builds a generalized collage of stories that might reduce uncertainties of newcomers. Another example involves people working together in crisis to fill in information gaps. Starbird and Palen [34], for example, describe the use of Twitter by "digital volunteers" to share emergency response information in the aftermath of the 2010 Haiti earthquake. This use of social media illustrates the power of shared wisdom for self-organizing groups in crisis for disaster relief.

Perhaps one of the most significant benefits of sharing personal health wisdom at the group level is taking part in something that is larger than oneself – indeed, the "sum" can be greater than it's "parts". Knowing that one is not alone, but is working as part of a team can provide purpose and meaning to an otherwise frustrating or negative health experience. Furthermore, compiling the specialized and varied experiences of many into a collage of illness experiences can greatly enrich our understanding of the breadth and complexity of that illness, allowing room for increased completeness as various sides of the story are assimilated. At the same time, these advantages of shared wisdom at the group level can also raise critical challenges, including domination by the more powerful to sway or bias the group (cf. Sect. 3.3.1.2) and dangers of "group think" [19].

6.3.3 Crowd Level: From Collaborative Bricolage to Collective Discovery

At the crowd level, people work collectively to discover and build knowledge. Rather than executing on a known objective together, decentralized workers contribute in concert to crowd-source emergent knowledge as a product of their collective action. In citizen science, for example, a large group of volunteer amateurs is called upon to capture and analyze data en masse rather than relying solely on the traditional scientist. One long-standing project is Galaxy Zoo (http://www.galaxyzoo.org), which invites the public to answer questions about telescope images on the Internet. Answers are aggregated to help classify galaxies. The value of sharing wisdom at the crowd level is in discovery of emergent knowledge that can result from low cost and efficient aggregation of experiences shared en mass among distributed volunteers.

In the health domain, the trend of crowdsourcing personal health data is taking shape in which everyday people take part in large-scale research by sharing their personal health experiences en masse. From PatientsLikeMe (http://www.patientslikeme.com) to DIYgenomics (http://www.diygenomics.org), Internet-based tools are leveraging the sharing and collaboration features of social media to accrue volunteers, conduct trials by aggregating personal health experiences, and report results comparable to traditional clinical trials. For example, patient-reported data collected on PatientsLikeMe has been analyzed to investigate off-label prescribing and the effect of lithium carbonate on progression of amyotrophic lateral sclerosis [39]. Similarly, Swan [35] describes the use of Genomera (http://www.genomera.com) to crowd source health research studies that link genetic and behavioral data en masse. Other examples include the use of patient-generated data to spawn hypotheses about links between clinical observations, drugs, genetics, and disease [38] or to discover new adverse drug effects [3].

Emergent knowledge that advances personalized medicine, translational science, and biomedicine more broadly is one of the significant benefits of sharing personal health wisdom at the crowd level. Although crowdsourcing can lower costs to research participation, collection of large data sets, and efficient knowledge discovery, this trend towards democratization of science is not without concerns about data quality, bias, reproducibility, and other impacts on traditional approaches to scientific research. Patient-generated health data shared through social media can be suspect, focused on individual experiences whether contributed by an outlier or one in the norm. However, by aggregating such data en masse, critical patterns can emerge – widely recurring patterns offer a kind of 'majority vote' through which unprecedented insights may emerge. This potential for discovery is the true marvel of this new medium of wisdom in the crowds: through a bird's eye perspective on apparently unrelated individual experiences new general rules emerge.

6.4 Conclusion

In this chapter, we discussed the personal health wisdom of patients – its characteristics, the social media tools people use to share this wisdom, and the benefits and challenges of using personal health wisdom at multiple levels from individual, to group and crowd. Through this discussion, we illustrate the growing ubiquity of personal health wisdom on the Internet and its great potential to shape the health of individuals and biomedicine more broadly. Growing interest in the use of patient-generated health data on the Web among researchers and practitioners in a range of disciplines underscores the importance of considering the role that personal health wisdom will play in our future health care infrastructure. Whether the wisdom of patients is used to aid individual health management, groups with specialized interests, or society at large, challenges to information quality and personal privacy remain salient. However, the multifaceted role of personal health wisdom presents a paramount opportunity for interdisciplinary collaboration that has great potential to overcome those challenges and spread the benefits of patient power across the web.

References

1. Ackerman MS, Halverson CA. Organizational memory as objects, processes, and trajectories: an examination of organizational memory in use. CSCW. 2004;13:155–89. doi: 10.1023/B:COSU.0000045805.77534.2a.
2. Bender JL, Jimenez-Marroquin MC, Jadad AR. Seeking support on facebook: a content analysis of breast cancer groups. J Med Internet Res. 2011;13(1):e16. doi: 10.2196/jmir.1560.
3. Benton A, Ungar L, Hill S, Hennessy S, Maoa J, Chung A, Leonard CE, Holmes JH. Identifying potential adverse effects using the web: a new approach to medical hypothesis generation. J Biomed Inform. 2011;44(6):989–96. doi: 10.1016/j.jbi.2011.07.005.
4. Burdick D. Rehabilitation of the breast cancer patient. Cancer. 1975;36(2):645–8. doi: 10.1002/1097-0142(197508)36:2+<645::AID-CNCR2820360806>3.0.CO;2-X.

5. Civan-Hartzler A, McDonald D, Powell C, Skeels M, Mukai M, Pratt W. Bringing the field into focus: user-centered design of a patient expertise locator. In: CHI'10; 2010. pp. 1675–84. doi: 10.1145/1753326.1753577.
6. Campbell HS, Phaneuf MR, Deane K. Cancer peer support programs – do they work? Patient Educ Couns. 2004;55(1):3–15.
7. Crespo R. Virtual community health promotion. Prev Chronic Dis. 2007;4(3):A73.
8. Esquivel A, Meric-Bernstam F, Bernstam EV. Accuracy and self correction of information received from an internet breast cancer list: content analysis. Br Med J. 2006;332(7547):939–42. doi: 10.1136/bmj.38753.524201.7C.
9. Eysenbach G, Powell J, Englesakis M, Rizo C, Stern A. Health-related virtual communities and electronic support groups: systematic review of the effects of online peer-to-peer interactions. Br Med J. 2004;328(7449):1166. doi: 10.1136/bmj.328.7449.1166.
10. Frost JL, Massagli MP. Social uses of personal health information within PatientsLikeMe, an online patient community: what can happen when patients have access to one another's data. J Med Internet Res. 2008;10(3):e15. doi: 10.2196/jmir.1053.
11. Giese-Davis J, Bliss-Isberg C, Carson K, Star P, Donaghy J, Cordova, N Stevens MJ, Wittenberg L, Batten C, Spiegel D. The effect of peer counseling on quality of life following diagnosis of breast carcinoma: an observational study. Psycho-Oncology. 2006;15(11):1014–22. doi: 10.1002/pon.1037.
12. Granovetter MS. The strength of weak ties. Am J Sociol. 2006;78(6):1360–80. doi: 10.1086/268018.
13. Huh J, Ackerman MS. Collaborative help in chronic disease management: supporting individualized problems. In: CSCW'12; 2012. pp. 853–62. doi: 10.1145/2145204.2145331.
14. Hardey M. The story of my illness. Personal accounts of illness on the internet. Health. 2002;6(1):31–46. doi: 10.1177/136345930200600103.
15. Hoey LM, Ieropoli SC, White VM, Jefford M. Systematic review of peer-support programs for people with cancer. Patient Educ Couns. 2008;70(3):315–37. doi: 10.1016/j.pec.2007.11.016.
16. Hoch DB, Norris D, Lester JE, Marcus AD. Information exchange in an epilepsy forum on the world wide web. Seizure. 1999;8(1):30–34. doi: 10.1053/seiz.1998.0217.
17. Hartzler A, Pratt W. Managing the personal side of health: how patient expertise differs from the expertise of clinicians. J Med Internet Res. 2011;13(3):e62. doi: 10.2196/jmir.1728.
18. Horrigan JB, Rainie L, Fox S. Online communities: networks that nurture long-distance relationships and local ties. http://www.pewinternet.org/~/media//Files/Reports/2001/PIP_Communities_Report.pdf.pdf, Oct 2001.
19. Janis IL. Groupthink. Psychol Today. 1971;5(6):43–6, 74–6.
20. Khan SA, Cohall A, Kukafka R. A tag based recommendation engine to suggest information resources in an online community for health promotion. In: AMIA annual symposium proceedings. Bethesda: American Medical Informatics Association; 2008. p. 1002.
21. Lorenzi NM, Weiss JB. Synthesizing community wisdom: a model for sharing cancer-related resources through social networking and collaborative partnership. AMIA Annu Symp Proc. 2008;2008:793–7.
22. Lorig KR, Sobel DS, Stewart AL, Brown Jr BW, Bandura A, Ritter P, Gonzalez VM, Laurent DD, Holman HR. Evidence suggesting that a chronic disease self-management program can improve health status while reducing hospitalization: a randomized trial. Med Care. 1999;37(1):5–14.
23. Luks A. Helper's high: volunteering makes people feel good, physically and emotionally. Psychol Today. 1988;22(10):34–42.
24. Lutters WG. Storytelling in collaborative work: the challenge of preserving sensitive interactions. ACM SIGGROUP Bull. 2002;23(2):22–23. doi: 10.1145/962185.962194.
25. McDonald DW. Supporting nuance in groupware design: moving from naturalistic expertise location to expertise recommendation. Dissertation, University of California, Irvine, 2000. http://www.pensivepuffin.com/dwmcphd/papers/McDonald.Dissertation.2S.pdf.

26. Meier A, Lyons EJ, Frydman G, Forlenza M, Rimer BK. How cancer survivors provide support on cancer-related internet mailing lists. J Med Internet Res. 2007;9(2):e12. doi: 10.2196/jmir.9.2.e12.
27. Newman MW, Lauterbach D, Munson SA, Resnick P, Morris ME. It's not that I don't have problems, I'm just not putting them on facebook: challenges and opportunities in using online social networks for health. In: CSCW '11; 2011. pp. 341–50 doi: 10.1145/1958824.1958876.
28. Palen L, Hiltz SR, Liu SB. Online forums supporting grassroots participation in emergency preparedness and response. Commun ACM. 2007;50(3):54–8.
29. Potts WW. Is e-health progressing faster than e-health researchers? J Med Internet Res. 2006;8(3):e24. doi: 10.2196/jmir.8.3.e24.
30. Reissman F. The "helper" therapy principle. Soc. Work. 1965;10(2):27–32. doi: 10.1093/sw/10.2.27.
31. Swift TL, Dieppe PA. Using expert patients' narratives as an educational resource. Patient Educ Couns. 2005;57(1):115–21. doi: 10.1016/j.pec.2004.05.004.
32. Sarasohn-Kahn J. The wisdom of patients: health care meets online social media. http://www.chcf.org/publications/2008/04/the-wisdom-of-patients-health-care-meets-online-social-media, Apr 2008.
33. Schwartz CE, Sendor M. Helping others helps oneself: response shift effects in peer support. Soc Sci Med. 1999;48(11):1563–75. doi: 10.1016/S0277-9536(99)00049-0.
34. Starbird K, Palen L. "voluntweeters": self-organizing by digital volunteers in times of crisis. In: Proceeding CHI'11. New York: ACM; 2011. pp. 1071–80. doi: 10.1145/1978942.1979102.
35. Swan M. Crowdsourced health research studies: an important emerging complement to clinical trials in the public health research ecosystem. JMIR. 2012;14(2):e46. doi: 10.2196/jmir.1988.
36. Terveen LG, Hill W. Beyond recommender systems: helping people help each other. In: HCI in the new Millennium. Boston: Addison-Wesley; 2001. pp. 487–509
37. White M, Dorman SM. Receiving social support online: implications for health education. Health Educ Res. 2001;16(6):693–707. doi: 10.1093/her/16.6.693.
38. Webster YW, Dow ER, Koehler J, Gudivada RC, Palakal MJ. Leveraging health social networking communities in translational research. J Biomed Inform. 2011;44(4):536–44. doi: 10.1016/j.jbi.2011.01.010.
39. Wicks P, Vaughan TE, Massagli MP, Heywood J. Accelerated clinical discovery using self-reported patient data collected online and a patient-matching algorithm. Nat Biotechnol. 2011;29:411–4. doi: 10.1038/nbt.1837.

Chapter 7
Distinctive Features of Services Conveyed Through Mobile Apps

7.1 Introduction

Mobile apps or apps for short are one carrier technology for Consumer Health Informatics services, as are text messages and the Internet. Since this volume is about services rather than about technology we approach the field from character of services, methods of evaluation, deployment etc., as outlined in Chap. 1, mostly disregarding or just mentioning the carrier technology. Mobile apps are gaining ground so fast and some aspects are so distinctive, however, that we briefly address these here. For deeper specific insights the reader may check Siau and Chen who provided an early assessment from the perspective of technology and care process engineering [4]. A more recent and broader outline how smart phone technology and client needs can be brought to fit has been provided by Klasnja and Pratt [1].

7.2 Values Added Through the Technology

Laptop and desktop applications can employ of a large screen, a pointing device, keyboard, multichannel sound input and output and video input and output. What appears as an advantage alone at first has a downside. Since this diversity of options invites to design ever new fancy interaction patterns and display styles, clients who are at odds with technology may feel puzzled if not frightened and hence not fully exploit opportunities that are principally contained in a web based Consumer Health Informatics service. In contrast, the limitations in size and input capacity of smartphones have led to a quasi-standard of interaction pattern within few years. Most providers of services comply with the standards (home key, touch an input field of the screen to bring up keyboard, gestures for recover from standby and for synchronize, icons for mailing, erasing etc.) and hence also infrequent users can feel comfortable after a short while. It is the appeal of simplicity and the playful nature which can attract individuals who would not touch a classical computer.

Therefore, growing numbers of citizens need not be ushered to use smart phones and apps. The name that Google™ uses for its distribution channel, Google Play™, is a message about the whole field. Google Play™ store, App Store by Apple and Amazon®'s App store are the largest distributors of apps.[1] Apple has installed an exclusive distribution mechanism for iOS through the App Store whereas Google™ also tolerates other distribution channels and serves the Android™ platform. Amazon® distributes for the Android™ and Fire OS platforms.

Besides playful nature, ubiquity is another promise of apps. Wherever and whenever the client wants information, has data to enter or relies on reminders they are right there. He need not wait, memorize, or use proxies that remind him instead. These features together establish an atmosphere of trust and a feeling of convenience that makes people like and continuously use their apps, not only medical ones.

Ubiquity is essentially valuable for all medical conditions that require timely recording or decision support. Smoking cessation, anxiety disorders, metabolic diseases such as diabetes, where challenges have to be met when they are there, not at home or in the office when back at the computer, benefit most from assistance in the pocket.

The fact that smart phones can operate as measuring and recording devices for various modalities adds to the feelings of trust and convenience. Such measuring and recording includes GPS positioning for emergency reporting or dispatching functions but equally for identifying facilities such as hospitals or pharmacies in the vicinity of the present location. Smart phones can also detect acceleration and can, therefore, to some extent function as fall detectors. They can detect and record sound and imagery. So physically they are equipped for wide ranging screening, diagnostic and educational purposes.

Besides technical selling points smart phones also add to and benefit from new developments in the way people communicate and perform activities of daily life. This reaches from momentary quasi synchronous exchange of chitchat with distant company – sometimes interfering with the communication with local company – to organizing revolutions. In the middle ground it provides all kinds of functions from convenience and joy, such as video telephony, to mastering serious logistics challenges such as purchasing 24/7 or finding and booking a new means of transportation when a planned one fails. The growing feeling that it works, adds to habituation and, again, trust which extends to the medium and its services. Why should that stop when it gets medical?

---

[1] Various other providers offer apps, including but without claiming completeness BlackBerry®, Windows Phone Store by Microsoft®, Nokia® Store. The analysis concentrates on those three providers which together have a market share of more than 80 % in January 2015.

> **Take Home**
>
> Smart-phones and smart-phone apps have unique enticing features, including
>
> - Standards of handling
> - Playful appeal
> - Ubiquity
> - Built-in measuring devices
> - Virtually unlimited community
> - 24/7 reliable convenience
>
> These make them an easy access point to Consumer Health Informatics also for technology neutral or adverse citizens.

7.3 Distributors' Take on Medical Quality

All the major distributors apply some diligence for harmful apps not to be distributed and installed. The criteria for "harmful" are not or not easily accessible to the general public. Interested individuals have to become developers to the price of \$25 (Google^{TM}, one time) or \$99 (Apple, yearly) and search for a while at all three. In the "Amazon Distribution Agreement" (http://developer.amazon.com/public/support/legal/da) "harm" is used for malevolent software and financial loss, including through tax violations. Only well hidden under "Distribution schedule", "Additional Distribution Terms", "Embedded Advertising" an app developer must guarantee for embedded ads that they do not "cause injury to any person or damage to any property...".

Harm at Google^{TM} used to be technical and material only in summer 2013: at its "Protect against harmful apps", http://support.google.com/accounts/answer/2812853, the warning used to read: "Installing this app may harm your device". By February 2015 this was changed to "harm *you* (emphasis by the author) or your device". Lots of settings for software verification against technical harm are subsequently outlined. However, how harm to the user will be safeguarded against remains in the dark.

The Google Play Developer Distribution Agreement at http://play.google.com/intl/ALL_us/about/developer-distribution-agreement.html (only visible after registration) gives Google^{TM} the right to disable an app if it "could cause serious harm to user devices or data", unchanged in February 2015. Apple declined to provide information – mentioning that it is the "company's policy not to participate in surveys and research" – whether they are establishing patient safeguards in their developer requirements.

It is out of Amazon$^{®}$'s, Google^{TM}'s and Apple's consideration whether an app might harm the user's body or mind although medical apps in their stores are galore. The mainly technical approach to safety of apps supports the proliferation of multiple contents conveyed through the same technology, such as multiple textbooks, checklists for various purposes, charting and graphical display of diverse trends etc. If a developer did a checklist for Christmas presents and a monitor for sunshine hours why not do a checklist for medications and a monitor for depression scores? If your technology passes Amazon®'s, Apple's or Google™'s criteria with one contents it will do for any, no matter whether you have the least knowledge of a domain. Replication of a technology with different contents is the business model of many nameless companies or individuals such as http://limbua.com/, and http://macropinch.com/ or World Apps,[2] a developer that is so secretive that neither Google™ nor Yahoo!™ nor Bing® finds it in an Internet search. World Apps' apps exist for Asthma, Herbs, Aromatherapy, Chiropractic, Buddha, and Creative Writing, with no medical credentials and no accountability.

The presence of lots of entertaining contents next to serious – including medical – contents may have an enhancing and trailing effect: having collected entertaining rather than intimidating experiences with fun applications the threshold may be lower to try serious ones. However, notions of trust that develop through entertainment apps that have been checked technically and never fail, may unconsciously transfer to medical contents, not realizing that providers such as Amazon®, Apple and Google™ do not care about medical correctness, safety or effectiveness. Methods of checking trustworthiness (cf. Sects. 3.4.3 and 3.5) and safety (cf. Chaps. 8 or 12) may find themselves outside their field of vision.

Take Home

Major app distributors have each set up similar stereotypical procedures including

- rules for developers to register
- policies and technical guidelines for technically safe app operation
- sales processes

This gives developers and hence distributors opportunities for business of scale because guideline compliant technologies can be developed and multiply re-used.

The respective market place is characterized through feelings of smooth operation and safety which unconsciously transfers to medical apps although no Consumer Health Informatics methods to actively check trustworthiness or medical safety are in place.

---

[2] Just as examples that the reader may try to replicate and which do not stand out in any aspect pertinent to Consumer Health Informatics; explicitly: they are not meant as negative but as typical examples. Many others work similarly.

7.4 Clients' Traps and Barriers in Checking Quality

Regarded as a medical place, however, matter of fact quality is a necessary ingredient and we look into handles for clients to assess quality. App distributors have large shelves of offers. Each individual offer comes with some information about the developer and versions, client reviews and client ratings. Client reviews are mostly short and fast to read and graphical displays of ratings are instantly appealing. If the app stores were nothing but a fun place quality could be defined as what other customers like and following reviews and ratings could be a workable heuristics to find quality. We have, however, seen examples and investigations where what the clients like most is not what has the highest medical quality (Sects. 5.3.4.1, 3.3.1.2 and 6.3.2). Mechanically following check-mark ratings turns out a weak heuristics. This appears in contrast to the value that is assigned to personal health wisdom in Chap. 6. However, volunteering to outline individual advice from own experience and expose it to the community is a different matter than anonymously check-marking an app in passing.

Approaching quality through face credentials of the providing source or developer information is even harder for the client of apps than for classical Internet-based services. We have seen in Sect. 3.4 that there are no safe criteria to find out trustworthiness of arbitrary providers. HON has only recently started to certify apps. Many apps not even have "face" information such as authors, scientific sources used, or a legal notice. If any, the reference often is the website of the developer. This is a deficiency in structure quality in its own right because the client who seeks a service in the apps world is referred to the Internet world to inquire about indicators of quality.

What he may then find varies enormously. Provider "institutions" for the world wide market include individual programmers residing somewhere, some of whom are in command of English – and some are not – who boast themselves of specializing in programming wonderful checklists for Christmas gifts or medications. At the upper end there are some world-renowned health care providers or scientific institutions such as the Mayo Clinic. The NLM has not entered the field, they do not author apps. A noteworthy good service, though, is an Internet based search function for apps. Apart from the fact that the seeker needs both media – Internet and mobile device – and is not intimidated through the suggestion "appendicitis" when he enters the search term app he receives a large number of suggestions that all are medical and apparently of good quality. CDC has some apps, e.g. vaccination schedules, alerts and travel health coaches.

Not all legal notices or "About us" are easy to read. Some provide professional credentials in the form of impressive multi letter abbreviations that actually point to academic qualifications which, however, the layperson is unlikely to know and needs to do more research to appropriately assess and differentiate (cf. Sect. 5.3.4.1). In general, a comprehensive approach to quality assurance for apps is still due as has also been highlighted in a comment to the influential British Medical Journal [2]. Individual evaluations exist, though, cf. [3].

Quality deficiencies may show as accidental utilization of clearly inferior while missing a clearly superior resource. A client who relies on Fitforfravel may miss life-saving quality information because he does not become aware of the true specialists he needs (cf. Sect. 5.3.1). Clients who are skeptical of scientific medicine or inclined to deny certain procedures due to rules of religious or cultural communities (cf. Sect. 8.4.2.3) easily find themselves re-enforced through apps such as Gesundheitsirrtümer[3], http://www.appsundco.de/iphone/apps/medizin/gesundheits-irrtuemer-wissenswertes-aus-gesundheit-medizin/ or Health Remedy - Heal Using Natural Medicine which has breast cancer on its list of conditions and lures the prospective medicine sceptic with "Why take tablets and chemicals with lots of side-effects when there are natural ways ...". Therefore, risks already outlined in Chaps. 8 and 3 materialize here as well, in a place where trust towards the medium is the prevailing attitude.

> **Take Home**
> Customer rankings which are a common instrument to assess apps are a hazardous heuristics to check medical quality.
> Individual investigations of quality through literature search or legal notice and provider credentials follow up is often hampered through lack of references, hard to find and delusive information.
> Consequently clients may hit inferior or ideologically misguided rather than existing high quality Consumer Health Informatics services.

7.5 Further Necessary Precautions When It Becomes Serious Medicine

When smart-phone or tablet apps become constituents of regular Consumer Health Informatics services, precautions have to be in place that fend off two kind of risks. Risk one is the instantaneous denial of service due to – in a wider sense – physical reasons. Battery management must make sure that either batteries are charged or exchanged in time or that the client becomes aware of a closing down routine that allows him to take precautions until the next charging opportunity comes. Unfortunately, highly encapsulated batteries in newest generation smart-phones prohibit the "exchange battery" option.

Cell phone coverage can also not be taken for granted. Exceptions are not so rare when one thinks of nature disasters such as blizzards, volcano eruptions or floodings, and of places such as remote areas in the Rocky Mountains, let alone Third World countries. Paradoxically, medical and other apps may be required desperately when the situation is bizarre or the location is far from any personal help.

---

[3] German for Health misconceptions.

7.5 Further Necessary Precautions When It Becomes Serious Medicine

To compensate for failing cellular network coverage smart-phone apps in the medical domain have to have a fallback local solution for essential functions. The fallback may not achieve optimal solutions but must definitely avoid the actual risk of not providing any required information and the emotional risk of deteriorating trust into a service. Such fallbacks may for instance provide 1 week trends of locally stored variables such as blood glucose concentration rather than months' or years' trends.

Risk two is the loss of data due to discontinuation of service through cellular network providers or any other third parties without whom the whole Consumer Health Informatics service does not work. To prevent such kind of risk enforceable contracts have to be closed that guarantee for data to be migrated even in the case of bankruptcy of some of the providers. Contracts should better also make sure that clients of a Consumer Health Informatics service cannot be taken hostage by a cellular network provider which insists on continuation of an unfair base contract as a prerequisite to further transport the added value medical service. Such demands cannot be met through boards of medical self administration (cf. Sect. 17.4) or state legislation. Nationwide and ultimately international safeguards for the continuous availability of infrastructures underlying Consumer Health Informatics apps are required.

Various other risks are associated with the handsome floating nature of the device itself, some of which also pertain to classical cellular phones. Many cell phones respective SIM cards are not permanently and continually associated with one person. Therefore confidential health information cannot be transmitted without session authentication. Smart-phones may also be lost in which case session authentication also helps to protect privacy. Continuation of a service after loss of a smart-phone also requires precautions. For the one the amount and duration of data storage in the device must be kept at a minimum. If a smart-phone and its SIM card or other unique identification is also used as part of a two factor authentication method as described in Sect. 13.4 fallbacks have to be in place to re-establish access.

Take Home

For sustained safe operation of smart-phone based Consumer Health Informatics services two major types of risks must be managed.

Technology Both device and network may fail. Fall-backs must be in place such as closing down routines for battery low or local kernel functions at network down and subsequent recovery and synchronization.

Business Providers may merge or default and successors in law wish to discontinue the medical operation. Or clients may lose SIM cards or any other interference with regular service delivery may happen. Precautions must be made and respective legislation may be advised to protect medical data and services against all such risks of discontinuation.

References

1. Klasnja P, Pratt W. Healthcare in the pocket: mapping the space of mobile-phone health interventions. J Biomed Inform. 2012;445(1):184–98. doi: 10.1016/j.jbi.2011.08.017.
2. McCartney M. How do we know whether medical apps work? Br Med J. 2013;346:f1811. doi: 10.1136/bmj.f1811.
3. Singh P. Orthodontic apps for smartphones. J Orthod. 2013;40:249–55. doi: 10.1179/1465313313Y.0000000052.
4. Siau K, Shen Z. Mobile healthcare informatics. Med Inform Internet Med. 2006;31(2):89–99. doi: 10.1080/14639230500095651.

Part II
Building Safety Nets Around the Active Client

Chapter 8
Dimensions of Patient Risks and Requirements for Patient Safety

8.1 The Client as Resource

The focal point of any Consumer Health Informatics approach is the consumer or client. He has been called the least utilized resource in terms of efficient health services. He may, however, as well be the least reliable and the most fragile or vulnerable part of the system because he is a severely ill patient or emotionally stressed through the disease and acts in an environment that may hold additional noxious stressors [2], not to speak of actual limitations in rational decision making caused by the disease process itself. In any case, knowing your client is as key a factor here as it is in any other service. Therefore, next to medical and quality of life outcomes safeguarding of risks and adverse events must be among the criteria that deserve paramount attention within Consumer Health Informatics .

To illustrate and underline this latter claim we will contrast two ways of managing a case. Let us consider a responsible family physician and a patient he knows. In a new visit the patient complains being short of breath. The doctor confirms the complaint and stages the shortness of breath as moderate to medium. The doctor notices that the patient is more overweight than before. He senses recent alcohol consumption and some depressive mood, and he knows that the patient lives in a problematic family situation.

He will start with the routine of a physical examination (blood pressure, auscultation, lung function, ECG). In case of no findings he will turn his attention towards the weight increase, to the family situation and behaviors and emotions. He may be sending the patient home without any medication and encourage a follow up visit if symptoms persist. He may – reluctantly if at all – prescribe a bronchodilatating aerosol because he knows that the shortness of breath is the excuse to see the doctor but not the most pressing problem and that the easily sold bronchodilatating aerosol may not be the best cure but – knowing his patient's other circumstances of life – may rather put the patient's heart at risk. He will certainly not prescribe an aerosol refill without thorough investigation of the causes of the shortness of breath.

Let us in contrast consider a competitive sales oriented online pharmacy that mails prescription drugs without requesting a valid prescription from the client and generally establishes very low barriers for the patient to get his order approved. They will likely ask for immediate contraindications such as known allergic reactions against the broncho-dilatating substance but rely on the patient to know and to report accurately. They will request that the client clears them of any liability for damage incurred. They will unlikely notice, let alone follow up upon, all the other personal and behavioral risks. Easy to imagine that they neglect cardiovascular risks and ship cortisone or ephedrine and advertise discounts for larger packages. Some have "99% approval guarantee" (cf. Sect. 5.2.4 and [15]).

8.2 High Stakes and High Demands

Regarding the difference between the potential of services offered responsibly and the risk of services being offered irresponsibly we will formulate high demands on service design to protect the client. We maintain that the client be regarded and respected as an agent rather than as a target of providers' actions. Services should nevertheless be governed through legal maximes of medicine rather than from trade in general. Concretely the noli nocere maxim outlined in Sect. 17.11.5 should hold throughout rather than the caveat emptor maxim, cf. Sect. 17.7.1.

This demand must the more be made the more clients on the web or mobile web face long disclaimers where they are required to accept that the service provider waves liability for all kinds of negative consequences of using the service. In Sects. 17.4 and 17.6 we analyze the legality of such disclaimers. Here we address the farther ranging responsibility of providers of Consumer Health Informatics services. Since Masys [12] used the term "information toxicity" we are aware of the fact that bad results brought to a patient's knowledge unfiltered may cause harm. Consumer Health Informatics service providers should, therefore, either be sufficiently secure that their clients are mentally capable of receiving bad news without decompensating or they must redirect "bad news" towards a person-to-person setting. In the first place this is a matter of ethics: not to cause harm is a maxime of any medical service since the times of Hippocrates. Apart from the ethical obligation to apply the best conceivable measure to prevent harm, it also is a matter of credibility of the whole field of Consumer Health Informatics. Once it becomes publicly known that such services cause a considerable share of harmful outcomes the whole field of Consumer Health Informatics is at stake (see also Sect. 11.4).

For the sake of argument we take a very ambitious, demanding position concerning the comprehensiveness of assessing the client of a Consumer Health Informatics service. The ambition is to make Consumer Health Informatics services as personalized and as safe as they would be if offered through a family physician who involves specialists upon need. We should be aware that these ambitions will not be met under all circumstances. Nevertheless should they guide our efforts.

The ambitions will come as several sections and a table of desirable data and information that warrant the most comprehensive assessment and the most appropriate management of a case (cf. Table 8.1). Depending on the medical problem assessment can mean diagnosis but also need for screening and prevention. Management can mean therapy but also to do nothing – when an apparent excess risk is so marginal that follow up is not recommended.

> **Take Home**
> Responsible Consumer Health Informatics combines best active involvement of the client with utmost attention to potential threats and limitations to the client's capability to cooperate.
> Like a responsible family physician and unlike a sales driven enterprise does responsible Consumer Health Informatics strive at exploring each client's opportunities and risks before engaging in the management of the client's problem.
> Responsible Consumer Health Informatics's sophistication lies in actual prevention of harm rather than in waiving accountability for the consequences of harm.
> Responsible Consumer Health Informatics in its full consequences is not a final state that can be reached but an everlasting goal.

8.3 Outline of the Assessment Scheme

The assessment scheme that guides the structure of the following sections is organized as follows: We introduce mayor dimensions such as cognition. A mayor dimension typically has several sub dimensions such as health literacy, medical knowledge, etc. Every sub dimension is introduced through its name and an explanation about its purpose, and through which resource or method to capture an individual's state along the sub dimension. The distinction we are making between resource and method is not always crystal clear. Generally we will speak of a method when it requests cooperation through the client, e.g. filling a questionnaire. We will speak of a resource if it a material tool (flow-meter, ...) or an existing data collection that can now be used for this purpose, e.g. and ER or PHR or a social network trace. As an Example for the sub-dimension "Functional health literacy", often just "Health literacy" of the dimension "Cognition" high school levels from 1 to 12 and college and university degrees appear as a natural choices but will below be shown to be noisy and not valid. Clear cut as this and other dimensions may appear first, finding out a client's actual value may be very intricate and will be treated below.

The assessment of the person on the one hand is not so broad as personality psychology. It excludes aspects such as developmental psychology, psychoanalysis, heritability versus environmental coining and many others. We rather concentrate on

Table 8.1 Dimensions of client assessment. Column "Reference" points to text pages with further details

Dimension / Sub-dimension	Purpose	Resource/method	Comment	Reference
Medical risk				
Medical state	Appropriate clinical management	Client narrative /NLP	Not feasible	
		Forms, scales	Risk to overlook	163, 257
		Images, signals		163, 255
Medical history		Electronic record	Various types, ownership	255, 259 281
		Client memory	Limited validity	
Genetic risk		Client memory	Limited validity	259
		Family tree	Temptation to over-utilize	71, 261
		Gene, marker scan		
Exposure, physical/social	Context-aware management	Forms, scales	Risk to overlook	165, 166
		Social network traces	Ethical concern	
Personality				
Emotions	Personally appropriate management	Social network traces	Ethical concern	
Mental health				
Attitudes, values				
Emotions		Psychometric instruments	Co-"morbidity"	264
Mental health				265
Attitudes, values		Sophisticated consent forms	Risk of fraud	266
Culture, religion			No general method	170
Physical impairment	Ability-aware management	Checklist		171
Cognition				257
Literacy	Discreet client-provider communication	Curricular level	Low validity	176, 177, 266
Health literacy		Tests	Culture dependent	176, 176, 178
Digital literacy		Self-assessment		180
eHealth literacy		Self-assessment	Low validity	73, 179
Medical knowledge	Meeting client expectations		No general method	182
Identity, authentication				
	Secure client-provider communication	Physical token	Inconvenience	184
		Electronic signature		184
		Biometric identifier	Privacy concern	185

8.3 Outline of the Assessment Scheme

present traits that are pertinent to handling health-related information and instruction and to performing requested activities. Such traits include knowledge, attitudes and preferences. Such may originate from a religious or alike background and hence knowing the latter may be instrumental to assessing clients. On the other hand it is not confined to personality traits: it includes such mundane facts as authentication, legal guardianship to cover situations of childhood vaccinations, nursing care for elderly etc., medical insurance or other payment information, existence of a medical history, etc.

Before going into the depth of the dimensions we will further outline the use for the assessment dimension cognition and at the same time demonstrate that even dimensions that appear very straightforward may offer challenges to actually determine a client's state. The sub-dimensions of cognition include general comprehension capabilities, specific medical knowledge about the approach of the planned service but also computer, cell phone etc. handling skills.

Assuming we had a general education sub dimension of the dimension cognition and seek for methods or resources to determine its state for a prospective Consumer Health Informatics client, knowing that subsequently the service relies on the accuracy of this probing and may be missing the client if the state was not assessed appropriately. Concerning education level, years spent in school and degrees awarded may appear as the indicator of choice. However, graduating from a public high school in an under-served industrial suburb differs widely from graduating from a private school in an academic town. Actually, a survey 20 years ago demonstrated that 25 % of those achieving the lowest of five levels in a literacy test were high school graduates [8]. Furthermore, the college degree that a now 62-year-old client received 40 years ago may be totally over-, but also underestimating his present cognitive abilities. Therefore, asking the individual for the highest degree received on the one hand is simple and easy to perform but on the other hand may deliver very noisy results. We will have to look at more specific and at the same time narrower assessments and to relate their expected accuracies to necessary client and provider efforts. After all, such assessment may become a necessary prerequisite before contracting with a client.

The whole assessment scheme is broad, but meant as open-ended. It is a large set of dimensions and sub dimensions that became apparent from analyzing a variety of Consumer Health Informatics services. For any individual service only a subset is actually required. Some present or future services may require other dimensions or sub dimensions that are not covered here. Therefore, the assessment scheme presented here should be regarded as a checklist from which to pick required dimensions but also as a mental tool to look out for more dimensions that a newly planned service may have to cover.

In agreement with the general outline and emphasis of the book we address one necessary dimension only marginally: the client's information and communication technology environment and equipment. The scheme should include such simple-looking distinctions whether the client has DSL-Internet access or still needs a dial-up-connection first, using a telephone line and hence cannot place a hotline call at the same time. For other services cell phone network access must be guaranteed for persons whose cardiac arrhythmias are to be diagnosed from the distance. Being connected of course is a necessary requirement for most services introduced in this volume to work. It is, however, too wide a field to allow in-depth treatment here.

We establish all these ambitions because the long-term goal is that services conveyed in-person today can be replaced through services fully conveyed through the distance with the client playing an active part, i.e. Level 2 services.[1] It goes without saying that this cannot be achieved for every condition with every client under all circumstances. Unsatisfiable requirements will become apparent as we keep going. Therefore, another purpose of the ambitious list that will follow is to identify situations that will necessarily have to fall back to Level 1 with a face-to-face component.

Causes for unsatisfactory probing and assessment may be factual but also legal or ethical. Concretely, can we take correct answers to medically complex questions or questions about the distant past or to direct questions about embarrassing facts such as problematic alcohol consumption for granted? Would it help to search a client's social network personas, e-mail-correspondence or chat, tweet etc. appearance of prospective clients for respective cues? Would that be legal or should it be legalized in the best interest of the client, as further outlined in Sect. 17.11?

There are no easy answers. But in this chapter we will at least try to ask necessary questions. In a later Chap. 12, when more concrete examples of Consumer Health Informatics services have been analyzed we will present a few sophisticated resources or methods that have already been used in contexts of concrete Consumer Health Informatics services and will point to others that suggest themselves for future use.

> **Take Home**
> Responsible assessment of a citizen's potential and limitations to cooperate as a client of a Consumer Health Informatics service addresses various dimensions of the person and his context of living. Not all apparently appropriate methods and resources deliver trustworthy client assessments.
>
> The included assembly of dimensions and methods is meant as an open ended mental tool for planned Consumer Health Informatics services: Dimensions included here may or may not be pertinent and others may be required.

---

[1] Level 0 and Level 3 need not be considered here according to their different role assignments. Level 1 services preserve the initializing face-to-face encounter and its opportunities to assess all kinds of limitations of a patient. For more details on the distinction between the levels cf. Sect. 1.8.1 and Chaps. 3, 4, 5, and 6.

8.4 Overview of Assessment Dimensions

8.4.1 Medical Risk

The by far most important dimension is the client's medical risk. It comprises present complaints and respective diseases, including co-morbidities, but also his medical history and enabling factors such as familial or genetic dispositions or environmental exposures. Mental problems or psychiatric diseases could also be handled here but will rather be addressed in the "Personality" section (see Sect. 8.4.2).

8.4.1.1 Medical State

The client's present medical state is the immediate target of personalized advice and treatment. The better we know his core problem and vulnerabilities the more targeted the advice. His presumably preferred way to communicate complaints and observations comprehensively through natural language narrative – written or spoken – is mostly not feasible presently due to limitations of automated NLP. We have seen in Chap. 3 how badly search engines fail as reliable and reproducible providers of matching information when clients use decontextualized chunks of natural language in search for their health concerns. We therefore concentrate on structured and automated probing methods.

8.4.1.1.1 Form Filling and Numeric Scales

The client can check-mark symptoms in online forms, identify affected body parts through pointing to torso images, record severity or duration of problems on Likert or visual analogue scales etc. This allows apparently precise and unambiguous communication of the present state mapped to values of variables that the Consumer Health Informatics service makes use of. Examples are in Sect. 4.5.2 for COPD and in Sect. 4.4.2 for chronic pain. Limitations of such structured probing concern biased perception of symptom severity (cf. Sect. 12.2.1.1) or data entry errors due to all kinds of usability flaws of the forms, images or scales.

8.4.1.1.2 Images

Digital photography images and videos from laptop and more so tablets and smart phone cameras have reached a market penetration that for many Consumer Health Informatics clients they are a fact of life. For diseases that show through signs visible at the body surface photographs or video recordings can be transmitted to Consumer Health Informatics service providers that specialize in automatic image processing and classification leading to a diagnosis or staging of a condition, cf. `Skinvision` in Sect. 5.3.4.5.

8.4.1.1.3 Physical Signals

Some instruments such as blood pressure cuffs, cell phone heart sound recorders, blood glucose or airflow meters have gradually moved from the medical to the well being and lifestyle sector. Although presently the latter are not typically purchased by consumers spontaneously but prescribed by physicians they might also be used at places such as pharmacies. If applied correctly they deliver a sound account of a vital sign which may precisely capture an important aspect of a client's conditions.

8.4.1.2 Medical History

Next to the present medical state the history of the present problem and the presence and history of other problems plays a prominent role in correctly assessing the situation and evaluating management options.

8.4.1.2.1 General Purpose Electronic Record

In the favorable situation of the existence and accessibility of a longitudinal all encompassing Electronic Record (ER) in one of the forms described in Sects. 4.3.3 and 4.5, and further outlined in Chap. 14 it undoubtedly is the best resource as such. Presently comprehensive ERs still are an emerging and promising asset for the field of Consumer Health Informatics. Their context aware use as outlined in Sect. 14.3 has to develop in parallel to the deployment of the technology. It should, however be noted that the perspective taken in other places in this volume is client *participation*, while here it is client *assessment* or *surveillance*.

8.4.1.2.2 Service Specific Partial Electronic Records

Consumer Health Informatics services designed for prolonged health management in general or for chronic conditions may benefit from hosting a longitudinal record themselves. Examples are DrEd (http://www.dred.com) in Sect. 5.2.5.4 for a virtual provider that offers services for numerous diseases, the chronic pain management program in Sect. 4.4.2 and various chronic respiratory disease services discussed in Sect. 12.2.1.1. It should be noted that the quality of client provided data in a provider maintained record must be regarded in the light of limitations outlined in Sect. 8.4.1.1.

8.4.1.2.3 Client Memory

Past subjective complaints and findings can principally be queried from the client but all limitations in precision and reliability raised in Sect. 8.4.1.1.1 hold here as well, the more so the farther distant the past. Obviously reconstruction of past images and physical signals is not possible.

8.4.1.3 Genetic Risk

Only rarely does genetic disposition inevitably determine disease but it may influence likelihoods significantly. Knowing a genetic disposition may direct attention and focus such as to intensify screening or – in the case of onset – to apply more aggressive therapy. It may also stress the client and drive him into over-utilization of diagnostic or therapeutic services. Wisely used knowledge about inherited risk may, however, benefit the client through a personalized management of his risk or problem.

8.4.1.3.1 Personal Ancestry Forms and Family Trees

For prominently showing diseases such as myocardial infarction or breast cancer client memory is a reliable resource. Things differ for diseases that have varying etiologies, such as stroke or diabetes, or diseases that are conceived embarrassing or taboo such as prostate cancer. The precision that can be expected and examples of concrete family history of diseases online forms are outlined in Sect. 12.2.2. It should already be noted here that one fact affects the validity of familial risk information: The set of persons that the client spontaneously envisions as kin are not necessarily biological family. In law, out of wedlock, adoptive, foster or other relations may blur on his mind with biological family, the more so the larger or the more dispersed the family and the farther distant past ancestry.

8.4.1.3.2 Gene and Gene Expression Scan

A full gene scan is now possible. A continuously increasing number of SNPs is discovered. Micro-arrays can show the expression of selected genes or the concentration of other biologically active substances. Procedures to deliver huge amounts of highly accurate data are gaining ground. As outlined in other places (e.g. Sects. 3.3.2 and 9.4.2) interpretation of the data and management of the consequences of positive findings are equally pressing problems.

8.4.1.4 Physical Exposure

Physical exposure shows in various forms. It can be body posture at work ranging from typical white collar static office work to heavy load nursing or construction work. It can be exposure to UV radiation, workplace or home environment exposure to allergens, dusts, toxic substances, etc. Such exposures play a role in management of back pain, skin cancer screening etc. In a face-to-face encounter a family physician has a fair chance to notice consequences of some exposure or to infer related risks from demographic data and ask follow up questions.

8.4.1.4.1 Form Filling

Client narrative as primary data faces equal limitations as it does for the medical state. Online forms for types of exposure are principally appropriate but they may get rather large because exposures can be manifold. Online forms may be developed to unfold personalized shorter versions where sub-domains are skipped when entry questions have been negated and are presented at increasing depth as long as questions are affirmed. However, exposure can be so subtle and go unnoticed that the client does not even know. An infamous present example is the exposure to radioactive radiation in the consequence of nuclear power plant disasters the spread of which nobody can tell for sure. Together, both the client's limited willingness to work through long lists most of which does not apply for himself and the limited validity of client provided data, mainly the limited validity of negative answers, limit the whole endeavor of capturing physical exposure. The family physician might have an inspiration....

8.4.1.4.2 Social Network Traces

Harvesting hints to exposures from the client's profile in online sites is a dim future hope which would, however, require legal and ethical consent to a respective breach of privacy, the different flavors of which are addressed in Sect. 4.3.2.

8.4.1.5 Social Exposure

Much like physical, social exposure has various facets and narratives for automatic identification are not feasible. Exposure can be an individual life story with losses, violence suffered, etc. present familial, financial, workplace situation. It may coincide with being part of an under-served community such as ethnic minority. A family physician – if the socially exposed client has the opportunity to see one – would have a fair chance to identify cues and follow up. Confirmed exposures influence treatment decisions.

8.4.1.5.1 Form Filling

Basically the situation resembles the physical exposure one. But some social exposures are more conscious than subtle physical ones. Depending on their personality clients may appreciate the apparently anonymous nature of an online form to communicate embarrassing social exposures which they tend to conceal in face-to-face visits.

8.4 Overview of Assessment Dimensions

8.4.1.5.2 Social Network Traces

Here as well analogies with physical exposures hold. However, some social networks have formal "switches" for indicators of social states. If e.g. a client's relational state changes from married to divorced health related consequences must be considered.

To summarize, much more information turns out as desirable than can be determined with sufficient accuracy and reliability. This remains a weakness of Consumer Health Informatics that will only gradually be cured when text and data mining methods gain power. Chapter 6 demonstrates that at the population level automatic methods generate new health insights. At the individual level Karmen and coworkers demonstrate preliminary insights into using client posts for depression staging (cf. [7]).

Take Home

The client's medical symptoms, symptom history, and excess inherited or contextual risks are necessary core data for responsible ConsHI.

All generally feasible types of resources

- online forms and scales
- imagery
- physical signals/vitals
- gene or tumor marker scans

should be considered and their advantages and disadvantages weighed.

Access to the medical history and genetic or environmental exposures is often hampered through limitation and imprecision of the client's memories. Inasmuch as available general of service specific electronic records should be used or built.

Client traces in social networks as a resource to reveal contextual risks or risk prone behaviors promise authenticity but raise strong privacy concerns.

8.4.2 Personality

All sub-dimensions of the dimension "Medical risk" describe aspects of the client's health as such, assuming to be clearly communicated and equally meant by client and Consumer Health Informatics service provider. If it were about communication between information processing machines we would call it semantic interoperability. One of the communicators, however, is a human being endowed with a personality that adds beliefs and preferences, but also limitations to the equation. These are not medical by themselves but influence the behavior as a Consumer Health Informatics client. Immediately obvious example that we will return to are cognitive limitations – he simply does not understand – or convictions – he simply rejects an intervention such as a vaccination.

8.4.2.1 Emotional Stability

By emotional stability we mean that a person can pursue reasonably sized plans and endure some extent of delay, adversity and frightening information without decomposing. To abandon a weight reduction program if a weight loss does not show on the first day or suicidal ideations when receiving a pathological lab finding are examples of doubtful emotional stability. Both examples demonstrate that absence of emotional stability is a neighbor to mild psychiatric diseases: depression could be the cause for both behaviors. For various reasons, however, we will distinguish emotional stability from mental healthiness. Among the reasons is that methods to determine the two differ and that mental diseases can themselves be the target of Consumer Health Informatics services.

The family physician would know and take the degree of emotional stability into account when enrolling patients into long running therapies or when clearing their access to their lab data in an ER. Enacting similar precautions online is desirable for Consumer Health Informatics services.

8.4.2.1.1 Personality Inventories

The human personality has been the target of research, mainly in psychology, for long. Competing models of personality exist and questionnaires have been developed to substantiate the models and to classify subjects. In Sect. 12.3 models and questionnaires will be analyzed whether they can stage individuals' capabilities to play their assigned roles as clients of a Consumer Health Informatics service.

The use of social network profile traces may play a future role here as well but less than for social exposure because personality is too much woven into a person's fabric to show through profile "switches" discussed above.

8.4.2.2 Mental Healthiness

Mental health resp. mental conditions come in a double role. In one role they are the diseases for which help is sought from dedicated Consumer Health Informatics services for this disease. In the second role they are potential modifiers of behavior of a person who seeks a Consumer Health Informatics service for another primary disease and where the modifier needs to be known to warrant or exclude Consumer Health Informatics treatment for the primary disease. Typical combinations are depression as potential behavior modifier in treatment of anxiety (Sect. 5.2.2.3), diabetes mellitus 2 (Sect. 9.8) etc. In Sect. 9.4.1.2 we see that a lack of self affirmation leads to irrational decision making re glucose testing.

8.4.2.2.1 Psychometric Instruments and Social Network Traces

Much alike personality inventories structured instruments to be filled by the client exist in large numbers and their psychometric properties have been analyzed. Many date back to the times of paper and pencil in the psychiatrist's office and few have been validated for home computer, cf. Sect. 5.2.2.3. But they exist at least as valuable assets to start with. Calibrations may have to be redone for online versions.

These as well as social network traces are a future option. Compared to the personality sub-dimension monitoring traces for signs of psychiatric diseases has a better starting point. It can draw upon the vocabulary that questionnaires use to characterize the facets of the disease and spot the traces of respective words and their synonyms in a trace. A first indication that this can be brought to bear is [7].

8.4.2.3 Attitudes

Resistance towards and distrust of methods of scientific medicine are an undercurrent of prevention, diagnosis, and treatment of diseases. Such an attitude may develop individually or, as discussed in the next section, through habits and group pressure of cultural or religious communities. In either case, persons who refuse treatment the effectiveness of which is scientifically proven risk their health and their life. Ethically they claim the principle of autonomy for themselves to outweigh other principles (cf. Sect. 17.11). But still providers of Consumer Health Informatics services should be aware of resistance and distrust. A situation where the client silently declines a therapy while the logs of the provider show that the client cooperates is difficult to judge legally and morally. Regarding Sect. 17.5 the provider may be legally cleared by claiming that the "encounter ... (closed with) foreseeable reliance by the patient". In case of a negative outcome the provider may nevertheless be held morally accountable and face respective inquiry. This is extremely important when parents or other legal guardians decline on behalf of their entrusted minors or adult wards, cf. Sect. 8.4.4.

The family physician would know or notice, at least when we are dealing with an outspoken minority whose members would rather boast themselves than trying to conceal their conviction. That does not mean that the family physician can generally change attitudes. But he can at least search for alternative management of the patient's problem or convey utmost clarity about incurred risk. In contrasts to a Level 2 Consumer Health Informatics service a responsible physician can also assume the role of an advocate for a minor and apply for the guardianship to be withdrawn from those who deny a necessary treatment.

8.4.2.3.1 Sophisticated Informed Consent Forms

Informed consent is required in whatsoever Consumer Health Informatics service that goes beyond plain well-being logistics such as sports studio or healthy recipe recommendation. Informed consent can be requested through straightforward binary yes/no check mark, with "no" terminating the transaction. It can be a sophisticated walk through the steps of a decision making process which borrows from Shared Decision Making methodology, cf. [4]. It may be wishful thinking, though, that such an attempt can successfully untangle client fancies about the hostile nature of scientific medicine.

8.4.2.3.2 Online Behavior Pattern

The most outspoken among the prospective clients who end up declining an offered Consumer Health Informatics service may stand out in actively contributing to anti medicine online activities such as forums or blogs. If clients use true names or identities which can be matched across their diverse online activities clear cues are there to follow up upon active participation.

8.4.2.4 Cultural or Religious Background

Religious or cultural convictions or regulations issued by leaders of respective communities request members to decline certain services irrespective whether offered face-to-face or as Consumer Health Informatics service. This phenomenon is not confined to strange minorities. The reader may think of the world wide influence of the Roman Catholic Church and its impact on the abstinence from contraception.

If membership in a community can be found out it gives reason to follow up when a diagnostic or therapeutic strategy is considered that is banned in that community. In some countries membership with a church is part of demographic data (e.g. Germany) while in others it has to be thoroughly concealed to avoid prosecution (such as being Christian in some regions under siege of Islamic terror groups). Therefore, there are no universal approaches.

8.4.2.5 Physical Impairment

By physical impairment we mean all kinds of inborn or disease related restriction of performing bodily functions that most humans can perform and do not even think about it. Visual impairment can make it impossible for an asthma patient to read flow-meter data. Hard of hearing persons will not hear alarms and extremely left handed persons cannot manage devices designed for right handed use.

Impairments can often be seen in relation to characteristics of a home environment of living. A visually impaired client living together with a trusted caring spouse can have him do flow-meter readings for her. Conversely, a client with moderate restrictions in mobility, who lives alone in a remote place, will not be able to go buy pharmaceuticals and respective fall-backs have to be set up.

8.4.2.5.1 Online Checklists

Since the impairments are very well known to the prospective clients and they can well judge their limitations the responsibility is mainly with service providers. In designing a service they have the obligation to analyze, maybe simulate, all activities later expected to be taken over by the client, what kind of physical impairment would preclude a person from playing his role. When this is done properly and foresightfully most obstacles can be checked in structured online forms in the phase of enrollment.

Take Home

For a client to cooperate effectively with a Consumer Health Informatics service provider he must be fully sane, free in his decisions and physically capable of the acts that are his part.

Physical impairments may be faithfully detected through sophisticated online checklist.

For limitations residing in the person alone psychometric instruments may help. Social network traces may become of great help, if legally cleared.

Adverse attitudes imposed through or inbred with cultural or religious (pressure) groups maybe very obvious or very hard to identify.

8.4.3 Cognition

Most dimensions above are somewhat diffuse and hard to get one's hands around. Yet they are important because it is by far not warranted that a client contributes his part for a Consumer Health Informatics service to achieve its aim. The dimensions of cognition as such are as wide as the dimensions of personality but society has developed and widely uses procedures and scores to stage a person's cognitive reach and to analyze the difficulty of material for comprehension by humans of different educational levels. Although there is evidence that seekers of health information on the Internet follow advice without understanding its rationale (cf. Sect. 3.2.2) comprehension of conveyed information certainly is a factor that fosters success of a therapy. While the family physician may use his authority and trusted relation to establish treatment adherence even in the absence of comprehension, it certainly helps in Consumer Health Informatics if material presented to the client and his cognitive capabilities match.

Structurally the match between properties of material provided and capabilities requested of the clients can start from both ends. Material can be delivered as is and client enrollment can happen under the premise that the client proves his understanding of the material. Or client capabilities can be checked and the material adapted accordingly. By material we mean all the variety of text to read, probabilities to interpret, devices to handle, etc. A core element of adapting material to the user's capacities is adjusting text readability.

8.4.3.1 Text Readability

Empirical text readability research dates back to the 1920s. Very roughly, readability formulas are weighted sums of measurable properties of a text such as average number of words in a sentence, average number of syllables in a word, number of "hard" words where hard means known to a certain small percentage of the population only etc. Score values are then calibrated against empirically determined reading comprehension capabilities at different high school levels (or beyond) e.g. sixth grade. DuBay [5], available at http://www.impact-information.com/impactinfo/readability02.pdf provides a clear account of the history, methods, importance and impact. A stunning example comes from injury prevention: In articles in the journal *Pediatrics* it is shown that numerous child casualties in car accidents are owed to insufficient readability of the instructions for use of child-safety seats. The average reading level in the cited instructions was 10th grade – too hard for 80 % of the adult readers.

Readability scores exist for several languages. Among the most widely used for English are the Flesch Reading Ease, the Flesch-Kincade Grade Level and the Gunning fog formula. The child-safety seat example already hints to the importance of readability in medicine and even more so in Consumer Health Informatics because inasmuch as written instructions play a role insufficient comprehension on the part of the reader is a risk in its own right. Consequently public health officers recommend 6th grade high school reading level for all patient directed medical contents (cf. [5]).

Readability of medical text poses extra challenges. Medical information mostly needs numerals like in dosage instructions or likelihoods; reader numeracy is, therefore, challenged as well and authors and service providers must find easy to comprehend ways to convey the meaning and implications of numbers. Furthermore medical language is full of long "hard" specialty language terms which serve their purpose in communication between specialist but exclude lay persons (cf. Sect. 4.3.3). Therefore, many reading levels have to be bridged to reach the majority of readers.

Moderately good news is that the reading level of a given text can be automatically calculated through medium level complexity algorithms of Natural Language

Processing (NLP) named in Sect. 8.4.3.1 which mainly need lexicons and morphological analysis including rules for words of Latin or Greek origin. Texts can be continually adapted manually until they reach a criterion. They can even be delivered in different variants including more compact ones for advanced readers. Patients who have long suffered from chronic disease and have already gathered profound knowledge of both the condition itself and the sub-specialty terminology may prefer such compact concise information which by far exceeds their general text comprehension level. They do not want to be bothered more than absolutely necessary, as becomes evident in several investigations with diabetics, cf. Sect. 9.6.

8.4.3.2 Functional Health Literacy

8.4.3.2.1 Basic Definitions

Functional health literacy, or health literacy for short, has been defined as "the degree to which individuals have the capacity to obtain, process, and understand basic health information and services needed to make appropriate health decisions", as [9, p. 475] cites from an IOM publication.

The specification "functional" denotes the capability to not just marginally understand information acquired but "to use and interpret text, documents, and numbers effectively" [18, p. 514] and to bring them in concordance with one's intentions and make respective medical decisions. The use of numbers in medical contexts (quantities, dosages, ...) is also called medical numeracy but to the most part both concepts are regarded as intertwined in their enabling role for making informed decisions.

Although the NLM has not added Health Literacy as a MeSH-keyword until 2010, health literacy has since long been discussed as a modifier of compliance. Reduced or absent health literacy is a risk factor for worse outcomes (see various sources cited in [17]).

Health literacy necessarily builds on general literacy. Estimates from the US National Adult Literacy Survey suggest that 40–44 million of the US adult population are functionally illiterate, another 50 million have only marginal literacy skills. Taken together, Consumer Health Informatics service providers have to be aware that nearly one third of the adult Americans are at risk to not understand the information provided. In Sect. 1.9.2 we address the specific needs when presumably illiterate or marginally literate sub-populations are the dedicated target groups of a service. In this chapter here we pursue what can be done when the target group is a random sample from the general population and a provider tries to tell the literate apart from the illiterate.

8.4.3.2.2 Epistemic Foundation

Assignment of meaning to information draws on capabilities at all levels of the mind. It goes beyond the semiotic triangle of Ogden and Richards (1923) cf. [14] for the most recent facsimile edition.[2]

As a prerequisite before entering the semiotic analysis we must claim that a person commands the lower level cultural technique of mapping visual input of atomic signs to units according to the conventions of notation in a cultural environment. More plainly speaking: he knows letters and composes them into words. Most westerners do not command this technique for Chinese writing. They are illiterate in this very basic sense.

For a person who is capable of aligning signs to words in visual input material we can use Ogden's and Richard's distinction: Words – or more generally in semiotics: symbols – stand for entities in the world – physical such as a scalpel or all kinds of other such as anesthesia. Semiotics contends that this relation objectively holds between a symbol and an entity or does not hold, although there is no procedure to determine which of the two is the case. This relation serves as a foundation which exists irrespective of a person under consideration. In the person, however, the symbol evokes a thought, imagination, etc. i.e. causes a change in mindset – and be it: "sorry, no idea" which may actually be better than the wrong idea. Thoughts, imaginations on the person's mind – unless they are pure fantasy – are grounded in entities in the world. This grounding is or is not adequate: What the person envisions holds or does not hold for the entity in the world.

For a person to benefit from written material conveyed in Consumer Health Informatics services he must, therefore, assign an imagination to symbols and the imagination must not be totally of the mark. Using *surgery* for illustration: the person must

- compose s u r g e r y into the English word surgery,
- which must evoke imaginations of sharp instruments incising tissues of living beings for the purpose of healing and
- which allows him to subsume observations of open surgeries under the symbol, to be in doubt with minimally invasive surgery but not to subsume vaccinations or autopsies.

The example allows to demonstrate farther reaching implications for full comprehension of written material. It goes without saying that when a client mistakes surgery for purgatory and evokes respective imaginations he is likely to associate religious eschatologic expectations rather than real life clinical procedures with what he reads. This is of course an extreme case but for those readers who do not

---

[2]The following arguments are not meant as a lesson on semiotics. They rather use very basic notions of semiotics for illustration. The coverage of the topic at http://en.wikipedia.org/wiki/Semiotic_triangle is sufficient to follow the arguments.

know the words purgatory[3] and eschatologic[4] it may feel realistic. In any case a Consumer Health Informatics client may be misguided through a false imagination. The example also demonstrates that this may be more likely in biographies in certain cultural or religious backgrounds. Structurally, it is a more intricate and risk prone form of illiteracy: the client believes he understands but he does not and will act rationally from his perspective which, however, is irrational under correct assignment of meaning in the semiotic triangle.

Even if we assume that the client has correct imaginations which appropriately subsume entities in the world, there may still be risk prone higher level gaps above the semiotic triangle. Using the surgery example again if a person does not know the concept of anesthesia and that it is routinely and successfully applied during surgeries he may be scared to death to give his consent to undergo even minor surgery.

This last example demonstrates that using imagery – be it naturalistic or iconic – rather than written text does not really help. If a client has no acquaintance with the entity surgery and the cultural habits of typical clothing of surgeons at work an image of one masked person cutting into the other certainly evokes misleading imaginations. And intuitively appealing imagery for anesthesia that works without appealing to culturally learnt knowledge is a challenge at best.

Some of this is cultural, some is common sense, some is school teaching. The German language has a word "Bildung" for all that and more while the English "education" falls short. The phenomenon, however, is the same: That which a client knows, at the bottom, within and above the semiotic triangle is the essence of a biography rather than the result of a circumscribed curriculum. That is why the subsequently presented methods to determine "Bildung" or "education" have hard times to cover what we would actually wish to know about the client to safely convey information and advice. The family physician would probably know ....

Take Home

Cognitive load imposed through a Consumer Health Informatics service and cognitive reach of a prospective client must be in accordance.

If the cognitive load is not within and cannot be adapted to the client's reach a service should not be offered.

Up to one third of the populations of countries such as the USA are thereby excluded from many Consumer Health Informatics services.

Understanding cognitive load and reach requires semiotics. Reading level formulas, curricular achievements and the likes fall short of a valid match.

---

[3] According to Roman Catholic teaching, the state or place of purification or temporary punishment ... suffering and torment ... source: Wikipedia.

[4] Eschatology = ... part of theology ... the study of ... final events, ... the ultimate destiny; source: Wikipedia.

8.4.3.2.3 Curriculum Based Staging

The apparently straightforward approach to stage a prospective client's comprehension of information conveyed as part of a Consumer Health Informatics service is to ask for curricular levels achieved, such as n-th grade highschool, graduation, BSc degree, etc. This may be appropriate in populations with equity in access to education and where education happens at equal quality, or to identify extreme groups of very limited and very wide knowledge. But in regard of extracurricular factors of "Bildung" pure curricular staging will be very hard to calibrate for the large intermediate range that benefits most from personalization. An empirical example for varying congruence between curricular staging and literacy on a simple medical task is provided in Sect. 8.4.3.2.6.

Various tests are in use to determine literacy irrespective of grades awarded. Their psychometric properties are promising. The question, therefore, is whether they can be used for the online assessment of literacy as an indicator for the required "Bildung" and hence as an enabler for the client to benefit from supplied information for his medical outcome.

8.4.3.2.4 REALM

The oldest and most widely quoted test REALM (Rapid Estimate of Adult Literacy in Medicine, available at http://adultmeducation.com/AssessmentTools_1.html) cannot be used. It uses correct pronunciation of six or more of the eight medical terms in the test as criterion. The criterion is judged by a trained human arbitrator. The arbitrator also acts as an moderator who determines the speed of moving to the next term when the subject hesitates too long and who is instructed to judge as "pass" when accent overlays a morphologically correct pronunciation and to judge genuine native American yet false pronunciations as "fail". Since these distinctions are so subtle and the variations of accent can be very wide voice recognition will take a while to validly and reliably replicate the human arbitrator and hence to make REALM usable for presentation online.

8.4.3.2.5 TOFHLA

The (Test of Functional Literacy in Adults) family of tests has also been in use since the mid 1990s. A short form S-TOFHLA (also STOFHLA) consists of four numeracy items and two prose passages.[5]

---

[5] Availability of REALM and TOFHLA versions can be found at http://www.rcmar.ucla.edu/rcmar_wiki/Literacy_S-TOFHLA.html

8.4 Overview of Assessment Dimensions

The literacy part consists of two texts with overall 36 Cloze items.[6] Text one is a readability 4th grade (Gunning fog) (cf. Sect. 8.4.3.1) preparation for an upper gastrointestinal X-ray examination and text two (10th grade Gunning fog) a rights and responsibilities in a Medicaid application instruction. Numeracy items are as elementary as determining the next time to take a tablet if you took one at 7 am and should take them every 6 hours.

Filling S-TOFHLA takes 7 min. Thresholds have been established to distinguish literacy classes inadequate (<54 % correct), marginal (54 % to <66 % correct) and adequate. According to [3] correlation between S-TOFHLA and REALM is good (Spearman rank correlation 0.8 for different classes of the tools). Data are, however, more scattered for the medium than for the extreme ranges. In Sect. 12.4 we see an example of a limited external validation.

8.4.3.2.6 NVS

NVS (Newest Vital Sign) is a more recent development of testing different aspects of utilizing health information in an integrated setting that has nothing to do with vital signs [18]. It rather presents a nutrition label with quantities, percentages, and other numerical information imbedded into instructions which themselves include medical ("cholesterol") and plain language ("amount") terms. The subject can process the six questions which each have a non mistakable correct answer in appr. 3 min (range 1.5–6.2 min) and can score between 0 and 6. NVS has been tested against the presumable gold standard long version of TOFHLA in English and Spanish. Less than 2 correct answers and less than 4 correct answers were both analyzed as to their discriminating power between adequate versus marginal or inadequate health literacy. Sensitivity resp. specificity in the English speaking cohort (55 male, 195 female) were 72 % resp. 87 % with cut off <2 and 100 % resp. 64 % with cutoff <4. In other words: with NVS <4 all presumably limited literacy clients would be identified, but one third (36 %) of those receiving the "limited/no literacy" tag actually are literate – always assuming that TOFHLA stages health literacy perfectly.

For the USA a strong point of NVS is that it exists in parallel English and Spanish versions which underwent the same investigation of psychometric properties. The Spanish speaking cohort (29 male, 221 female) results are not so clear cut, though. For the <4 cutoff sensitivity resp. specificity are 100 % – as above – resp. 19 %: 4 out of 5 tagged "limited/no literacy" are literate. The <2 cutoff errs differently: it only identifies 77 % of the presumable limited or inadequately literate subjects (specificity = 57 %). The proponents of NVS argue that the more blurred results

---

[6]A Cloze item is a one word gap in a text for which the subject has four alternative words from which to select the one that best matches the meaning of the text. In one such sentence "The doctor will send you to a _____ X-ray" the correct selection from 'stomach, diabetes, stitches, germs' is 'stomach'.

among the subjects choosing the Spanish version is due to the "greater heterogeneity of language and *culture (emphasis by the author)* among our Spanish-speaking patients" [18, p. 521]. This is in line with the considerations above that full functional literacy includes things that life rather than school teaches. It also means that equal opportunities for ethnic minorities requires more than high quality translation. For more on under-served sub-populations cf. Sect. 1.9.2.

Weiss and coworkers also asked the question whether plain demographic or curricular data come close to predicting health literacy equally well as NVS. Again, the English speaking cohort had clearer results and a clear advantage for NVS, with an area under the ROC-curve of 0.88 for NVS, compared to 0.72 for educational level (in years of formal training), and to 0.71 for age. In the English cohort the 95 % confidence interval of NVS does not overlap with those of formal training and age, while in the Spanish speaking one it does; mean values are 0.72 for NVS, 0.69 for education, and 0.64. It may be asked whether prospective Spanish clients of a Consumer Health Informatics service should not just be asked for their age and years in school.

In the investigation that provides the characteristics of NVS there were more female subjects and females scored better in both populations. This bears the risks of two biases. One is a gender selection bias; the subjects are not representative of the population. There is certainly some truth to this but we found in some other places that women are a majority in the health information seeking community anyway (Sects. 3.2.1 and 5.2.3.3). Therefore, the samples are less biased in their representing the health information seeking sub-population. The second is a familiarity bias. Scoring on a food label interpretation may favor those who read food labels more frequently. Could this be women? A recent publication by Stran and Krol [16] shows that indeed women use food labels significantly more frequently and more intensely than men.

On the other hand Weiss and coworkers mention one more advantage of NVS in terms of literacy understood broadly: Solving an NVS food label task on food allergies requires the classical literacy skill of reading, such as deciphering peanut oil, the semiotic skill of having the right imagination of the substance, plus common sense that who is allergic against peanuts is affected by peanut oil. Another task within NVS requires numeracy by knowing that number of servings and calories per serving have to be multiplied, and the basic arithmetics; plus orientation, namely to find the base figures which are scattered around the label. NVS therefore tries to cover *functional* health literacy: the "capacity to obtain, process, and understand basic health information".

8.4.3.2.7 Using REALM, TOFHLA, and NVS Outside the USA

Neither REALM nor TOFHLA are suitable for replication in other cultures through straightforward translation while NVS comes close.

REALM's challenge is to map orthography to pronunciation. This test is a true challenge in languages where the orthography to pronunciation mapping has lots of variations such as in English or French. In iconographic languages such as Chinese it draws on having explicitly learnt the icon and its meaning. In languages with highly regular orthography to pronunciation relation such as German or Spanish it is not a true challenge: a test subject has a fair chance to pass by applying heuristics of composing patterns of letters into sound (English anemia vs. Spanish la anemia, German Anämie). In the concrete case of the eight items of the "English" REALM Greek (e.g. jaundice) or Latin (constipation) roots have made it into common language while the respective German common language words are German rooted (Gelbsucht, Verstopfung), i.e. not a problem to pronounce correctly for a literate who has no idea of medicine.

The second S-TOFHLA literacy part on rights and responsibilities in a Medicaid application instruction tests a capacity of vital importance for US patients: make sure you get the treatment covered; do not mess the procedures. Since no other country has the same procedures and some countries have all-encompassing (derogatively called "socialized" by proponents of an autonomy centered organization of health care, cf. Sect. 17.11.4) coverage without any financial obligations imposed on the prospective patient national (S-)TOFHLA's need to be conceived from scratch.

The skills tested in NVS are required in similar ways in different cultures and different languages. Finding the key information, knowing which arithmetic is required, doing the arithmetic is not confined to English speaking individuals living in the USA. It should, however, be noted that food labels may not be so widely available and concretely used in other cultures. This lets expect that sensitivity and specificity are different for similar items, as we have already seen between English and Spanish native speakers and between men and women.

8.4.3.2.8 eHEALS

Another approach by Norman and Skinner [13] should also be briefly mentioned because it claims to measure health literacy in an electronic media context. eHEALS (eHealth Literacy Scale) is based on eight five-point Likert scale self assessments of the style "I know how to find helpful health resources on the internet". The final set of eight items emerged from a biometrically guided selection process that had started with a much larger seed of items prima-facie approved by eHealth specialists. The instrument achieved good internal consistency and test-retest reliability over month. eHEALS scores did, however, not correlate significantly with subjects' intensity of using the carrier technologies such as WWW, instant messages etc.

eHEALS may appear as the instrument of choice because it combines the test of media or digital literacy with the test of health literacy. However, the methods cast quite some doubt on this claim. First, all empirical "validation" was achieved with 664 9th through 11th grade presumably healthy students. Less representative for the health information seeking population can a sample hardly be. Second, rather than an external validation eHEALS presents a flavor of the opposite: the lack of correlation with use of the technology. In other words: eHEALS-scored literacy does not grow with media literacy. Third and most critical: In light of all the evidence from thousands of adults that establishes wide ranging insufficient self perception of health information seeking capacities (cf. Sects. 3.3.1.2, 3.3.1.5, or 3.4.2.1) self-assessment cannot be recommended as an approach to stage eHealth literacy.

> **Take Home**
> The validity of self assessed eHealth literacy is moderate, at best. Often named tests for health or eHealth literacy (REALM, TOFHLA, eHEALS) cannot be recommended for Consumer Health Informatics for lack of specific resources or insufficient validation. NVS (Newest Vital Sign) shows some promise of validity and international adaptability.

8.4.3.3 Digital Literacy

If determination of a prospective client's eHealth literacy is so insecure, how about the base level, media or digital literacy, alone? In a time when the term "digital native" is about to get rid of its quotation marks it may appear untimely to challenge whether persons in need of health information may get stuck with not navigating the Internet itself productively. Actually few recent scholarly publications address the topic alone but rather investigate the problem of access to information resources among under-served populations, as we briefly do in Sect. 1.9.2. But some of us were born before 1996[7] and may still be struggling and feel uncomfortable and disoriented. So it is worth to address at least briefly how to assess the capacity of getting around in digital space. Eszter Hargittai has published an investigation in 2005 that nicely relates actual capacity to navigate the web, as measured in her own small investigation, to existing self rating instruments taken from GSS (General Social Survey) [6].

A random sample of 100 citizens from a county in New Jersey came to a lab to work on eight distinct search tasks from various aspects of daily life (jobs, purchasing, local events, ...). Number of correctly performed searches – measured as applying one search strategy from a large portfolio of strategies identified in a preliminary investigation – and time required to finish were the two proxy variables to indicate internet literacy. Determining Hargittai's score takes ~10 min. It measures a mixture of search efforts towards and navigation within resources.

The number of correct searches (effectiveness) and time required (efficiency) correlate more or less with numerous items of the type "Do you know how to <some activity in a web browser>?" (yes/know); "How familiar are you with <some activity in a web browser>?" (5-point-Likert scale). Hargittai ends up suggesting a score

---

[7]The year when John Perry Barlow coined the terms "native" in versus "immigrants" to Cyberspace, cf. http://w2.eff.org/Censorship/Internet_censorship_bills/barlow_0296.declaration

combined of her objectively determined proxies and selected self assessed ratings to achieve a highly coherent (Cronbach's $\alpha = 0.89$) measure of internet literacy.

> **Take Home**
> In contrast to the widely poor self-assessment of eHealth literacy, a small study on self-assessment of digital literacy suggests good validity.

Search skills are a center stage capacity for prospective clients of Level 0 Consumer Health Informatics services. Testing how well Hargittai's Internet literacy correlates with the quality of found health related websites is a question of scientific interest. However, even if the answer were clearly positive it is hard to imagine how to implement the consequences: Who would legitimize and enforce that he who wants to search health information on the web first has to get a Hargittai type internet "driver license"?

Both, Hargittai's [6] and Norman's and Skinner's [13] investigations are a decade old and the penetration of every-day life with digital media has dramatically increased. Different results can be expected in the years 2015 and later. However, what has actually increased most is media, not so much spread of disease and lay persons' need of and familiarity with health related information. Therefore, Hargittai's results on web and digital literacy may hold more now than 10 years earlier as a predictor of media literacy but that does not transform into eHealth literacy. Actually, Hargittai's instrument does not include any medical item. Therefore, a need for assuring eHealth literacy persists.

Navigation within sites plays a role at all four levels of Consumer Health Informatics services and it can be essential. If a service offers all types of acoustic cues, graphical displays and handles for manipulation, maybe recording of acoustic or other signs a digitally illiterate client may miss the best and we need not wonder why a treatment has no effect for him. For assuring those aspects of digital literacy required for a service specific tests and instructions are probably more effective. It goes without saying that basic principles of Human-Computer-Interaction should be respected. Hands on training – actual hands in the face-to-face initiation of a Level 1 service or "virtual hands" in terms of well made tutorials[8] – as intro into a Level 2 service should make sure that a client has at least seen everything he is supposed to use subsequently. For mission critical navigations or manipulations keystroke/mouse-click logging may be warranted as part of a provider's responsibility to assure that the treatment reaches the client. Kaye and coworkers [10] show for a different medical purpose how basic logging of users' handling patterns can be used diagnostically, to detect incoherent activities.

---

[8]The tutorials provided by the NLM at http://www.nlm.nih.gov/bsd/disted/pubmed.html to teach PubMed search are a very positive example, at least for users with medium or better health literacy.

8.4.3.4 Medical Knowledge

Although systematic investigations do not seem to exist physicians report that patients who manage a chronic disease over extended periods of time gather a fair amount of pertinent knowledge, be it names of pharmaceuticals, their active agents and their therapeutic targets, treatment side effects etc. including the specialty language. This goes beyond the sharing of valuable behavioral experiences outlined in Chap. 6. Examples are patients with renal insufficiency and failure including those having received a kidney transplant, rare metabolic diseases, etc. For those patients having achieved this nearly specialist state, we kind of have a reverse health literacy problem: They are willing and capable to digest information at or near physician specialist level. Being dumped with basic simplified or lengthy material will bore them. The question is whether the (knowledgeable) provider – (ignorant) client role distinction that mostly underlies Consumer Health Informatics makes any sense here or whether it should give way to an at par communication between provider and client that does not need pre-designed flows of initiative and information but rather high level sharing of up to date knowledge and current comprehensive data.

8.4.3.4.1 Disease Specific Literacy Check

For a prospective client to reach near specialist level command of the specialty language is a must. Therefore, condition specific functional tests of word meaning assignment should work to identify knowledgeable individuals. Here functional means to not only ask for the meaning of terms in lay language but what discriminatory power a symptom has, the value range of a pertinent lab or the difference between the targets of two pharmaceuticals. Consumer Health Informatics services for "patient specialists" presently are a niche where, however, high level client expectations can be met. DASH for Health (cf. Sect. 9.4.2.3) has one such service element: having started with one behavioral article per week posted for their clients [11] they responded to client requests for a second more basic scientific article on another day of the week. The regular pattern and high quality of the reading material has been and still is in the 14th year of the existence of DASH for Health an attractor for the whole service (Tom Moore, personal communication November 2014).

> **Take Home**
> Patients who have long been living with a chronic disease may have collected knowledge at near expert level and respective expectations towards a Consumer Health Informatics service provider.
> Testing client level of expertise includes, but is not limited to specialty language terms.

8.4.4 Identity and Authentication

8.4.4.1 Need for Secure Verification of Identity and Authorization

Finally we want to safeguard the whereabouts of a client as a human identity. Unless more sophisticated authentication of provider and client identities is set up the only identifying information – if any – that a Level 2 Consumer Health Informatics service provider sees of a client is the log-in ID while the client only sees a URI or app name and with some luck finds a legal notice. A fully virtual persona in a second life like scenario may go unnoticed and appear as a real client indefinitely unless we find ways to establish a true identity and achieve authentication of transactions and hence establish legal accountability of and towards a client.

The agent that a Consumer Health Informatics service providers deals with may be acting for himself or on behalf of a minor, an elderly, or other not capable to communicate. He may do so legally, legitimately or fraudulently, where legitimately means that ex post legal inquiry would conclude that in the absence of a power of attorney or an advance directive[9] it was in the best interest of the person for whom a service was used. Similarly, Consumer Health Informatics services where parents play a necessary crucial role in decision support for minors, need further elaboration of a legal framework. In the future when Consumer Health Informatics services are covered by private or public health insurance the client will have to prove his identity to achieve eligibility and coverage.

An ethical dilemma derives from the fact that an imbedding of Consumer Health Informatics in regular care necessitates a pervasive personal identity through all processes. That includes the opportunities of billing and payment through health plans, a longitudinal ER, and targeted deployment of emergency care when need be. Equity – in this case: access for all, with or without health insurance, with or without a legal identity – however, may require admission for fake personas irrespective of a known real identity. All opportunities above are harder to achieve now, if not out of reach. Only PHRs or PCHRs (cf. Sect. 14.1 ff) can be tried for a longitudinal ER. They may be more sparsely populated, though, than in the personal identity situation because providers are likely reluctant to grant access to their internal records or open their patient portals to users who do not come with a legal identity. Therefore, their patient safety potential will be lower.

We will subsequently only pursue the known legal identity situation.

8.4.4.2 Approaches for Secure Verification of Identity

Safe methods for either of the demands, to establish ones identity, ones legitimacy of acting on behalf of oneself or of someone else or ones eligibility for insurance

---

[9](also: advance health care directive) written instructions ... that specify what actions should be taken for ... health, if ... no longer able to make decisions ... ; source: Wikipedia.

coverage, draw on similar principles. They are now briefly introduced with their pros and cons. A detailed account can be found in Chap. 13.

8.4.4.2.1 Building on Classical Instruments of Identity Proof

Authenticating documents, tokens, instruments can be exchanged through certified mail where the identity of the recipient can be verified and notarized documents can be requested as need be. To establish coverage through insurance, policy numbers or SSN can be mailed classically before endowing the partners with methods to access electronically conveyed services. In case that proof of identity has been established through approved procedures from the paper era the partners are cleared to exchange entities that support smooth electronic authentication and ratification. These include – at different levels of safety – TAN lists, different forms of local TAN generators, TAN transmissions through parallel channels (e.g. cell phone TAN when main transaction is through Internet), chip cards and combinations thereof. Ideally they come as a pair of a token that only an authorized actor can possess and something that only he can know, cf. Sect. 13.4.

8.4.4.2.2 Electronic Signatures

Predecessors of the electronic signature have existed as digital methods of encryption for more than two decades.[10] They are slowly moving into the arena of public governance and probative force. When the encryption keys are issued by government certified trust centers and partners and procedures are in place, transactions such as closing contracts can be executed fully legally through qualified electronic signatures, without any paper changing hands. Apparently simple transaction such as prescriptions can greatly profit. A prescription has contract character because the physician assures and is accountable for applying the accepted state of medical knowledge while the patient is responsible for compliance (for a more detailed analysis see the whole Chap. 17 and specifically Sect. 17.6.2.3). With the prescription sheet handed over such a contract is implicitly closed. As long as the signed paper is a mandatory element of legal prescription and Consumer Health Informatics service provider and client are geographically apart the signed paper has to take the snail way. And when a drug is required immediately it is mailed

---

[10]Phil Zimmermann provided the first version of PGP – Pretty Good Privacy – to allow civil rights movements to communicate without authorities getting access. So the initiative initially served the purposes of civil disobedience rather than governance. Source: Wikipedia.

8.4 Overview of Assessment Dimensions   185

ahead of time upon telephone notice.[11] The paper prescription follows as FAX and the deal is finally legalized and the file closed when the letter with the signed paper prescription arrives.[12]

8.4.4.2.3 Biometric Authentication

The approach of biometric authentication to secure the identity of an individual has attracted recent scientific attention. By biometric authentication we mean "a method of differentiating individuals based on the analysis of qualitative or quantitative biological patterns" (MeSH-definition). It includes hand fingerprints, automated facial recognition, retinal scan and voice pattern recognition to name some that can be considered in Consumer Health Informatics services of the near future, but also vascular patterns and DNA profiles or fingerprints (MeSH-definition).

Using biometric patterns alone in Consumer Health Informatics and other medical scenarios has more disadvantages than advantages. First they are not safe against intrusion and identity theft. Artifacts such as fingerprint foils have already been faked successfully to get access. Second if Consumer Health Informatics client biometric authentication profiles are held in a database at the provider they are a welcome target for intrusion attacks because they are universal and do not expire under any normal circumstances. It is the same fingerprint that authorizes immigration, banking, health etc. Once stolen it cannot be stopped. Third and most critical in medical application: if a critical lab result or diagnosis leaks out under an artificial identifier assigned to an individual a new identifier can be assigned and the history can be left behind. If that same lab or diagnosis leaks out under a biometric authentication pattern it is forever associated with the holder of that pattern.

More sophisticated approaches are under way to increase the effort necessary to steal biometric authentication patterns.[13] But the problem remains that once exposed, an identity can never be made forgotten again.

---

[11]Between parties who mutually trust they are who they claim they are, without legally safe authentication either.

[12]A pervasive migration of the prescription process in Germany to the Telematik Infrastruktur the security/confidentiality strategy of which is outlined in Chap. 13 will presumable reduce cost by 400 Million US$ per year.

[13]Searching PubMed with `Biometric Identification[MeSH]` and `authentication` delivers increasing numbers of publications. Quite a few target, however, at secure identification of and diagnosis from bio-materials.

> **Take Home**
> Under regular circumstances Consumer Health Informatics are offered by accountable providers to sane responsible clients whose identities are known. In that case secure methods of probative force need to be applied on both ends.
> Methods of secure authentication include two way protocols where an individual requires knowledge and possession of a token and electronic signatures.
> Classical methods of proving identity and secure transport can be used to initiate secure electronic methods.
> Biometric patterns as identifiers have the highest need for protecting the true identity to become known to unauthorized intruders.
> From a perspective of equity offering Consumer Health Informatics services to personas without caring about their human identity is an option whose logistic, legal and ethical implications are not further considered here.

8.5 Further Reading

In a white paper summarizing a round table at the AMIA 2007 Spring Congress Keselman and coauthors [9] come to similar distinctions and potential risks that have to be assessed. However, we organize the dimensions differently. In this chapter we have distinguished the core problem in Sect. 8.4.1 from personal and societal influences that modify and blur the communication about the core problem, aiming at a checklist of what to pay attention to under what circumstances. The white paper distinguishes properties of communication channels towards the client/recipient, the recipient's high dimensional internal state which ranges from emotions to cognitions, his social influences which are somewhat broader than our cultural and religious background in Sect. 8.4.2.4 and his nation's or region's health resources aspects that we partially address in Sect. 8.4.4. The white paper also has a section on barriers which we address to some part here in the Cognition Sect. 8.4.3 but more deeply in Chaps. 3, 17, and 15 and Sect. 1.9.2.

In a 2004 review Butcher and coworkers summarize the state of the art of computers in clinical assessment [1]. They address both new opportunities of computerized instruments with their potential of personalization, animation etc. and new methodological challenges to validate the results.

References

1. Butcher JN, Perry J, Hahn J. Computers in clinical assessment: historical developments, present status, and future challenges. J Clin Psychol. 2004;60. doi: 10.1002/jclp.10267.
2. Brennan PF, Safran C. Patient safety remember who it's really for. Int J Med Inform. 2004;73:547–50. doi: 10.1016/j.ijmedinf.2004.05.005.

3. Baker DW, Williams MV, Parker RM, Gazmararian JA, Nurss J. Development of a brief test to measure functional health literacy. Patient Educ Couns. 1999;38:33–43.
4. Charles C, Gafni A, Whelan T. Decision-making in the physician-patient encounter: revisiting the shared treatment decision-making model. Soc Sci Med. 1999;49:651–61. doi: 10.1016/S0277-9536(99)00145-8.
5. DuBay WH. The principles of readability. http://www.impact-information.com/impactinfo/readability02.pdf, 2004.
6. Hargittai E. Survey measures of web-oriented digital literacy. Soc Sci Comput Rev. 2005;23. doi: 0.1177/0894439305275911.
7. Karmen C, Hsiung RC, Wetter T. Screening internet forum participants for depression symptoms by assembling and enhancing multiple NLP methods. Comput Methods Programs Biomed. 2015;120(1):27–36. doi: 10.1016/j.cmpb.2015.03.008.
8. Kirsch IS, Jungeblut A, Jenkins L, Kolstad A. Adult literacy in america: a first look at the results of the national adult literacy survey. www.ncjrs.gov/pdffiles1/Digitization/144980NCJRS.pdf, 1993.
9. Keselman A, Logan R, Smith CA, Leroy G, Zeng-Treitler Q. Developing informatics tools and strategies for consumer-centered health communication. JAMIA. 2008;15(4):473–83. doi: 10.1197/jamia.M2744; http://jamia.bmj.com/content/15/4/473.short.
10. Kaye J, Mattek N, Dodge HH, Campbell I, Hayes T, Austin D, Hatt W, Wild K, Jimison H, Pavel M. Unobtrusive measurement of daily computer use to detect mild cognitive impairment. Alzheimers Dement. 2014;10(1). doi: 10.1016/j.jalz.2013.01.011.
11. Moore TJ, Alsabeeh N, Apovian CM, Murphy MC, Coffman GA, Cullum-Dugan D, Jenkins M, Cabral H. Weight, blood pressure, and dietary benefits after 12 months of a web-based nutrition education program (DASH for Health): longitudinal observational study. J Med Internet Res. 2008;10(4):52. doi: 10.2196/jmir.1114.
12. Masys D, Baker D, Butros A, Cowles KE. Giving patients access to their medical records via the internet: the PCASSO experiment. JAMIA. 2002;9(2):181–91. doi: 10.1197/jamia.M1005.
13. Norman CD, Skinner HA. eHEALS: the eHealth literacy scale. JMIR. 2006;8(4):e27.
14. Ogden CK, Richards IA. The meaning of meaning: a study of the influence of language upon thought and of the science of symbolism, volume 3 of C. K. Ogden & Linguistics. London: Routledge/Thoemmes Press; 2013.
15. Orizio G, Schulz P, Domenighini S, Bressanelli M, Rubinelli S, Caimi L, Gelatti U. Online consultations in cyberpharmacies: completeness and patient safety. Telemed e-Health. 2009;15(10):1022–5. doi: 10.1089/tmj.2009.0069.
16. Stran KA, Knol LL. Determinants of food label use differ by sex. J Acad Nutr Diet. 2013;113(5):673–9. doi: 10.1016/j.jand.2012.12.014.
17. Vargas PA, Robles E, Harris J, Radford P. Using information technology to reduce asthma disparities in underserved populations: a pilot study. J Asthma. 2010;47(8):889–94. doi: 10.3109/02770903.2010.497887.
18. Weiss BD, Mays MZ, Martz W, Castro KM, DeWalt DA, Pignone MP, Mockbee J, Hale FA. Quick assessment of literacy in primary care: the newest vital sign. Ann Fam Med. 2005;3(6):514–22. doi: 10.1370/afm.405.

Chapter 9
Services for All Stages of the Metabolic Syndrome and Its Consequences

9.1 Introduction

We take the "Metabolic syndrome" as an example where diverse technologies and service types gather around a medical problem. MeSH lists as components of the metabolic syndrome

- excess abdominal fat
- atherogenic dyslipidemia
- hypertension
- hyperglycemia
- insulin resistance
- proinflammatory state
- prothrombic state

The topic is broad enough to fill a volume of its own if going into depth. As opposed to most other chapters we will, therefore, stay at a more superficial level medically but strive to demonstrate the diversity of Consumer Health Informatics services for the diversity of problems. Among the diseases for which the metabolic syndrome is a risk factor we will concentrate on diabetes mellitus 2.

9.2 Diabetes Pioneers: The IDEATel Project

Diabetes mellitus 2, which often is the offspring of an enduring metabolic syndrome lifestyle is a pioneer field of application of Consumer Health Informatics. As early as 2002 a group from Columbia University designed, implemented, and pursued for more than a decade an intervention of *"telemedicine in the management of older patients with diabetes ... resid(ing) in federally designated medically underserved areas"* (cf. [25, p. 49], where the study design was first presented). In absence of a consolidated expression Consumer Health Informatics in 2002 the term telemedicine was used but IDEATel had sufficient activity on the part of the patient to warrant the newer term. It is a Level 1 extension of services offered to patients in one urban and one rural target region. According to the available equipment in 2002 participants received 8 frames/sec videoconferencing equipment, blood glucose and blood pressure measurement devices for automated upload of data, and dial in Internet connection to the study server where they could view data. The approach was driven through concepts such as behavioral theory, patient empowerment, frequent interactions through the distance with study personnel, higher frequency monitoring of pertinent vitals than can be achieved in face to face care, and allowing the patient to choose his speed and process of learning.

IDEATel was implemented and launched. Numerous investigations delivered data on the design of the material, effective and not so effective program elements, patient cognitions including computer literacy, patient behavior modifications, relation to Medicare, etc. and most recently on the social impact of the program [24]. The more than 30 publications in between are a worthwhile read on sustained development and investigation in Consumer Health Informatics.

9.3 Outline of Chapter

For a treatment of more recent advances we will explore the topic along three major axes:

- Time course of the disease from risk assessment and primary prevention to treatment of complications (of diabetes mellitus 2)
- The four levels of Consumer Health Informatics services
- The types of information used from risk awareness information through automated capture of vital signs to active behavioral or treatment advice offered to the client

A prevailing theme of this analysis will be that the burden of the disease is low if non-existent *early* while it can be grave *late*. Therefore, even small improvements are hard to achieve but may be worth the effort. Another aspect will be lurking for many services: If regarded as a combination of a genetic disposition and a pattern of unhealthy behaviors the metabolic syndrome is the target for lifestyle changes. These can be achieved through behavioral guidance provided by dietary assistants, trainers etc., and resides in the sphere of well-being which is not regulated through medical professional codes. If the metabolic syndrome is regarded as a diagnosis therapists act in their capacity as medical professionals and have to comply with respective regulations. Details of this distinction are the topic of Chap. 17. Presently in ICD-10 the metabolic syndrome is not a diagnosis.

In the first major section we will follow the time course of the disease from awareness of the risks of the metabolic syndrome through treatment of one of its incurred diagnoses – diabetes – and finally management of complications of diabetes. For the different states of the disease we will present services at different levels in the sense of Chaps. 3, 4, 5, and 6. The information resources and in some case devices required for the respective Consumer Health Informatics services will also be outlined.

When this collection of opportunities has unfolded and some positive and some mixed results have been presented we will point to adjacent topics, other risks of the metabolic syndrome and creative services for juvenile diabetics. Regarding the mixed results throughout the chapter we cannot but conclude with some deep rooted skepticism about the prognosis to attenuate the metabolic syndrome epidemic through behavioral coaching.

9.4 Risk Awareness and Primary Prevention

For a condition that comes as silently and covertly as diabetes and cardiovascular disease do awareness of an existing risk and consequential lifestyle change and screening and monitoring of early signs are the most powerful management activities. Clients can then delay and potentially avoid the manifestation of the disease.

Awareness is not anxiety. It is the openness of mind to collect information from the environment and about oneself and to draw rational conclusions and to follow up if and only if the conclusions arrive at a tangible risk. To create awareness, so to speak to turn the client into "should I start collecting information" mode, can happen in various ways including public health programs, general practitioner observations and communications etc. But at a certain point in time the client must embrace his role of positioning himself, to actively collect and assess information and to draw conclusions for himself. He will draw on the communication sources and channels of his era which for many elderly still is family, friends and journals [27] while electronic media and primarily the Internet are gaining ground for the younger generations and where both professionals and virtual communities provide information. Therefore, seeking information about one's personal risk is a typical Level 0 situation (cf. Chap. 3).

9.4.1 Fostering Awareness

Risk awareness is not a one-way road: only those who likely are at high risk should draw that conclusion for themselves while those with no identifiable risk should not be talked into unnecessary behavior changes or utilizations of health care resources.

9.4.1.1 The Role of Knowledge

Genz and coworkers [4] investigated 1120 unsolicited visitors to the websites of a diabetes research institution and a social insurance company in Germany.[1] Visitors were checked for no known diagnosis of diabetes. The investigation shows that knowledge and awareness develop differently dependent on the quality of the information that clients access. A random half of the sample (intervention arm) was directed to the newly developed certified quality website of the diabetes research institution while the other half (control arm) could browse few selected information services as they existed on the Internet at the time of the investigation. So for the control arm the situation was like a Level 0 search (cf. Chap. 3) under the more favorable condition that attention was directed to good quality information, like in Sect. 9.4.2.1.

Subjects in both conditions were asked right after studying the material and 2 weeks after their first visits to their information source about their knowledge on glucose metabolism and their attitudes and intentions concerning metabolic testing. The intervention arm had significantly higher knowledge scores but a significantly lower intention and a more critical attitude towards metabolic testing. This is in agreement with an also observed more intense feeling of conflict about personal health decisions in the intervention. However, these observations should not at all be regarded as negative outcome. We are not making a pre-post comparison and do not know the percentage willing to test in the "untreated" subjects. Even if we tried to poll for a baseline metabolic testing willingless before exposing the subjects to their intervention we would have to be aware of Hawthorne or social desirability type biases, cf. Sect. 15.2.3.3. We can only relate the post willingness to test in the two arms to the prevalence of diabetes mellitus 2 in the population. It is 6 % population wide and at most 12 % in the age cohort (average ~50 years). Willingness to test turns out as ~25 % in the intervention and more than 30 % in the control arm. Of course population statistics do not inform about individual behaviors and diagnoses. If they would, however, only 12 of 25 in the intervention vs. only 12 of 30 in the control arm actually face the diagnosis. The intervention arm predicts over-utilization of 25/12, the control arm of 30/12, i.e. we have an apparent over-utilization by a factor of more than two if those who self-report that they will take metabolic testing actually do. However, to add to the required precautions of interpretation when base rates are not known: regarding that around 80 % of all study cohort visitors to the two web sites reported having already undergone glucose testing before the study they do not appear to be representative for the German population with their 12 % prevalence but rather a non random aggregation of higher risks. Then proportions of willingness to test demonstrate a good sense for reality rather than an encouragement to over-utilize. If this is so the service presented here does what it should: arouse risk awareness and thought processes. It avoids what it

---

[1]Deutsches Diabetes-Zentrum, http://ddz.uni-duesseldorf.de/en/ and Techniker Krankenkasse, http://www.tk.de/ (in German).

should avoid: to drive scores into unwarranted testing and utilization of resources. This does not say a word whether individual decisions to test or not to test are correct.

9.4.1.2 The Role of Personality

A strong – affirmed – personality is a good determinant of appropriate health risk awareness while anxiety is not. Van Koningsbruggen and Das [28] designed an experimental setup where self affirmation was stimulated in an experimental arm and left unaffected in a control. In both arms actual risk of diabetes was estimated through a battery of questions on behavior, medication, own and family medical history. Responses were then collected after presenting a health message "What everybody should know about type 2 diabetes" that described the disease and its risks and finally encouraged to take a diabetes mellitus 2 risk test.

Having been self affirmed let a majority of persons apparently at risk embrace the risk assignment and encouragement to test while a majority of persons apparently not at risk derogated the message and did not consider testing. In contrast the control arm participants' attitudes towards risk and intention to test was equally scattered in at risk and not at risk individuals. Therefore, exaggerated perception of health risks as cartooned in Molière's Imaginary Invalid can be due to lack of knowledge and a weak personality.

Take Home
- Proper risk awareness lies between the extremes of negligence of health risks and Imaginary Invalid like anxiety.
- Good knowledge and an affirmed personality foster proper risk awareness.
- Consumer Health Informatics service can be instrumental to convey good knowledge and to affirm clients' personality.

9.4.2 Turning Awareness into Risk Avoiding Behavior

While the section above emphasizes the aspect of awareness of one's potential risk and the indication for lab screening we now investigate how awareness transforms into behavior change. For most individuals who eat too much and too unhealthily and exercise too little eating better and exercising more offers a whole bunch of health benefits and only marginal risks. We therefore concentrate on benefits and how we can assess whether they materialize and sustain.

9.4.2.1 Small Impact Behavior Modification Services

In an investigation at a military base Hunter and coworkers [6] pursue the humble goal to stop weight increase but also accept clients who want to reduce weight. In a Level 1 Consumer Health Informatics service where the target population is a clinically known 2.5 % subset of the most severely overweight clients (average BMI 29) an Internet program (BIT, Behavioral Internet Therapy, which consists of behavioral, diet and exercise recommendations; calory calculations, diary) is randomly assigned to 227 of the study population of 222 men and 224 women; the other 219 receive the usual care at the military base (subsequently: the control). In this high-risk population Internet outperforms control with statistical significance. The effect sizes, however, first stir doubt about the meaningfulness. Average weight loss after 6 months is 1.3 kg in the Internet arm, compared to 0.6 kg weight increase in control. BMI performs similarly. Nothing is known whether the program sustains its effects after the end of the 6 month study. So, Much ado about (almost) nothing (Shakespeare, 1598–1599?)?

It should be in mind that "Much ado" is not actually true. The service used only marginal in-person initiation and could be transformed into Level 2 virtual only through mailing or e-mail outreach. It does not apply any measurement device or specific instrumentation. It can be nearly effortless without losing functionality or increasing hazards. Those invited to enroll would only have to find out their risk level by using their own scales at home with the major remaining challenge being correct BMI calculation. Sadly enough this *is* a challenge for quite a few, as outlined in Sect. 8.4.3.2 but for the sake of argument we assume that it can be mastered. "Nothing" is not true, either: as argued in Sect. 9.2 small improvements can have valuable long term effects.

Therefore, cost-effectiveness is worth an investigation and has been reported in a separate publication [17]. The differences in outcome between BIT and control arms (for instance 1.3 kg weight loss in BIT versus 0.6 kg weight gain in control makes up 1.9 kg difference) are related to the additional cost of the Level 1 BIT service. The figures reported (for instance \$36.44 per kg weight loss under the least favorable cost assumptions for BIT) are a valuable first step. They inform decision makers what health behavior effect can be achieved at what price. For a comprehensive assessment we would have to know the future savings in terms of saved treatment cost and other indirect gains of weighing 1.9 kg less.

Carr and coworkers [2] also have a structured program underpinned by a theoretical model of human motivation that comes in 16 lessons for 16 weeks. It is available as classroom or as Internet service, and meanwhile also as book. For the Internet variant Active Living Every Day (ALED-I) Carr's group investigates the increase in physical activity – primarily defined as pedometer-measured steps done per day – in a similarly high risk group (BMI in lower 30s) and compares with intent-to-treat (control). In the treatment arm steps per day increased significantly by 1384 – but it also increased by more than 800 in control. A "nice" subject expectancy effect (cf. Sect. 15.2.3.3.2) presumably invoked through the fact that treatment and control arms equally received the pedometer measuring device. By contrast, target

9.4 Risk Awareness and Primary Prevention

variables that characterize metabolic risk more comprehensively than step counts improved in treatment and remained unchanged in control.

In an 8 month follow-up [3] the researchers have to concede that the physical activity effects do not sustain while the more complex indicators of metabolic state preserve their 16 week values. So this is another unidirectional Internet delivered educational service that loses its appeal and stimulating power after the end of the trial. Nevertheless, ALED-I and a similar service that focuses on nutrition can since be purchased from http://www.activeliving.info/ or http://amazon.com for $39.95. Since the services do not target a diagnosed disease but rather are lifestyle or well-being products they do not fall under the verdict of Sect. 17.4 that finds practicing of medicine without in-person contact illegal but rather match the characteristics of lifestyle and well-being outlined in Sect. 17.7.1 where services may be legally sold and purchased, no matter whether they do or do not have an effect.

Take Home

The effects of low intensity unidirectional informational and educational services are moderate at best and hard to quantify.

- Mild interventions through Internet based education and convenience functions can help control weight.
- The calculated cost per kg weight reduction is moderate.
- True cost-effectiveness cannot be established because the financial gain of an achieved weight reduction can under most circumstances not be quantified with reasonable effort.
- Client-reported outcomes such as pedometer counts may be compromised through various biases.

9.4.2.2 The Role of Being Part of a Community

The services presented next achieve more by adding community to the purely educational and diary/feedback functionality.

Stewart and coworkers [21] also have the setting of a military base and regulations for weight (AWCP[2]) and physical fitness for the soldiers that a majority do not meet. As opposed to [6] in Sect. 9.4.2.1 they make active use of the community by advertising through an intranet that is a prevailing resource of information sharing at the base. Within that website the H.E.A.L.T.H. (Healthy Eating, Activity, and Lifestyle Training Headquarters) was advertised and everybody could enroll anonymously. H.E.A.L.T.H. is an Internet-based tailored CBT concept meant to be used anonymously in order to prevent the stigma of being overweight. It has a comprehensive overview and feedback functions ("dashboard" of goals and performance). Lots of self reported data can be entered and viewed. Among all who

---

[2] Army Weight Control Program.

enrolled the study concentrated on those with weights above AWCP limit minus 5 % (soldiers) or above 25 BMI (civilians). The researchers got approval to the exempt from study participant informed consent i.e. actually nobody knew that those who enrolled and where above inclusion criteria thresholds were surveyed as to their weight development. Therefore, it can be expected that all the biases described in Sect. 15.2.3 are not present here and weights that participants chart can by and large be taken for granted.

It is not surprising that a Consumer Health Informatics service that is just there and that is only made known concurrently with other information in the military base intranet does not receive skyrocketing attention upfront. In 2 years of mild advertising plus 1 year of cooling down the number of subscribers kept climbing and eventually reached more than 4500, most of whom, however, only stopped by once. The following analysis concentrates on the 298 medium (2–7 visits) and the 58 high (more than 7 visits) utilizers. The demographics of the groups do not surprise except that the soldier participants – as opposed to most studies of voluntary enrollment to health programs – were male in majority.

The central outcome target was "above 5 % weight loss". Since enrollment as well as dropping out could happen anytime and the anonymous nature of the whole investigation precluded reminders to be sent different time schemas were applied. Among the medium utilizers 12 % achieved the target at some time, 9 % at their last login. For the high utilizers efficacy was much higher: one third were down 5 % or more at some time and almost as many (28 %) at last log-in. Regression analysis between the three classes of utilization and the percentage of 5 % target achievement was significant for these two time schemas as well as for a first log-in versus half a year later weight recordings.

Generally, these results are not overwhelming either, but they demonstrate that a service can survive and maintain momentum if it is embedded in the shared web resource that a closed community uses and that in the absence of all biasing factors discussed in Sect. 15.2.3 true effects actually materialize.

9.4.2.3 Cost-Effectiveness Stratified by Risk Group

An employer sponsored program gets out some more and finds differential effects between different risk groups. The DASH for Health program is a Level 2 Internet delivered Consumer Health Informatics service provided in a common effort by Boston University and EMC Corporation, offered to EMC^2®'s US based employees and adult family.

DASH for Health has two main components: a regular service of two articles on health, exercise, nutrition etc. published per week and announced through e-mail notification and a dashboard for participants to record progress reports on body weight, blood pressure, eating and exercising habits. DASH for Health conveys a very liberal motivational attitude: At onset it is mildly advertised through EMC^2® management who declare that they will not access any health-related data. At

9.4 Risk Awareness and Primary Prevention

EMC^2® DASH for Health meets an enterprise with a health aware and caring culture. The wording used in the service, like in "Progress report", gives the whole endeavor a positive optimistic appearance.

The being embedded in the health plan infrastructure of a major employer offers the opportunity to link the effects of the Level 2 service to the tangible medical reality of the participants. They were seen and keep being seen by doctors under contract with their employer's health plan and claims data and medical outcome values emerged naturally. These were analyzed with respect to condition specific clinical outcomes [10] and as to overall yearly health care costs [20]. Actual values from two consecutive calendar years could, therefore, be used for the reporting.

In the first investigation, a historical comparison, cf. Sect. 15.3, with 2834 enrolled of which 735 were still actively using at the end of the year average weight reduction was significant for the overweight clients (1.9 kg, $p < .001$, $n = 151$), systolic blood pressure reduction was significant for the hypertensive (6.8 mmHG, $p < .001$, $n = 62$), and self reported diet was healthier for everybody. Only for the last outcome variable a subject expectancy effect (Sect. 15.2.3.3.2) may bias the result.

In the second investigation a bird's eye view on the yearly cost of a cohort of 1967 participants was taken. While there is no cost reduction for the whole cohort the authors find a reduction of $827 per year among the 729 cardiovasular risk participants. The authors find a reduction of cost per year of $14 per visit to DASH for Health among all those who visit frequently (more than nine times per year). In the combination of any medical condition with high frequency of visits the cost reduction per visit reaches $55.

In a personal communication [12] the lead author for the DASH for Health program confirmed in December 2013 that more than 10 years after initiation the program was still in use at EMC. Throughout the years more than 11,000 employees had enrolled and 18 % of the first year participants were still using it.

Take Home
- A behavior modification program can operate with tangible benefit and no obvious harm as a Level 2 service.
- Cost reductions mainly materialize for high-risk groups.
- Being associated with an employer can be a means for long-term sustainable operation.

9.4.2.4 Adding Virtual Community

In the next increment in terms of Consumer Health Informatics virtual rather than local community can be added, as reported by Kuwata and coworkers [9]. Next to advice on diet and exercise for patients with metabolic syndrome it purposefully includes a social network service. A pilot study showed that the latter contributed to client adherence, although long-term experiences are still missing.

While in Kuwata the social network functions are just there and "see what happens" they are an active component in [16]. The intent of the Consumer Health Informatics service is to increase physical activity, taken as step counts in sedentary metabolic syndrome adults. The target group extends from just BMI >25 to more progressed states of morbidity: diagnosed diabetes mellitus 2 or coronary artery disease.

For a clinical trial of the subsequent treatment concept a random subsample (appr. 6000) of patients of a University of Michigan Health System provider was drawn. Five hundred and twenty-five were eligible (sedentary, medical condition(s), Internet access). Three hundred and twenty-four enrolled after informed consent and a medical clearance form signed by their physician.

The hypothesis of the trial was that in comparison of two variants of a contents rich service, the variant with virtual community would fare better. Faring better was primarily taken as larger increase in step counts. Before onset all 324 recorded a 1 week baseline sample of daily steps with the display of the step counter being tape sealed.

The base contents shared between control and experimental arm were pedometer uploads, step-count feedback, individually calculated incremental goals, personalized (using various demographics) motivational messages. At onset a random subgroup received just this. The virtual community arm participants could also post and read messages.

The investigation itself has various methodological shortcomings and unconvincing results. The baseline step counts call for both Hawthorne and social desirability effects (Sect. 15.2.3.3): the upcoming experimental situation may have modified behaviors, as well as the habit to showcase the health aware citizen. For both reasons it is likely that baseline counts are higher than an unaffected baseline and hence observed increases in step counts underestimate the true effect.

It also happened (not the fault of the investigators) that the cohort randomized to the experimental virtual community arm was lower risk in various respects: lower percentages of all medical conditions and higher baseline step counts. The latter could be compensated for by not comparing endpoint steps/day between the groups but rather endpoint – baseline increase in steps/day.

The results hold good, mixed, and bad news. The good news certainly is that step counts increased in both arms. However, they increased almost equally in control and virtual community arm. Truly alarming is the fact that standard deviations of increases for both arms are larger than the increases themselves. It appears that we have more scatter than effect.

But we find potential explanations in the fact that within the virtual community arm only 65 % actually used posting and reading. So what was assumed to be the active ingredient that discriminates between control and experimental treatment was not present in one third of the subjects in the experimental arm.

Some other behavioral observations and outcomes are worth mentioning, though. A higher percentage in the virtual community arm (79 % vs. 66 %) stayed till the end. Participants who at baseline reported not receiving social support from family

9.4 Risk Awareness and Primary Prevention

or friends for their physical activity were more active online community members. Step counts increased moderately with number of posts, i.e. differentiating among those who found themselves in the online community arm shows some dose-response kind of behavior: the more participants embraced the opportunity the more they got out. However, those with real social support upfront also were more likely to increase their step counts.

Two more observations make the service a worthwhile object of study. In a separate paper [18] the authors describe their effort to get and keep the online community active. This included covertly providing seed posts before going public, injecting posts when the activity of a thread calmed down and contributing to the numbers of distinct threads not to become too large such that activity would not be dispersed over too many places.

The hooking up with the classical health care system sees this Consumer Health Informatics service on the borderline between Level 1 and Level 2. For the trial the major recruitment was through a classical provider but some word-of-mouth by-passers to the web site were also enrolled. All subsequent screening of eligibility (for the trial, but the same would hold for a regular service) happened online. Only finally the prospective clients had to provide clearance through their physician. The trial would certainly not have been approved without such safeguard. However, between a physician and a client who the physician knows and who asks for clearance this could be provided without an extra face-to-face encounter.

Take Home

The general attempt to demonstrate that adding messaging between clients improves physical exercise (step count) outcome of a coaching service fails, because

- baselines cannot be safely established
- the outcomes scatter widely
- the messaging is not used by one third

Some other interesting insights on individual benefits emerge:

- The amount of individual utilization of the messaging is correlated with
    - exercise outcome
    - lack of real social support
    - perseverance of visiting the service
- Real social support is correlated with exercise outcome.

With more experience and figures on adverse events from a large population the service may end up asking prospective clients for either physician clearance or declaration that they understand the risk and waive liability. It would then be a Level 2 service which has a potential to scale up: once large enough online community traffic will require less human effort and attention towards not drying out. And pedometers are approaching the status of lifestyle gadgets, so the investment may be in the reach of the target group. As long as it only targets healthy person at excess risks for a certain disease and only recommends behavioral modifications it resides in the legal arena of well-being and lifestyle and is not subject to the request of in-person initiation for Level 2 services established in Sect. 17.4 for practicing medicine.

9.5 Treatment Support and Coaching

9.5.1 Simple Tight Medical Guidance

A Consumer Health Informatics service by Avdal and coworkers [1] developed in Turkey is very basic Level 1. It addresses computer literate insulin dependent type 2 diabetics. Compared to a control arm that received face-to-face education and blood glucose related monitoring at intervals of up to 3 months through a diabetes nurse in a polyclinic, experimental arm clients accepted the burden to upload glucose values daily and enjoyed the convenience to do it from home and to receive initial education and regular coaching information at home through the Internet. On the part of the provider the major distinction also is convenience: Analyzing patient data at the computer in due course and communicating the result when done rather than fast track under the pressure of a busy clinic while the patient is waiting. Since for the experimental arm the nurses can generate graphical displays of glucose level time courses and make them available to patients, the service has an element of feedback of past behavior and its effects. But apart from that control and experimental arm received the same quality of information which was equally provided through clinical professionals. The only element of using IT typical functions to increase efficiency was a FAQs collection to be filled by the nurses and available in both study arms.

The encouraging result is that the experimental arm achieves significantly more reduced HbA1c values and significantly more often attends health checks. Which could be interpreted as the Consumer Health Informatics arm providing *superior quality* of service. However, the article is not detailed enough to exclude that it is an effect of *increased quantity* of exposure. While control arm participants contact their nurses at long intervals, Internet arm participants record and send daily glucose values and presumably receive feedback and advice more frequently. What can at least be safely said is that some convenience for patient and provider and workload balancing for the provider can be achieved without losing on quality.

9.5.2 Medical Guidance and Tailored Behavioral Information

Drawing on a long history in the field of Consumer Health Informatics in diabetes mellitus 2, McMahon and coworkers [11] present results from a more sophisticated and data intensive 1 year investigation. Their subjects were badly controlled diabetics (HbA1c > 8.5 %) of whom about one half had been diagnosed more than 10 years ago. They were mostly male and mostly well-educated. Recruiting went through the Department of Veterans Affairs Boston Health care System.

In an attempt to investigate factors that help to decrease HbA1c as major outcome variable 151 patients were assigned to one of three treatment arms. In two of the three conditions patients were actively coached, either through telephone or Internet, while in the third condition ("self management") they were pointed to selected vetted information resources on diabetes management including some that offered peer sharing and mutual support.

All three arms underwent the same face-to-face initiation which included the use of a blood glucose and a blood pressure measuring device. They were also instructed about an approved diabetes management regime which was the basis of all subsequent coaching in coached arms. All arms underwent a detailed baseline assessment of various medical and one diabetes distress measures.

For both coached arms the attempt was made to establish an equal quantity of exposure by implementing a biweekly reporting scheme. The telephone arm, therefore, had biweekly phone calls while the online coaching arm was encouraged to upload glucose and blood pressure readings biweekly and then receive feedback and advice asynchronously through messages to their computers. Telephone reminders were issued to those who did not log into their portal every 2 weeks. Advice that coaches recommended and made available to their clients included information about the disease such as medications, glucose monitoring, and others including nutrition, exercise, well-being. Inasmuch as advice included the variation in pharmaceutical treatment it had to be affirmed by the patient's primary care provider in order to take effect. The face-to-face initiation and this double checking with the classical provider clearly classifies both coached approaches as Level 1.

Compared to this straight case management scheme clients in the third arm just received a user ID and access for the dedicated website which linked forward to approved resources and then were left to themselves except that their pre-existing relations to health care providers were not affected and they could seek advice from them when they felt the need.

Members in all three arms underwent quarterly checks of nine medical indicators. Diabetes distress was probed through a standardized questionnaire at onset and after the end of the year.

A heap of data emerged which show improvement in all variables, some significant, with no clear pattern whether certain target domains (nutrition, blood pressure, glucose etc.) fared best under one of the three arms. Only decrease in HbA1c was consistently highly significant through all treatment arms and all four quarters. The strongest decline was in the first quarter for all three arms but values kept improving throughout the year. The decrease did not differ significantly among the three groups. Patients with highest baseline HbA1c values (>10 %) had strongest declines in all three therapy arms. Dose-response effects could not be identified: the number of logins in the online coaching arm or the number of phone calls in the respective arm did not correlate with the decrease in HbA1c. Therefore, the average amount of time that the providers spent with their clients equally in the two coached groups – approximately 2 hours of specialized nurse working time per patient throughout the year – only helps to get an idea of the gross human workload when turning the experiment into a regular service. Compared to that the effort is nearly zero for the third, the self management arm. Perseverance also appeared strongest here. Although not significant 43 % of participants in that arm were still visiting into the last quarter, compared to 10 % respectively 12 % in the telephone and online coaching arms. This supports the hope that the method that empowers the patient the most is the most sustainable, compared with the ones where the initiative remains with the provider. The third treatment arm could even be set up as a Level 2 service because the underlying regular care keeps flowing, mutually agnostic, though, of the Consumer Health Informatics service. Since the Consumer Health Informatics service provider does not actually offer personalized care the third arm can also be regarded as a Level 0 situation under the more favorable condition that attention was directed to good quality information, like in Sect. 9.4.1.1. The arm three self management portal then plays the role of a trustworthy provider as described in Sect. 3.5. If patients mainly stay because the linked services they reach through the portal are peer support services we find ourselves in the vicinity of Level 3.

9.5.3 Tight Medical Guidance and Behavioral Coaching

An investigation from Korea resembles [11] in Sect. 9.5.2 in various respects. Kim and coworkers [8] also target obese diabetics – where notably obesity starts at BMI > 23 in Korea – and offer weekly advice provided through a nurse who specializes in diabetes mellitus 2. Here as well the medical history and risk factors are taken into account, partially from patient reporting, partially from the EHR of the tertiary care hospital where the study is affiliated. They are visible and made use of by the provider who is one of the researchers as well. When advice consists of medication changes the patient's primary care provider is notified. Patients in the intervention arm receive their advice once per week through the Internet and can read them on mobile phones or at land-line Internet access points. The control arm just keeps going and measurements of various labs pertinent to diabetes are collected equally in control and intervention arm.

Two major differences should be noted compared to [11]: First, the advice to the patient can relate to insulin or other medication dosage but it can equally be behavioral such as that bad glucose control can result from lack of exercise. Second, the patients in the experimental arm have to record blood glucose readings several times per day, fasting in the morning and postprandial i.e. after every meal.

Although the sample was smaller here (18 intervention and 16 control out of 40 enrolled finished the half year study period) significant improvements materialize in the intervention arm alone. The control remains unaffected. The major point of concern, however, is that the effect is by far stronger after the first 3 months

9.5 Treatment Support and Coaching

than after half a year. HbA1c arm average falls from 8.16 % to 6.94 % and then rebounds to 7.07 %. There is no medical explanation for that in the data such that an explanation that lends itself is that the researchers are just demanding too much of a good thing: while in [11] experimental arm participants were requested to note the fasting glucose once per day and to report every 2 weeks participants here do several measurements and data transmissions every day. They may just get tired of the effort, despite convenience of using ubiquitous cell phone technology.

In summary we find a Level 1 service which can turn Level 2 when offered through a 3rd party that has existing personal treatment relation with the patient. Legal procedures for medication changes must, however, be found. The service does not have Level 0 or Level 3 elements. Human effort is not reduced – it may even increase – but workload balancing can be a benefit. To avoid wearing and reduced adherence an adaptive data capture scheme with longer intervals when glucose is in good control and tightening when control fades could be considered (cf. Sect. 4.5.2 for a similar strategy in COPD management).

Take Home

Compared to regular care Consumer Health Informatics services achieve better control of HbA1c throughout.
Perseverance

- increases with patient empowerment
- decreases beyond a certain intensity of the intervention

To make medication changes a legal part of a service requires clear procedures to involve classical care providers.

9.5.4 On the Way to Automated Insulin Dosing

Simon and coworkers [22] in the Netherlands are at an early stage of what may become a Level 2 Consumer Health Informatics service. In a small scale in-depth investigation they test whether the core functionality of treating diabetes – insulin dose adaption based on recent history of glucose level and insulin dosage – can be done and safely communicated to patients at home through a fully automated clinical decision support system. The PANDIT prototype interface mimics a diary for fasting blood glucose readings, insulin advice and insulin taken, further remarks and binary selection whether the patient experienced hypoglycemic symptoms. The interface has been tested intensely with no catastrophic and two major (according to [14]) usability errors showing. We now take a deeper look at the safety of the advice itself and the consequential question whether PANDIT could be released as a Level 2 service with human supervision taken out of the loop.

In the 4-week-long test with 10 insulin-dependent diabetics acting from home patient uploading of diary entries and consequential insulin dosing adaptation advice was actually provided and conveyed to the patients by diabetes nurses while in the background the PANDIT clinical decision support algorithm also calculated its advice. Afterward, human and machine advice were compared and the 27 out of 74 (36.5 %) situations where PANDIT calculation differed from nurse recommendation were resolved in a three-step expert judgment process. One of 74 ended up being judged as a safety issue, i.e. risk of a hypoglycemic incident.

The closed loop decision support where PANDIT rather than a nurse provides insulin dosage advice would at that stage certainly not be judged safe enough. The risk of one in 74 dosages potentially leading into hypoglycemia would likely not pass a medical devices safety check or get approval through professional associations. However, what are the alternatives? Of course the PANDIT advice can be fine-tuned towards on the average lower insulin dosage and hence reduce the likelihood of the short term risk of hypoglycemia for some. The price would be slightly higher glucose concentrations on the average for many, hence increasing the risk of long-term damages and complications of the hyperglycemic state. This is a typical situation where utilitarian weighing of benefits and risks as described in detail in Sects. 17.11.6 or 17.11.8 might lead society into judging that few hypoglycemic incidents can be tolerated if the population of diabetics as a whole profits from tightly knit dosing advice. This may be the more so if it turns out that both, hypoglycemic incidents and unfavorably high long term glucose concentrations are more likely with unmonitored constant doses, i.e. without PANDIT style continuous timely dosage advice. In other words: besides investigating how to make PANDIT perfect it should be investigated whether even an imperfect PANDIT is superior to what we are facing with the numbers of diabetics increasing, health care funding under permanent scrutiny and staff decreasing (cf. Sect. 2.3).

Interestingly, even larger figures on insufficient control of the diabetic state have been provided in a US investigation, though with a widely different background and widely different objectives and results have therefore to be transferred with caution.

In a cross-sectional investigation in Northern California [23] with more than 14,000 diabetics, some on insulin, some on other medication, the two major questions were what percentage of that cohort had a severe hypoglycemic event within 12 months and whether the incidence was dependent on health literacy. For the first, incidence actually was significantly higher among health illiterate or marginally literate in the USA. To compare with the PANDIT cohort where health literacy had not been checked we make the assumption that all Dutch patients were health literate and estimate those Californian results that came out for the health literate, roughly half of the population. Within the full population 59 % of those where insulin was the medication – like the PANDIT cohort in [22] – had severe hypoglycemic events. The proportion in health illiterate subjects was highly significantly higher and therefore 30 % of the literate insulin dependent patients encountering a severe hypoglycemic event within 1 year is used as a rough estimate. This 30 % of severe hypoglycemic events "happening" to literate insulin dependent diabetics in regular care outnumbers the one out of 74 severe hypoglycemic events in 4 weeks equals 16 % in a year "caused through" unsafe

PANDIT advice by a factor of nearly two. I.e. the notion of PANDIT as a risk prone service becomes questionable. The argument for PANDIT turns even more favorable if the assumption is false that all PANDIT's subjects are literate and if the dependency between literacy and hypoglycemic incidents is the same in the Netherlands as in the USA. In that case the Dutch sub-cohort of literate would have even fewer than one of 74 incidents.

The circumstances of the two investigations are by far too different to claim the factor 2 of PANDIT being superior to classical care as soundly proved. It should, however, add substance to an ethics approach that, while rightly assessing risks of technology, risks of inaction should equally be assessed.

> **Take Home**
> An experimental closed loop insulin dosage adaptation service based on patient reported readings and self report of hypoglycemic states
>
> - would presently not be approved for routine use
> - achieves a 1 in 74 risk of leading into a hyperglycemic state
>
> Evidence from a different setting insinuates that the service's risk of hyperglycemic states is half as large as constant unmonitored insulin dosage.
> This is a paradigm for decision makers to weigh opportunities and marginal risks of Consumer Health Informatics services and under what circumstances services can be approved for routine use.

9.6 Fostering Self Management

Diabetes is a chronic disease the burden of which is moderate to low at early stages and mounts over time. Good management at early stages is key to delaying and to some part avoiding complications. This makes it necessary, however, to consequently take medications, monitor pertinent vitals and control diet and physical activity for a very long time, actually, lifelong. Since dealing with the disease is not fun in its own right, services that target at supporting patients in sustainably managing their disease have to be very well considered in terms of encouraging long-term use and being and remaining attractive.

In the following we see one systematic review that tries to identify features of services requested above and the design of one service by the same group that tries to map and experimentally test the insights from the review. Variations of this service in terms of design and used technology follow.

9.6.1 In Search of Factors for Services to Last

9.6.1.1 A Systematic Review

Yu's 2012 systematic review [31] analyzes the effects of educational tools on diabetes knowledge and diabetes related medical outcomes such as HbA1c. In a scrutinized selection of not more than the 57 best out of the 1541 retrieved articles they found quite some variation in methodology. Still they achieved some valuable insights, although not all positive: They identified various usability errors in the analyzed Consumer Health Informatics services. Inasmuch as they found outcome effects their determining factors were inconclusive and could not be related to clinical usefulness or usability in general. This review conveys the impression that online patient education of diabetics does not find common ground. This is in line with our argument in Sect. 15.7 about a Cochrane review of Consumer Health Informatics services for asthma: that the carrier technologies (internet, mobile phone, smart phone etc.) and their modes of interaction, positioning and locator services etc. develop so fast that systematic reviews almost inevitably are outdated when they are published. This puts the usefulness of an investigation such as [31] under doubt and it also affects the subsequent analysis of selected services.

> **Take Home**
> A systematic review on web tools for management of diabetes is inconclusive concerning enablers of lasting use and effectiveness. Systematic surveys in fields driven by technologies developing as fast as those underlying Consumer Health Informatics are likely outdated when they are appear.

9.6.1.2 An Implementation and Evaluation Based on the Systematic Review

Yu's group has set up and tested an experimental Internet based Consumer Health Informatics service for diabetes self management that tries to combine the best lessons from the above review [32]. It puts the psychological construct of self-efficacy center stage because it has been shown in various general and diabetes related approaches as a driver of better self-management. It builds on a Knowledge to Action framework which emphasizes involvement of users and stakeholders, adaptation to local needs etc. which in the Canadian Institutes of Health Research funded setting means adaption to provincial health care systems.

Service elements that were planned as consequences or implementations of the theoretical constructs or review results include

- multimedia diabetes education modules to better reach persons with limited literacy,

- service elements to cope with diabetes, reduce stress and improve management,
- a sophisticated scheme to combine passive receipt and active retrieval of the information,
- a forum to communicate with peers and
- various tips to foster communication with the patient's health care provider.

The resulting service prototype was tested and explored with 81 adult diabetics in a 9 months pre-exposure and 9 months concurrent data collection [33] during use of the service. Clinical data were collected every 3 months, questionnaires to calculate a self-efficacy score every 3 weeks throughout. Finally appraisals of enablers and concerns about risks to use and adoption were collected in interviews.

Neither self-efficacy scores nor clinical outcomes improved to an extent that would warrant the effort. If any, messaging between clients made the service attractive for sustained visits and reliability and e-mail reminders were positively mentioned. However, the authors concede to have learnt from their subjects that the Consumer Health Informatics service is perceived as yet another chore to keep up with, beside the struggle with the disease itself and other priorities of their lives, and that it will not succeed until it is seamlessly integrated with daily routines.

> **Take Home**
> A multifaceted Consumer Health Informatics service to improve clinical outcome through better self-management does not show lasting effects in a nine plus 9 months pre-post trial.
> The major obstacle is the lack of integration of the service in daily routines and hence additional effort on top of the onerous life with diabetes.

9.6.2 Building a Service That Reflects Own Experiences

Compared to Yu's and coworkers' attempt to harvest from published observations (cf. Sect. 9.6.1.2) Glasgow's group [5] rather turns long lasting own experience with Consumer Health Informatics in diabetes self management into a fully operational experimental service which has been tested in two variants against control in a 1 year investigation. Psychological constructs also play a role here, such as RE-AIM, a self-efficacy related structured approach to uphold motivation when the enthusiasm of the first months is over. We will see that many design decisions reflect concrete experiences of threats to continuous utilization.

Four hundred and sixty-three overweight patients with diabetes mellitus 2 and at least one more cardiovascular risk factor were enrolled for a trial. Participants also had to have telephone and to have Internet access at least biweekly. An Internet portal was available to all three treatment arms. Two Internet arms were compared to enhanced usual care (EUC; where enhanced "means computer-based health risk appraisal feedback and recommended preventive care behaviors", [5, p. 3]). All arms first received an individual risk assessment and recommended prevention regime communicated in person, and instructions about the Internet portal and the advice to start with easily achievable goals for medication adherence, eating and physical activity. The CASM (Computer Assisted Self Management) and CASM+ intervention arms could record their daily observations in a tracking part of the software. They could see graphical displays of the time course of few diabetes related labs (HbA1c, cholesterol) and of blood pressure. They had a moderated forum, community resource sharing, and teasers such as a quiz. This is not so much different from Yu above [32], except more sophistication in knowledge management here.

Glasgow's and coworkers program has been worked out in numerous steps that reflect their experiences with what puts self-management at risk. After having worked with the portal for 6 weeks participants were supposed to create their personalized "action plans" where the portal helped to specify the medication, eating and activity related plans, for each action to identify barriers and to choose from portal supplied problem solving strategies. Participants also received periodic computer generated motivating calls and could leave requests for being contacted there.

Within an otherwise Level 2 service the CASM+ arm had additional face-to-face i.e. Level 1 re-enforcement and knowledge building sessions. After 2 and 8 weeks participants received calls and they had three two hour group meetings. The first was scheduled so as to discuss the uploaded action plans with the participants and add hints e.g. re shopping, eating out, etc. The second went into depth of catching temptations and their consequences by introducing the concept "Behavior Chain". It cast light on how high risk situations to abandon ones plans can be turned in adhering behavior patterns. The third informed about community resources and how to benefit.

For all three arms Glasgow and co-workers picked numerous items from various validated instruments to establish outcome measures, which are all listed in [5] and would be by far too long to be covered here. Assuming that they were well selected the following are the results.

Twelve month attrition rates for EUC, CASM and CASM+ were 18.2% resp 31.4% and 25.3%. Variables considered as moderators for the medical and psychosocial outcomes turn out negligible. So subsequent results hold similarly for the three arms.

Web site visits were frequent in the first month (11 visits average per month) and declined continually to less than 3 at 12 months. The two interventions equally outperformed EUC significantly in day to day behavior (eating, fat intake, activity) but not in medication adherence. Since they are all self reported the precautions listed in Sect. 15.2.3.3 principally hold but regarding the scrutiny applied to select instruments hopefully keeps those biases small. Improvements were strongest at 4 months. The difference between experimental and control at 12 months was overshadowed by a hard to explain ongoing improvement in the EUC arm. Of course effects in the control arm always are candidates for Hawthorne type effects (Sect. 15.2.3.3.1). These should, however, materialize most in the beginning while here the effect is strongest in the end. Clinical outcomes differed amazingly little

9.6 Fostering Self Management

between the lumped Internet vs. the EUC condition, for 4 and 12 months. We find some ongoing improvements and some rebounds. Psychosocial outcomes rebound even more than clinical after 4 month.

This all holds equally for English and Spanish speaking patients, for patient with low literacy, for patients with the most cardiovascular risk factors, so at least do we have a mixture that helps with equity. Unfortunately the achievements are so minor and scattered such that we have to concede that keeping a disease at bay today whose debilitating consequences "feel" like ages away remains a challenge that we have not mastered yet. At the same time it is one of the challenges in the field of Consumer Health Informatics that deserves our attention because the prevalence, long term consequences, and cost are vast.

Take Home

A multifaceted Consumer Health Informatics service with emphasis on knowledge enhancement and personalized goal setting

- is superior to normal care plus static Internet information only initially and only for behavioral outcomes
- loses most of the 4 month improvements at later checkpoints
- equally underperforms for well served and underserved client subgroups

Face-to-face coaching on goal setting in the most intensive treatment arm does not improve outcomes.
Continuously decreasing visit frequencies may explain the lack of strong effects.

9.6.3 Exploring the Consequences of Smart Phone Ubiquity

Regarding the rebound after a few months that we see in various experimental services it appears a bit blue eyed to draw meaningful conclusions from a small experiment as the one from Norway by Nes and coworkers [15]. We still take a look because they introduce smart phones as core carrier technology. They equipped 11 type 2 diabetics (age 45–71 years, 7 male) with smart phones that carried a web portal with diary for blood glucose (automatically transferred), diet, medication, activities, feelings and evaluation of feedback they received regularly. Diary entries were due three times per day and were enforced through SMS reminders and repeat reminders that included a link that would open the personal portal. After 90 min an entry was prohibited. A human counselor delivered daily SMS feedback based on the ACT theory, i.e. CBT advanced towards values and value based mindful behavior. Participants received an introduction through one of the researchers and were given various instructional material about the equipment.

The researchers took pre and post data on the clinical variables monitored but were primarily interested in the assessment of the service through its users. Like

Glasgow (cf. Sect. 9.6.2) they used approved instruments for diabetes related quality of life and coping aspects and came up with own five point Likert scale questions about the concrete service.

General satisfaction was good, challenges of smart phone handling were mastered. Contents and diary design was positively approved, as well as the human conveyed daily feedback. Various details add to this impression but the most critical single results – no wonder – are diary response rates between 21 % and 97 % (average 68 %). Sixty-eight percent comes very close to the average that Glasgow could hold for *twelve* months. No wonder, because a very tense schedule (90 min delay means missed entry) supposedly raises problems for many active clients. While being in the best interest from the researchers perspective to collect timely data and to provide timely feedback on unfavorable situations it is a no brainer for many clients. Rather than managing they may feel like being overly managed.

Take Home

A smart phone based tight monitoring and psychologically founded feedback service achieves

- good usability and satisfaction ratings for the service design
- good ratings for the therapist generated SMS feedback, however,
- not more than two third of the three requested data uploads in time

A likely explanation is that ubiquity and convenience of the smart phone cannot outweigh the intrusiveness of requests to self report behaviors and emotions frequently.

9.7 Complications Management

Various complications are likely consequences of diabetes mellitus 2. They include conditions with little burden of disease upfront such as hyperlipidemia and others with debilitating signs such as diabetic foot, neuropathies, or retinopathies. Some investigations on the use of face-to-face or print media patient education programs on more stealthy complications, mainly for nephropaties, show some clinical improvements (cf. [26]), but Consumer Health Informatics services are lacking.

Consumer Health Informatics approaches have been tried for one of those complications with early "visible" signs, so to speak: for retinopathies. Their prevalence estimates range from 10 % to 60 % in patients with known diagnoses of diabetes mellitus 2. According to Joshi and Sivaswamy [7] early diagnosis and treatment can prevent visual loss and blindness. But the high volume of individuals requiring regular professional eye checks and the lack of qualified staff in India comes close to being prohibitive for serving all in need. Joshi and Sivaswamy [7] developed a Internet based service DrishtiCare that was tested as a telemedicine service (cf. Sect. 4.2) which contains some potential for future Consumer Health Informatics Level 2 deployment. In a setting with patients of three local primary eye hospitals in the authors' team offers decentralized eye screening, automated quality assessment, instructions to persons taking the fundus camera images in case of insufficient quality, and automated diagnosis from images when the quality is sufficient. Patients diagnosed with one of the complications of diabetes mellitus 2 are followed up upon by ophthalmologists.

In Joshi's and Sivaswamy's preliminary investigation the automatic classification of 119 patients' images delivered 27 diagnoses that required follow up. This share of 27/119 lies well in the middle of the epidemiologically known share of complications, but sensitivity or specificity are not reported. Before launching clinical routine such results are certainly required. Assuming that they can be provided DrishtiCare reduces the workload of ophthalmologists in central eye clinics to ~1/4 – a reduction in cost and effort that the authors list as a goal of their approach. However, DrishtiCare presently requires trained technicians in standby across the sites where patients show up for screening. A perspective worth checking is whether images can be taken in less controlled settings such as pharmacies without specially trained personnel. Up to date fundus cameras no longer need mydriasis i.e. the investigation is not the least intrusive any more. Quality is being checked anyway. So a lower effort telemedicine solution would be to let pharmacists, nurses, dieticians, etc. take the images. A Level 2 Consumer Health Informatics service would be patients taking the images themselves following instructions made lay person readable. Knowing that DrishtiCare quality control intercepts images of insufficient quality the medical risk would be small to non existent. The percentage of patients requiring in person consultation might increase somewhat, but patients would be empowered to take control of their eye vision.

9.8 Attenuation of Comorbidities

Depression is a common comorbidity of diabetes mellitus. According to a review by Roy and Lloyd [19] prevalence in diabetics is twice to three times as high as in persons without a known chronic disease. Prevalence estimates in diabetics range from 5% to 30% for diabetes mellitus 2 (compared to 4–28% in the matched control groups). Fewer studies exist for diabetes mellitus 1, but orders of magnitude are similar. Generally, up to one in three diabetics are in need of psychotherapy as well. For a respective Level 2 Consumer Health Informatics service the reader is referred Sect. 5.2.2.4.

> **Take Home**
> Consumer Health Informatics services for complications of diabetes mellitus 2 are rare and at an early stage.
> For some comorbidities services exist, such as depression.

9.9 Adding Level 3 Self Support

http://TuDiabetes.org is a patient self support portal devoted to the diverse forms of diabetes. It is offered world wide through the California based Diabetes Hands Foundation. Besides various articles in lay language with limited use of diabetes specific medical terms it offers diary and feedback, forums around devices, complications, management and coping. Therefore, it is broad in scope and not limited to one of the disease progression states organizing the sections before, although primary prevention plays a minor role. It has Level 2 virtual provider and Level 3 wisdom of patients characteristics.

http://TuDiabetes.org has demonstrated scientific value in an investigation on prevalence of mild and severe hypoglycemic events in insulin dependent patients. Weitzman and coworkers [29] report on probing members for self reports of events, plus various demographic and disease specific data. Absolute figures are not pertinent here because the majority of Tu.Diabetes.org members as well as study participants had diabetes forms other than diabetes mellitus 2. Valuable observations, though, are that among these long term "experienced" diabetics (median years since diagnosis 17 years) 5 % had not sensed hypoglycemic events. Of the whole sample, about 50 % self-reported more than 4 "lows" (mild hypoglycemias that the patients could control themselves) within the past two weeks. 30 % self-reported one or more severe events in the last year, where they needed third party assistance, often clinical care. The debilitating nature of insulin dependent diabetes becomes even clearer when reading that – based on self reports, therefore with all due caution concerning subject reflections biasing the result, cf. Sect. 15.2.3.3 – 15 % had car accidents or injuries, 37 % limited their driving activity, 23 % avoided sex, and other deprivations of a normal human life.

Browsing the forums of http://Tu.Diabetes.org demonstrates how readily questions and worries of some are picked up by others and how gratefully advice and encouragement from those who "have been there" (cf. Sect. 6.1) is taken up. The service displays a spirit of optimism and willingness to manage. This is also clearly reflected in [29]: Nearly all study participants permitted follow up contacts through the research team, more than 30 % permitted display of their HbA1c charts to be made visible to trusted others, and more than 40 % were interested in reviewing interim research results. What a contrast between this severely affected group of persons and the notorious psychology sophomores mentioned at the end of Sect. 12.2.2.1: They tested a family tree elicitation software, were offered their printed results – and all but one declined.

9.10 Concluding Remarks

9.10.1 Collateral Benefits

Behavioral achievements concerning diabetes mostly also reduce risk or burden of disease of hypertension, dyslipidemia and others. Therefore, whenever in this chapter behavioral or clinical improvements re diabetes mellitus 2 could be shown improvements re other facets of the metabolic syndrome are also likely.

9.10.2 New Options on the Horizon

While all services in previous sections by and large are a variation of the theme that the adult high risk person or diabetic provides reports of his state and receives advice, with community coaching and upholding perseverance here and there, two recent creative alternatives in support of juvenile diabetics demonstrate that the space is much wider. One is mySugr junior, the paired apps discussed in Sect. 5.3.4.4 where parents communicate with their children about eating and insulin dosing. The other is a virtual reality service that influences obese mothers to order less caloric food for their kindergarden age children [13].

9.10.3 Visitors and Responders: Research Questions

Mostly in the first section of this chapter we see success and failure next to each other. Success is often associated with community of different forms, real as well as virtual (cf. "Take Home" on pages 197, 199). Whether community actually helps, as suggested through [10, 16], or [29], or whether community functions as a source of novelty that satisfies curiosity and by that token fosters perseverance, as apparent from [9, 16], or [33] remains open in regard of the Consumer Health Informatics services presented here.

Throughout this chapter we see moderate if any effects that can doubtlessly be attributed to Consumer Health Informatics services. The reasons named to explain failures are manifold, one being that the required client effort is perceived as too high and integration into routines of daily living as insufficient, although it appears as technically solved in Sect. 9.6.3. We also see success rates lower at later stages of the metabolic syndrome. In earlier stages apparently high risk clients achieve weight reductions, irrespective of the design of a service (cf. "Take Home"s on pages 197 and 195). This applies to those that volunteer for the trials, which are a small share of the approached populations, as few as 58 of 4500 in [21]. Services that address diagnosed diabetics fail almost throughout. We have a moderate effect in [11] alone. Here, however, the effective Consumer Health Informatics service elements are hard to identify. The results are in accordance with the assumption that the mere fact of additional attention, i.e. Hawthorne or subject expectancy type effects (cf. Sect. 15.2.3.3) are sufficient to explain the better HbA1c control.

One hypothesis now is that further sophistication of the Consumer Health Informatics services is required to reach the diabetics in their later stages as efficiently as we reach the early stage high risk clients who have not yet been diagnosed. A competing hypothesis is that diabetics are a distinct sub-population which we cannot yet characterize but who are doomed to get the disease at some point in time – no matter whether they enroll and how they respond to our services – while others are protected upfront – equally no matter whether they enroll and how they respond. This is the hypothesis of a diabetic personality the exploration of which reaches far beyond Consumer Health Informatics. Presently it is not more than a hypothesis which finds, however, support through a clearly shown genetic component to the origin of diabetes mellitus 2 (cf. [30]).

References

1. Avdal EÜ, Kizilci S, Demirel N. The effects of web-based diabetes education on diabetes care results. A randomized control study. CIN: Comput Inform Nurs. 2011;29(TC2):TC29–34. doi: 10.1097/NCN.0b013e3182155318.
2. Carr LJ, Bartee RT, Dorozynski C, Broomfield JF, Smith ML, Smith DT. Internet-delivered behavior change program increases physical activity and improves cardiometabolic disease risk factors in sedentary adults: results of a randomized controlled trial. Prev Med. 2008;46:431–8. doi: 10.1016/j.ypmed.2007.12.005.
3. Carr LJ, Bartee RT, Dorozynski CM, Broomfield JF, Smith ML, Smith DT. Eight-month follow-up of physical activity and central adiposity: results from an internet-delivered randomized control trial intervention. J Phys Act Health. 2009;6(4):444.
4. Genz J, Haastert B, Müller H, Verheyen F, Cole D, Rathmann W, Nowotny B, Roden M, Giani G, Mielck A, Ohmann C, Icks A. Blood glucose testing and primary prevention of type 2 diabetes – evaluation of the effect of evidence-based patient information: a randomized controlled trial. Diabet Med. 2012;29:1011–20. doi: 10.1111/j.1464-5491.2011.03531.x.
5. Glasgow RE, Kurz D, King D, Dickman JM, Faber AJ, Halterman E, Woolley T, Toobert DJ, Strycker LA, Estabrooks PA, Osuna D, Ritzwoller D. Twelve-month outcomes of an internet-based diabetes self-management support program. Patient Educ Couns. 2012;87(1):81–92. doi: 10.1016/j.pec.2011.07.024.
6. Hunter CM, Peterson AL, Alvarez LM, Poston WC, Brundige AR, Haddock CK, Van Brunt DL, Foreyt JP. Weight management using the internet. A randomized controlled trial. Am J Prev Med. 2008;34(2):119–26. doi: 0.1016/j.amepre.2007.09.026.
7. Joshi GD, Sivaswamy J. DrishtiCare: a telescreening platform for diabetic retinopathy powered with fundus image analysis. J Diab Sci Technol. 2011;5(1):23–31.
8. Kim H-S, Song M-S. Technological intervention for obese patients with type 2 diabetes. Appl Nurs Res. 2008;21(84–9):84–9. doi: 10.1016/j.apnr.2007.01.007.
9. Kuwata S, Taniguchi S, Kato A, Inoue K, Yamamoto N, Ohkura T, Teramoto K, Shigemasa C, Kondoh H. Metaboli-Net: online groupware system providing counseling guidance for patients with metabolic syndrome. Stud Health Technol Inform. 2010;156:65–70. doi: 10.3233/978-1-60750-565-5-65.

10. Moore TJ, Alsabeeh N, Apovian CM, Murphy MC, Coffman GA, Cullum-Dugan D, Jenkins M, Cabral H. Weight, blood pressure, and dietary benefits after 12 months of a web-based nutrition education program (DASH for Health): longitudinal observational study. J Med Internet Res. 2008;10(4):52. doi: 10.2196/jmir.1114.
11. McMahon GT, Fonda SJ, Gomes HE, Alexis G, Conlin PR. A randomized comparison of online- and telephone- based care management with internet training alone in adult patients with poorly controlled type 2 diabetes. Diabetes Technol Ther. 2012;14(11):1060–7. doi: 10.1089/dia.2012.0137.
12. Moore TJ. e-mail Dec 2, 2013. Personal communication. Tom Moore is the initiator of DASH for Health.
13. McBride CM, Persky S, Wagner LK, Faith MS, Ward DS. Effects of providing personalized feedback of child's obesity risk on mothers' food choices using a virtual reality buffet. Int J Obes. 2013;37:1322–7. doi: 10.1038/ijo.2013.87.
14. Nielsen J, Mack R, editors. Usability inspection methods. New York: Wiley; 1994.
15. Nes AAG, van Dulmen S, Eide E, Finset A, ÓB Kristjánsdóttir, Synnove I, Eide H. The development and feasibility of a web-based intervention with diaries and situational feedback via smartphone to support self-management in patients with diabetes type 2. Diabetes Res Clin Pract. 2012;97:385–93. doi: 10.1016/j.diabres.2012.04.019.
16. Richardson CR, Buis LR, Janney AW, Goodrich DE, Sen A, Hess ML, Mehari KS, Fortlage LA, Resnick PJ, Zikmund-Fisher BJ, Strecher VJ, Piette JD. An online community improves adherence in an internet-mediated walking program. Part 1: results of a randomized controlled trial. J Med Internet Res. 2010;12(4):e71. doi: 10.2196/jmir.1338.
17. Rasu RS, Hunter CM, Peterson AL, Maruska HM, Foreyt JP. Economic evaluation of an internet-based weight management program. Am J Manag Care. 2010;16(4):e98–e104.
18. Resnick PJ, Janney AW, Buis LR, Richardson CR. An online community improves adherence in an internet-mediated walking program. Part 2: strategies for encouraging community participation. J Med Internet Res. 2010;12(4):e72. doi: 10.2196/jmir.1339.
19. Roy T, Lloyd CE. Epidemiology of depression and diabetes: a systematic review. J Affect Disord. 2012;143:S8–21. doi: 10.1016/S0165-0327(12)70004-6.
20. Sacks N, Cabral H, Kazis LE, Jarrett KM, Vetter D, Richmond R, Moore TJ. A web-based nutrition program reduces health care costs in employees with cardiac risk factors: before and after cost analysis. J Med Internet Res. 2009;11(4):e43. doi: 10.2196/jmir.1263.
21. Stewart T, Han H, Allen HR, Bathalon G, Ryan DH, Newton RL, Williamson DA. H.E.A.L.T.H.: efficacy of an internet/population-based behavioral weight management program for the U.S. army. J Diabetes Sci Technol. 2011;5(1):178–87.
22. Simon ACR, Holleman F, Gude WT, Hoekstra JBL, Peute LW, Jaspers MWM, Peek N. Safety and usability evaluation of a web-based insulin self-titration system for patients with type 2 diabetes mellitus. Artif Intell Med. 2013;59:23–31. doi: 10.1016/j.artmed.2013.04.009.
23. Sarkar U, Karter AJ, Liu JY, Moffet HH, Adler NE, Schillinger D. Hypoglycemia is more common among type 2 diabetes patients with limited health literacy: the diabetes study of northern California (DISTANCE). J Gen Intern Med. 2012;25(9).962–8. doi: 10.1007/s11606-010-1389-7.
24. Shea S, Kothari D, Teresi JA, Kong J, Eimicke JP, Lantigua RA, Palmas W, Weinstock RS. Social impact analysis of the effects of a telemedicine intervention to improve diabetes outcomes in an ethnically diverse, medically underserved population: findings from the IDEATel study. Am J Public Health. 2013;103:1888–94. doi: 10.2105/AJPH.2012.300909.
25. Shea S, Starren J, Weinstock RS, Knudson PE, Teresi J, Holmes D, Palmas W, Field L, Goland R, Tuck C, Hripcsak G, Capps L, Liss D. Columbia University's Informatics for Diabetes Education and Telemedicine (IDEATel) project: rationale and design. JAMIA. 2002; 9(1):49–62.
26. Thomas N, Bryar R. An evaluation of a self-management package for people with diabetes at risk of chronic kidney disease. Prim Health Care Res Dev. 2013;14:270–80. doi: 10.1017/S1463423612000588.

27. Tu HT. Surprising decline in consumers seeking health information. http://www.hschange.org/CONTENT/1260/1260.pdf, 2011. Tracking Report 26, Accessed 21 Sept 2013.
28. van Koningsbruggen GM, Das E. Don't derogate this message! Self-affirmation promotes online type 2 diabetes risk test taking. Psychol Health. 2009;24(6):635–49. doi: 10.1080/08870440802340156.
29. Weitzman ER, Kelemen S, Quinn M, Eggleston EM, Mandl KD. Participatory surveillance of hypoglycemia and harms in an online social network. JAMA Intern Med. 2013;173(5):345–51. doi: 10.1001/jamainternmed.2013.2512.
30. Weires MB, Tausch B, Haug PJ, Edwards CQ, Wetter T, Cannon-Albright LA. Familiality of diabetes mellitus. Exp Clin Endocrinol Diabetes. 2007;115:634–40. doi: 10.1055/s-2007-984443.
31. Yu CH, Bahniwal R, Laupacis A, Leung E, Orr MS, Straus SE. Systematic review and evaluation of web-accessible tools for management of diabetes and related cardiovascular risk factors by patients and healthcare providers. J Am Med Inform Assoc. 2012;19:514–22. doi: 10.1136/amiajnl-2011-000307.
32. Yu CH, Parsons J, Mamdani M, Lebovic G, Shah BR, Bhattacharyya O, Laupacis A, Straus SE. Designing and evaluating a web-based selfmanagement site for patients with type 2 diabetes – systematic website development and study protocol. BMC Med Inform Decis Mak. 2012;12(57). doi: 10.1186/1472-6947-12-57.
33. Yu CH, Parsons JA, Mandami M, Lebovic G, Hall S, Newton D, Shah BR, Bhattacharyya O, Laupacis A, Straus SE. A web-based intervention to support self-management of patients with type 2 diabetes mellitus: effect on self-efficacy, self-care and diabetes distress. BMC Med Inform Decis Mak. 2014;14:117. doi: 10.1186/s12911-014-0117-3.

Chapter 10
Basic Services Reach Out Towards Under-Served Populations

10.1 Introduction

Since mobile phone coverage is nearly universal and basic phones are equally available and present even in far out places, the technologies of short text messages (SMS) and Interactive Voice Response (IVR) suggest themselves as a low profile small investment carrier technology to exchange narrow band information in forms of reminders or alike with large populations. This chapter is driven through a technology which is specifically accessible and important for under-served vulnerable populations and their diverse medical problems.

10.2 Short Text Based Messages: SMS

The following section introduces the use, effectiveness, and important environmental factors for successful use of short text messages exchanged between Consumer Health Informatics service providers and clients. The subsequent shorter section covers Interactive Voice Responds (IVR)-based services. Finally, we address various environmental aspects to be considered for successful implementation of Consumer Health Informatics using mobile phones. The section is organized to start with simple unidirectional reminders or instructions stereotypically sent from providers to clients and ends with sophisticated extended dialogues in support of extended care or demanding decision-making.

Compared to services in most other chapters short text messages, subsequently called SMS, are rather basic technology. On the one hand this limits functionality in many ways. On the other hand SMS capable mobile phones are now so widely available that nearly everybody has access, even in the poorest Low and Middle Income Countries (LMIC) (see [8] for an overview). Smartphones are also gaining ground in LMIC. But neither bandwidth nor price tags of devices foster wide distribution in poorer countries as of now. Since this chapter is also devoted to Consumer Health Informatics for underprivileged populations we purposefully concentrate on classical mobile phones. Therefore, it should not come as a surprise that among the nearly 30 services used as teaching examples more than a half originate from poor, partially very poor countries. About half the examples from developed countries originate in the large scarcely populated Australia and Canada. Before we go into detail, there is another note about variation: as already analyzed in Sect. 1.6 for the whole discipline of Consumer Health Informatics the used articles are extremely widely spread; 34 cited articles are in are in 30 different journals.

> **Take Home**
> Mobile phones services and mobile phones, be they very basic in function, are widely and increasingly available not only in high income nations. Although severely limited in bandwidth and display they achieve health benefits. Low and middle income countries together with scarcely populated high income countries have a clear majority of projects.

10.2.1 Public Health Outreach

Public health campaigns used to employ and still employ paper pamphlets. These are, of course, limited in dissemination by the orders that can be printed, the places that can be used for distribution, address lists and budgets for mailing. The Internet has gained ground for dissemination. Both media share the advantage to easily include detailed explanations, imagery, and in the case of Internet sound and animation. Both media share the disadvantage of limited outreach to those in highest need: poorly educated underprivileged groups in rich countries and even more so the majority of populations in LMIC.

Of course, using SMS instead requires to confine oneself to very simple content, content that fits into 160 (in some countries only 128) characters which an individual SMS can carry.

Text to Change (TTC) is a service that a group from the Netherlands has brought to test in Uganda [2]. In the experiment of the years 2009 and 2010 described here TTC is used by more than 4000 employees of one rural and one urban company, most of whom had their mobile phone service from one of four providers. The idea of TTC is to increase population knowledge about important public health topics by appeal to the fun of a quiz competition with moderately sized incentives randomly given to a small percentage of the participants. To participate clients must answer short text questions following a simple syntax provided with the question (e.g. "BOTH 1", if two assertions made in the question part are both true).

The applied technology easily scales up: as long as network coverage is sufficient (which it apparently was not for some of the providers, since response rates varied dramatically between providers) prepared quiz texts can be automatically deployed to participants. Syntactically not matching replies can be handled through follow-up instructions, which ultimately led to mostly automatically analyzable replies. Participants then received immediate feedback whether their answer was correct, with some additional information.

It turned out that among the topics of a quiz (HIV, STI, malaria, tuberculosis, sexual behavior, medical male circumcision, and population demographics) clear winners in response rate were conditions that appeal to one's personal fate (HIV 79 %, malaria 78 %) while the lowest was with population demographics (37 %), the most abstract topic. It also turned out that incentives the size of a T-shirt, a mobile phone, or airtime worth one to 4 day daily incomes, or free HIV testing, influenced response: right after a publicized lottery win response rates were nearly three times as high than months later.

A deployment of services such as TTC to complete adult populations seems feasible although low socioeconomic status and illiteracy are likely factors to preclude some part of the population. The investigators did not test whether knowledge actually increased. Since quiz questions came at a rate of less than one every 2 weeks this cannot be taken for granted.

In a public health outreach investigation from Iran knowledge did increase, but behavioral consequences were hard to interpret. A project presented in [15] addresses a known public health concern: iodine deficiency which evidently affects brain development negatively in young children when present during mother's pregnancy or during the first years of life. The use of iodized salt in households is an approved method which, however, requires knowledge and awareness, including proper methods to store the salt.

In an RCT involving 205 women recruited in health centers in Tehran an experimental group received daily educational SMS for 6 weeks while both groups at onset received introductory information about the project and the importance of iodized salt. At an 8 weeks endpoint knowledge, awareness, behavior, and iodine metabolism were checked in both groups. The good news about the experimental group is that iodine urine concentration, concentration of iodine in salt samples taken from the homes, knowledge about medical and practical aspects of iodized salt, and attitudes towards its importance increased significantly, according to scrutinized tests and questionnaires. The apparently bad news is that there is nearly equally good news about the control group. It also improved on all outcomes although not significantly on attitude and urinary concentration of iodine. Therefore, effects between onset and endpoint are present in both experimental and control. In Sect. 15.2.3.3 possible explanations through biases for a group to show effects without receiving treatment are discussed.

The only significant differences when comparing the SMS and control groups were for knowledge resp. attitude: scores increased significantly ($P = 0.004$ resp $P = 0.027$) *more* in the SMS group than in the control group at the 8-week endpoint. This can be interpreted in different ways. The pessimistic way is to say that an increment in knowledge and attitude does not transform into equal increment in behavior, thereby challenging the cost effectiveness, i.e. the effort made to improve knowledge and attitudes by salvos of SMS sent over weeks in relation to the size of the medical outcome. In the light of the biases mentioned above an optimistic interpretation is that the effects in the control group are solely owed to the fact that an experiment is on and are transient while the knowledge collected and attitudes built in the SMS group last and lead to sustained improvement in behavior and metabolism. The latter is substantiated in a recent follow up investigation [16] of the same group from Tehran: insufficient urine iodine concentration correlated with low attitude scores highly significantly, independent of education level.

> **Take Home**
> Campaigns of series of SMSs to convey healthy attitudes show effects:
>
> **Healthy behavior quiz** Nearly 80 % answer the most appealing questions, with peaks after publicized lottery drawings.
> **Iodized salt utilization** An early increase in knowledge and attitudes eventually transforms into higher use.

10.2.2 Unidirectional Behavioral Stimuli

Many services use pretty simple SMS or series of SMS to remind clients of different aspects of their treatments. The largest share relates to appointments and compares effectiveness and sometimes cost-effectiveness of such services to no reminders or to phone reminders. The smaller but still large share relates to adherence to medications or other healthy behavior at home. Basics will be reported in this section and some farther ranging comparative assessments follow later in this chapter. With more than 25 pertinent publications in the last 4 years alone the reporting necessarily is highly selective and follows didactic considerations.

10.2.2.1 Visits

10.2.2.1.1 Reducing Missed Appointments

We first analyze two studies from developed countries where utilization of human resources resp. waste of scheduled and not used visits is the major outcome. Then we look at one from Australia and one from Tanzania where better delivery of care is the major target.

In a RCT with 6450 patients in an academic primary care clinic in Geneva, Switzerland automated SMS appointment reminders were compared with human telephone call reminders in a scrutinized non-inferiority design [21]. Non-attendance, defined as not showing and not rescheduling an appointment, was already moderate in rate. It could be lowered from 14 % before the intervention in the winter of 2010/2011 to 11.7 % in the SMS group and to 10.2 % in the telephone group. This difference in effect came out as SMS being statistically not inferior to telephone. The authors compare the absolute numbers of appointments that were *not* missed through the effect of the respective interventions, the very low costs for automatic SMS deployment and the notable costs for making phone calls. They come to the conclusion that although the absolute effect in the SMS group is smaller it is the only cost-effective intervention: Its net benefit amounts to €6410, compared to only €850 in the telephone group in half a year. Both amounts are not impressive but since a large subsample of the subjects of the study confirmed that it was helpful and not intrusive and since it can be implemented on a large scale easily it is worth a recommendation.

In a similar study from London, UK, researchers from a mental health clinic show larger effects in a less scrutinized research design [26]. In a pre-post analysis with nearly 2000 patients of a community mental health clinic in the years 2008 through 2010 they show that the number of missed appointments decreases from 36 % in the phase without alerts to the phase with alerts. Twenty-six percent respectively 27 % of appointments are now missed when two SMS alerts are sent seven and five resp 7 and 3 days ahead of a due appointment. The authors identified two other factors (gender, length of last inpatient admission) as also influencing the likelihood to miss an appointment. Of course other things may have changed between 2008 and 2010 which casts some doubt on the results when compared to a randomized controlled design. However, the effects are large enough to tolerate some imprecision. When extrapolating from the increased number of appointments attended in the two SMS patterns in the London clinic to the population of outpatient psychiatric patients in UK the authors arrive at yearly savings of $245 million.

The investigations from Geneva and London share the properties that simple SMS are automatically generated and sent and that the outcome targeted essentially is economic. The next two services are also based on simple SMS but now the outcomes are delivery of care.

10.2.2.1.2 Encouraging Utilization of Health Services

Regarding an epidemic of syphilis among Men having Sex with Men (MSM) the Melbourne (Australia) Sexual Health Centre tried to increase syphilis testing rates by making an online questionnaire about sexual behaviors and consequential automatic SMS reminders for MSM part of their standard procedures [32]. Those of their male patients who confirmed having sex with men were invited to the program and subsequently exerted choices whether and how they wanted to receive fully automated reminders for repeat syphilis testing. Choices included frequency and nearly half the patients opted for e-mail rather than SMS. In an opportunistic assignment of groups (the online questionnaire was not presented at certain times of the day and for some weeks the program didn't work because the computer had been stolen) it so happened that a certain part of the patients did not participate in the reminders program and served as a control group.

Patients in the experimental group had 3 times as many clinic visits than patients in the opportunistic control group. More important, their testing rate for syphilis was 67 % compared to 39.3 % in control. As a byproduct testing rates for various other STI also increased by factors of about two. Finally, the authors found double to triple detection rates of infections that might have gone unnoticed with incurred risks for patients and their partners as well. This was topped by a more than fourfold increase in detection of early highly contagious symptom-free syphilis.

Of course, the recruitment "methods" for control and reminder leave room for improvement and doubt. Mainly the variance in hours of the day when patients were or were not enrolled may have induced some selection bias. However, the size of the reminder (997) and control (1382) groups and the uniformity of results across different tests and infections suggest that there is indeed a medical effect which may multiply due to avoided infections of partners.

The last service discussed in this section has been tested in one of the poorest countries, Tanzania, and addresses one of their major health concerns: perinatal mortality. On one of Tanzania's islands investigators [13] set up a very pragmatic and realistic experiment to find out whether expecting mothers could be moved to seek skilled delivery attendance.

To combine the need for an experimental design with the logistic capabilities of the primary health centers they decided for block randomization where 12 centers and the mothers treated there were control while in 12 others the SMS intervention package was offered to all expecting mothers who could provide an own or close relation mobile phone number. No phones were given to any participants but rather were available resources purposefully used. Mothers did not even need to be literate as long as they could name a trusted relation who would receive the reminders on their part. Starting with their first antenatal visit they were registered and subsequently a web-based information system generated the calendar dates and the SMS content pertinent to the respective gestational age. Mothers in both control and experimental also received vouchers to call their health centers. Numerous SMS were actually sent in the experimental group, two per month until gestational age 36 weeks and thereafter two per week.

The dropout rate of the 2637 women assigned to either control or SMS was amazingly low: 2550 were followed until including the post study survey 6 weeks after giving birth. As a major apparently positive outcome the authors report 60 % births with skilled attendance in the SMS compared to 47 % in the control group. Since the absence of skilled birth attendants is among the major risk factors for perinatal casualties this appears like a large improvement. Unfortunately it turns out that it only materializes for mothers with urban residence. Here, even 82 % sought skilled attendance while mothers from rural places were stuck with a disenchanting 43 %, even less than the overall average in the control group. Sadly enough, in the poorest places on our planet delivering information is not enough. Programs are bound to fail if we cannot also offer logistics support.

> **Take Home**
>
> SMS that invite or remind to utilize health care resources show positive effects but also concerns:
>
> **Scheduled visits** Automated reminders increase appointments held or re-scheduled in time. Telephone calls achieve more although SMS are statistically not inferior. Since automated SMS scale up easily they are a clear choice.
>
> **Accepting professional help** SMS that encourage to seek needed medical help (STI testing in MSM, skilled birth attendant service) increase turnout significantly, with the worrying exception that mothers in distant places in poor countries such as Tanzania just do not make it to the regional health center.

10.2.2.2 Medication and Behavior

While all services introduced so far require that the patient moves, be it to the clinic next door or to a faraway health center, we now discuss one simple but highly successful service that reaches patients at their home and motivates for healthy behavior at home. Mostly this means drug adherence but there are also examples such as to encourage abstinence after male circumcision [17] or other behaviors not related to pharmaceuticals.

In a short term randomized controlled trial conducted in three medical centers in Taiwan the effect of medication reminders on rate of delayed and rate of missed medications was investigated [7]. Patients who reported having missed medications in the past and were receiving a new medication for at least 7 days were eligible. If consenting they were randomized at a two to one ratio to either experimental or control. Experimental arm subjects received SMSs that were automatically generated from prescription data in the health information system. On the first of 7 days the SMS was a detailed instruction which comprised the visit where the prescription was received, the brand names, doses and instructions how to apply. On all subsequent days it was just a reminder. Such SMS were send to patients in experimental for each prescription they had received. Patients in the control arm just got the prescription. Primary outcomes were percentages of delayed and missed medications. Before the first day and on the eighth day behaviors were investigated through structured telephone interviews. The first interview also covered various demographics which did not show any major differences between control and experimental arms and also established baselines as follows: 80.2 % respectively 84.7 % in control versus intervention arms reported having delayed medications in the past. 43.7 % versus 46.1 % in control versus intervention remembered that they had missed medications before. In the eighth day interview control and intervention arm reported reduction in both delayed and missed medications. Compared to the baseline values delayed doses decreased by 46.4 % versus 78.8 % for control and intervention and missed doses decreased by 61.1 % versus 90.1 %.

The large reductions in the control arm indicate strong biases as discussed in Sect. 15.2.3.3. However, the differences between the two arms are large enough and the controlled design and high turnout at post-test suggest that the SMS actually have an effect. An open question, not only in this investigation, is whether such effects sustain with ongoing routine SMS being sent, whether this depends on the content and logistics of the SMS, or whether clients develop routines of better medication adherence independently of ongoing SMS.

> **Take Home**
> A well considered strategy of educational and reminder SMSs can significantly increase adherence to a new medication in patients with chronic condition and a history of low adherence.

10.2.3 Client Initiated Request Processing

While the services presented so far are provider initiated, be it public health authorities outreaching to the general public or health care providers encouraging their patients for adherent behaviors we now come to services that hold themselves available for clients to take the initiative and that deliver personalized information in response.

An initiative of the Planned Parenthood Federation of America for teens and young adults started offering a service "designed to provide immediate answers to urgent sexual and reproductive health questions" [5, p. 1]. The service comes in an instant messaging (IM) and a text messaging (SMS) variant which share most of the content and dynamics. Concretely, interested clients can initiate the IM from the Federation's website (http://www.plannedparenthood.org/) or the SMS service through sending a text message to the service's mobile number. The service is manually operated daytime hours and far into the night all days of the week. Trained counselors read the request and select – and when need be modify – one or more chunks of text from a database of approximately 900 templates. They are prepared to answer medical questions about abortion, emergency contraception, pregnancy testing, STI testing and others, but also assist in identifying clinics and even making appointments. To make the service known it was advertised for on the homepage of the Federation and through ads adjacent to the TV shows "16 and Pregnant" and "Teen Mom".

An investigation of 1 year of use of the service (September 2010 until August 2011) tried to collect demographic and utilization data. For this purpose counselors collected basic data and degree of feeling worried before the service (pretest), then responded to the client's request, and then asked a few more questions about remaining worries and satisfaction with the service (post-test). Being taken to pretest and post-test survey collection was not compulsory and varied between IM and

SMS. Therefore, selection biases may be present and all statistical analysis has to be regarded with some caution. However, some results stand out. The first is the sheer number of 32,589 conversations recorded in the United States with about 50 million persons in the age groups addressed through the service. This means that about one out of 1700 young people not only felt the urge but found the place to be helped immediately and discreetly in a problem of sexual and reproductive health. We can also note that by and large the percentage of very worried clients did not essentially decrease from pretest to post-test. The percentage of female users (nearly 90 %) by far outperforms the gender imbalance that is anyway present in most health-related topics and searches. But since it is mostly the girls who have to handle the consequences of unplanned sexual intercourse we need not wonder, not to mention the TV series where the ads were placed. Finally, traditionally underserved ethnicities (Latino/Hispanic, Black) used the services over-proportionally compared to their share of the US population. Latino/Hispanics also profited over-proportionally from the SMS branch of the service i.e. compensated for their still lower access to the Internet.

The Mobile for Reproductive Health (m4RH) program in Kenya addresses an adjacent health management problem. It advises clients on contraceptive methods. Supported through some charities it was built to provide messages in basic language about nine different contraceptive methods without charging fees. Clients can select the method they want information about through a simple numerical key and then receive 2–3 concise messages. m4RH also has a searchable database to locate clinics. The service was made known through ads in a small number of clinics of two chains and in a radio campaign where family planning was promoted to young people.

During the pilot phase from January 2010 to June 2011 investigators solicited data from 4817 unique users [29]. With an average of 9 months after the initial query clients were asked through a simple battery of three SMSes to be answered for their age, gender, and whether they had changed their contraceptive method. Turnout for the demographic questions was order of magnitude 1/4 whereas nearly 1/2 for the change question. The male to female ratio was around 1/3 with higher percentage of male respondents in the younger age groups. The clear majority in age (60%) was between 20 and 29. In telephone interviews with 26 of the 4817 participants researchers tried to gain a deeper understanding of the effects and of the user satisfaction. Basically, the clear and simple language and anonymity were widely appraised. The quotes clearly demonstrated learning effects. Changes in behavior likely also happened: a clear majority of those who answered the respective SMS question actually confirmed to change. Those that gave more detail in addition to their standardized yes or no answer provided a clear picture how they had been affected by what they had learned.

Both services have a lot in common. They enter a niche where quality advice is needed, sometimes urgently and existentially, but where societal habits and taboos keep clients from seeking it from otherwise trusted parties. These are needs mostly of a generation that is familiar with the used technology. The fact that, when the client requests, both services offer the whole spectrum from matter of fact medical knowledge to clinic referral makes them highly convenient. No wonder that they are both still up and running although we have no objective evidence – only client self reports – that they have an effect and although the Planned Parenthood service must be manually staffed and hence sustainability depends on continuous flow of sufficient funding.

Take Home

Consumer Health Informatics services where advice can be collected instantly about sexual health, contraception and abortion achieve high numbers of requests and high satisfaction.

Short term help Through SMS to a "helpline" operated 7 days a week far into the night adolescents in the USA can get pertinent information about medical procedures but also logistics information about providers as reply SMS manually composed from canned text. The service is mostly used by females.

Long term planning In Kenya a similar helpline rather addresses planned contraception and advises all age groups and males and females about methods and their pros and cons.

Anonymity and convenience are success factors in this sensitive domain.

10.2.4 Closed Loop Services

We now come to more complex services where sophistication may lie in different places. The service presented next [25] is part of a closed loop vaccination registry process. It was established in clinics in New York (NY) where primarily minority mothers bring their children for checkups. Eighty-eight percent were publicly insured, 58 % Spanish-speaking.

For the winter season 2010–2011 the authors set up a program to send mothers whose children had not yet been vaccinated for influenza, SMS information of different kinds, carefully adapted to their individual situation. Early in the season it started with three educational SMS about vaccine safety and the risks of influenza, where the transmitted text was adapted to the age of the child or adolescent. Those mothers, where a vaccination had not been recorded in the registry, received another SMS later in the season including Saturday clinic dates where the timing of SMS tried to balance workload in the clinics; and the same again in January for as yet not vaccinated children. Altogether the mother would receive up to five SMS, each tailored to her personal situation and the logistic and calendar givens. Texts were available in English or Spanish, were automatically first sent in the language known about the mother from her EHR and she could change any time.

In an RCT with 7574 children the influenza vaccination rate could be increased from 39.9 % to 43.6 %. Not an amazing effect but it still means that some more than 100 anyway vulnerable children received appropriate protection that would not without the service. Another clear advantage is that the service can be offered again year-by-year with minimal effort and maintenance. Only educational material may need revision when major new insights affect vaccination safety or effectiveness and Saturday clinic schedules must be renewed. This low effort pragmatic approach is a strength that the authors also note, compared to more sophisticated more human resource intensive interventions.

> **Take Home**
> Am automated personalized scalable SMS launch plan to encourage mother for influenza vaccinations of their minors achieves increased vaccination rates through repeated follow up on non-responders and including place and opening hours information.

10.2.5 Enhancing Complex Therapies

When the medical problem is complex a complex therapy concept may be required. Ybarra and coworkers [31] present such a service in the complex field of addictions, concretely, smoking cessation. Drawing on the wealth of prior research attempts grounded in CBT, self-efficacy theory, relapse prevention, as well as empirical results about the time course and critical days in the typical career of a person wanting to quit smoking they build a complex intervention, SMS Turkey, mostly based on automated SMS. Clients who declare that they want to quit smoking receive messages that pertain to their stage in the quitting process. Before the declared quit day they are encouraged through five messages per day to clarify their reasons to quit for themselves. In the early phases of quitting common difficulties and discomforts are discussed through five or more messages per day while later the dangers of relapse are a major topic in a continually decreasing number of messages per day. In addition to this automatic part clients are asked on the most critical days known to be the second and the seventh day whether they are still smoke-free. Those who are failing are manually redirected to other content that tries to reinforce the intention of quitting.

SMS Turkey demonstrates that rather complex therapy regimes can be implemented nearly fully automated. In a RCT with 151 participants it shows again, however, how hard the challenge of smoking cessation actually is. Judging by the outcome measures of self-reported abstinence at a 3 month endpoint verified through carbon monoxide readings the experimental arm was not superior to a control arm who only received flyers with equal content as the SMS intervention arm. Only in two subgroups, females and light smokers, quit rates were significantly higher in the SMS arm and with 30 % in the order of magnitude that human conveyed therapies achieve. Therefore, SMS-based automated services are not the magic bullet where therapies conveyed in person also mostly fail.

10.2.6 Delivery of Test Results

While everything so far was either stereotypical or personalized to groups text messaging can obviously also be used to convey individual messages such as personal lab test results. In a survey with 500 clients of the Sydney Sexual Health Centre (SSHC) [14] polled participants as to their preferences whether they wanted results of STI and HIV testing through SMS, e-mail, a secure Internet site, or personally conveyed, which could be face to face or by telephone. For every outcome (HIV, STI; positive or negative) the participants were encouraged but not enforced to vote for one preferred communication mode. From an amazing 95 % respondents the authors found high percentages actually voting unanimously. Various subtle differences between outcomes or subgroups will not be discussed here. However, a few outstanding preferences respective objections became visible. Only 5 % preferred a secure Internet site, irrespective of the outcome. When tested negative, participants shared about equally around 1/3 between SMS, phone call and in-person. Assuming they were tested positive, however, participants would prefer in-person, at 40 % with STI and 56 % with HIV. Older participants were less likely to prefer SMS, and Men having Sex with Men (MSM) also clearly preferred in-person communication of a positive HIV finding.

What can be learnt from this investigation is that nothing can be learnt, it may appear. This is actually true if one is out for clear cut rules without exception. What we can learn, however, is threefold: First, providers of Consumer Health Informatics services should be aware that the trust in Internet security is too low for such delicate information as HIV or STI test results. Second, clients will want to have choices. Third, when offering the choice of a preferred channel a bulk of the negative test results can be automatically delivered to the client's satisfaction while personal contact is clearly preferred when there seems to be an infection. This is not really surprising because a positive test result requires follow-up anyway. The results as a whole, however, encourage efficient and presumably cost-effective and human resource saving transmission of negative results to a clear majority in populations like the clients at the SSHC.

Take Home

When SMS Consumer Health Informatics services are tried for complex or embarrassing conditions miracles cannot be expected and sensitivity for privacy issues must be high, allowing clients to make differentiated choices about channels which they trust.

10.3 Interactive Voice Response: IVR

Interactive Voice Response (IVR) is the branch of Human Computer Interaction where voice or telephone keypad serve as input and voice as output modality. On the client side it shares with SMS that the required technology and equipment is nearly ubiquitous and that the variability and bandwidth of information that can be conveyed is narrow. On the provider side voice-recognition technology is required for more convenient interaction, which, however requires more technical sophistication, is more error prone, and, consequently, fewer IVR than SMS based services presently exist.

10.3.1 Public Health Outreach

Two investigations describe IVR outreach to citizens eligible for colorectal cancer screening who had not had screening before [1, 12]. They are similar in many respects such that lessons can be learned from the differences. Both are offered by major health plans of their respective regions (Group Health® in Washington State, subsequently "Group Health", and Kaiser Permanente® Colorado, subsequently "Kaiser") which means that the targeted populations are as similar as populations from two distinct United States can be in terms of ethnicity, education, and wealth. The interventions targeted similar age groups (50s to lower 80s) and excluded according to similar criteria such as active colorectal cancer and various comorbidities; Kaiser also excluded patients known to be high risks due to family history. Both services encouraged for a test kit to be used at home and for colonoscopy, in accordance with the respective US guideline and let their clients choose the screening modality. Primary outcome in both investigations was whether some kind of screening test was taken within half a year. Both investigations invited all eligible individuals (approximately 8000 versus 50,000) to enroll and their 5 min long IVR dialogs both included education about the screening, the opportunity to order a test kit; Group Health also had recorded educational material about barriers to screening available for clients addressing such in the IVR call.

The two services differed in convenience of the testing, in perseverance of the outreach, and in achieved testing rates. Additionally, Kaiser provided distinction in screening rates among subpopulations.

Difference in convenience means that Group Health requested clients to personally deliver the test kit to their physician's office and that they used an older test kit FOBT (fecal occult blood test) which consists of three individual specimens while Kaiser supplied the FIT (fecal immunochemical test) one specimen kit and accepted mail return of the kit.

At Group Health the IVR call stood alone and a test kit was only mailed upon client request within the call. At Kaiser the IVR call was the first of several steps, depending on clients' behaviors. A test kit was mailed within 2 weeks if ordered and within 6 weeks if not ordered. Clients with test kits not mailed in within 4 weeks of delivery received a letter. In case of a positive test result Kaiser enacted active follow-up towards colonoscopy which is, however, beyond the primary outcome discussed here.

At Group Health appr 34 % initiated and appr. 20 % finished the IVR call half of whom underwent screening. At Kaiser 17 % finished the IVR call and than one half (7 %) screened through FIT sent back *before* Kaiser's follow up mailing began. Including all elements of followup, however, Kaiser finally achieved 45 % screening. The investigations applied different study designs and according to their respective statistical models the achieved screening rates of 10 % (Group Health) resp 45 % (Kaiser) demonstrate significant increases compared to usual care.

Kaiser's data also show low and high responders. Screening rates were significantly lower in members below 65 years of age, African Americans, Hispanics, active smokers, and persons with high BMI. A truism proves true once again: hard to reach target groups are hard to reach.

Here two other apparent truism also prove true: that more helps more and that convenience helps. Kaiser's perseverant package for the Colorado populations ends up at 45 % screening while Group Health's one IVR call impulse does not achieve more than 10 % for the structurally very similar Washington State population. We see kind of a dose response behavior. The convenience factor is confirmed in many other Consumer Health Informatics investigations.

Take Home

In comparison of two outreach programs where IVR calls were launched to similar populations the following factors let one service outperform the other by a factor of more than four in participation in colorectal cancer screening.

Information Medical *plus* how to master barriers in the process
Perseverance Depending on first response follow up calls and mailings
Convenience Return mail processing of the test kit (rather than required visit)
Logistics In case of positive test suggestions for follow up

At the same time notoriously hard to reach target groups (African Americans and Hispanics, smokers, overweight persons) underperform here as well.

10.3.2 Enhancing Complex Therapies

The group around John D Piette at the University of Michigan has collected quite some experience in offering IVR-based services to mostly elder, often lower social status patients who are being treated for chronic conditions, concretely diabetes, hypertension, heart failure, cancer, or depression. The services are all characterized through robust basic touch-tone or spoken yes/no answer based patient input and recorded voice advice personalized to the patient's symptoms, complaints, with some decision logic controlling the voice messages exchanged with the client. IVR calls are typically launched once a week automatically (with different repeat schemes in case of failed calls) at times designated as convenient by the patients. Typically, 6–12 week long experiments were monitored as to adherence to answering and completing IVR calls and to health and behavioral effects. All services were initiated through some kind of primary care medical service where eligible patients were encouraged to enroll. In some of the experiments primary care physicians received e-mail or fax alerts when the IVR calls revealed a condition that required urgent attention. Patients with diabetes or depression were encouraged to involve an informal caregiver (family or friend) who would then also receive an account of the patient's state and suggestions how he could be supportive. Therefore, although being basic in voice technology the Consumer Health Informatics services provided quite some sophistication in terms of integrating with the patient's home and medical environment.

From the richness of results we can only report a small part here. Originally in American English the service [22] was translated into Spanish for use in Honduras and Mexico, was double checked for translation accuracy, as well as for cultural fit by local health professionals and was well accepted in the Latin American countries. Mostly, telephone surveys after the end of the intervention were run and the majority of users in all settings attested ease-of-use and helpfulness. In all experiments IVR completion rates (calls where clients did not prematurely terminate an ongoing "conversation") started between upper 70 % (diabetes, depression) and lower 90 %. Completion rates decayed moderately in other conditions and remained constant for cardiac failure, with incidental differences in slope, such that we do not really know whether the services, when offered routinely for indefinite periods of time, will preserve their attraction. One consistently promoting factor is the involvement of informal caregivers to the patient's choice. Some other information on intensity of the intervention and long term use can be derived from Sect. 10.4.3.

> **Take Home**
> IVR based coaching can motivate usually under-served patient groups with chronic conditions in the USA and low income countries to actively manage their health. Effects improve when local health care providers and family or friends are involved in the design of the services.

10.3.3 Cognitive Assessment

Regarding the requests made in Sect. 12.4 about safeguarding clients capabilities to cooperate in Consumer Health Informatics services we find a low key-low effort partial solution to cognitive assessment of elderly citizens through automated IVR conveyed services [3].

10.4 A Closer Look at Effectivity

10.4.1 Intervention vs. Other Factors

We look at two investigations of effectiveness of SMS to foster healthy behavior where two co-factors cannot be neglected: Money and habits.

Wakadha et al. [30] attempt to achieve high vaccination rates by sending SMS reminders to designated cell phones (the mother's or some close relation's) 3 days before and on the day of a due pentagram vaccination. For that part of the mothers where no technological or logistic problem interfered 90 % coverage for the first and 86 % for the second vaccinations was achieved, certainly a high value in rural Kenya, although values for direct comparisons are not available. However, mothers received incentives worth a 1 day income in that region when they presented their babies for the vaccinations. Since no investigations have been made so far that compare an SMS-based motivational campaign with and without incentives we cannot know for sure which of the two was the major therapeutic agent.

Another investigation from rural Kenya, meant as clinical trial of SMS effectiveness, rather was successful as an epidemiological study of risk factors [17]. In the randomized controlled trial with 1200 males having undergone male circumcision the experimental group received SMS daily in the first week and weekly in the subsequent five postsurgical weeks reminding them not to resume sex before 6 weeks, to foster good wound healing and avoid the excess risks of HIV transmission. At the end of 6 weeks all participants were asked whether they had resumed sex prematurely.

Control and SMS group did not differ significantly in that primary outcome. However, demographic and behavioral subgroups clearly stood out compared to the rest of the population as to early resumption. In the sequence of significance of the subgroups as factors low education was the absolutely strongest, next and about equally strong were being married, living with a partner or having had more than one sexual partner in the month before the surgery. A sober insight into how hard it is to break strong habits and even more sober what a health hazard bad education still is.

> **Take Home**
> Causal effects of Consumer Health Informatics intervention are hard to show when other strong factors are present, such as incentives for desired behaviors or differences in education and habits.

10.4.2 Behavioral vs. Clinical Effect

In a typical medication adherence Consumer Health Informatics service (cf. Sect. 10.2.2) for patients with asthma a group from Denmark [28] tests in an experiment of four plus 8 weeks whether one simple reminder SMS per day to take a morning and a nighttime dosage of inhaled corticosteroid affects the patients.

10.4 A Closer Look at Effectivity

Participants were treated as usual in the first 4 weeks and then randomized. Primary outcome was dosages taken which was checked every 4 weeks where both experimental (SMS) and control arms came for a clinical checkup. The device to dispense the aerosol allows to precisely determine how many dosages have been taken such that the only factor of insecurity is that malevolent patients vaporize their medicine into the air. A second measure of medication adherence was taken in parallel: patients received a refill prescription for weeks 9–12 at the 4-week checkpoint. Percentage of refills claimed and time lag between expected exhaustion of the old prescription to claiming the new one were recorded. Clinical outcome was also measured in all relevant dimensions (airway inflammation, lung function, reactivity to airway constricting substances, general and specific allergic level).

In a small RCT with 26 subjects the authors clearly show that the adherence in the experimental arm increases strongly and decreases as strongly in the control arm, with the arms ending at 81.5 % (SMS) vs. 70.1 % (control). This behavioral effect is highly significant and one would expect that the SMS arm fares clearly, maybe significantly better clinically. But it does not. The two arms do not differ in any one clinical outcome measure at the end of the 12 week interval.

The explanation of this discrepancy that comes to mind first is a Shakespearean "Much ado about nothing": Leave the SMS service away and everything is fine. However, a closer look suggests that there may be some value to it anyway. First, the short intervals between clinical checkups for both control and experimental groups certainly causes some kind of subject reflection effect, most likely a Hawthorne or social desirability effect: control group participants react to the experimental setting and try to behave well in the awareness that their behavior will be evaluated (Sects. 15.2.3.3.1 or 15.2.3.3.2). If this is true, adherence in the real world, without an intervention, can be much lower than the present control arm figures suggest. Second, the decrease in adherence in the control arm from 84.2 % to 70.1 % in 8 weeks, i.e. nearly 2 % per week is alarming. We do not see a clinical difference between 84.2 % and 70.1 % because therapeutic schemas have some safety margin which tolerates, as it appears in this trial, underdosing of 30 %. The question is what is the critical threshold of underdosing that adherence should not fall short of. Maybe another 10 weeks and adherence approaching 50 % clinical effects would show and turn dramatic, since asthma still is a severe disease and needs regular treatment.

Shakespeare hits again in another medication adherence Consumer Health Informatics service for patients after routine cardiac surgery. A group in Canada [27] has set up and investigated an IVR service that makes IVR calls to patients weekly, later biweekly and than four weekly to check on various aspects of medication and for conditions that may require in person telephone follow-up or new hospitalization. In a RCT with 331 patients the control arm receives in person calls on days three and ten after discharge. In a telephone survey after 6 months in both experimental and control medication adherence, medical events in retrospect, and in the case of the IVR arm satisfaction with the service were collected. Example medication questions are whether refills were collected, whether there were problems in administering medications, adverse effects, problems with their primary care physician concerning continuation of medication etc. Patients could also request recorded text information about medications to be played to them during the automated call. Starting and recording the calls was fully automatic, including up to two repeats when the first call was not successful; client answers could be yes or no and were analyzed by basic voice-recognition.

The investigators recorded adherence with the IVR service, adherence with the medication, and events. The figures are disenchanting. Only 15 % of the calls concluded satisfactorily automatically. Thirty-one percent required nurse callbacks to clarify some issue the patient had brought up. Fifty-four percent were unsuccessful. I.e. by and large the "IVR dosage" was about half the planned one. Most frequently named reasons for callbacks were involvement of other providers and changes in medication (together 562 callbacks), incisive events (emergency department or hospital readmission) and could-be events (suspected adverse medication events) followed with 72 and 69 nominations. Adherence with the medication differed highly significantly, being 74.5 % in the experimental and 38.5 % in the control arm, according to patient memories. Subject reflections may also play a role here with some likelihood in the experimental arm to over-report, but since an almost twofold over-reporting in the experimental arm does not seem plausible, medication adherence likely differed. ER visits and hospitalizations, however, did not differ. I.e. such hard patient outcomes as events where memory can be trusted and self reports could be verified independently if severe biases were suspected were equal in both arms although the control group only took about one third or their medications.

Therefore, to justify the human effort of the about 670 calls to 164 patients in the IVR arm, more data to substantiate the necessity are required. The service might achieve equal effects which much fewer calls, generally or personalized to patients' risks (cf. Sect. 10.4.3). It might also be worth to offer more of the routine transactions (use of medications, how to get results) that now require callback, through automated answers such that human effort can concentrate on client answers that are either very unclear or point to critical developments.

Take Home

Associating clinical outcomes with Consumer Health Informatics service induced behavioral changes can be challenging.

- The confusing momentary observation that a control arm with 70 % asthma therapy adherence has equal clinical outcome as the SMS intervention arm with 80 % tempts to interpret that the service advises to overdose. A closer look at the decay in adherence in the control arm rather suggests that patients there are on the verge of a clinically relevant under-dosage.
- The confusing observation that post-surgical patients who were offered intensive IVR coaching did not differ from a control arm in clinical outcomes (clinical and medication events) tempts to be interpreted as not warranting the necessary high human effort in follow up. A closer look at the logging of IVR initiated contact attempts shows that a large part either did not reach the client or involved human effort that could be automated.

10.4.3 Size and Format of the Intervention Effort

Some investigations address the question of "dosage": the frequency of messages or calls and the extent of the individual message or call. A prevailing lesson from these investigations is that much does not necessarily effect much.

A first glimpse at an investigation in New York City [9] demonstrates the limited effect of a massive educational campaign of a family planning center with a population where Caucasians were the minority (29 %). In a randomized comparison with an arm that had access to the usual educational material of the center the experimental arm received one SMS per day for half a year each carrying some piece of information of the mechanisms, risks, benefits etc. of oral contraceptive methods. All 659 participants underwent a knowledge test before and after the 6 months.

The experimental arm fared significantly better than the control arm. However, both arms improved: from a baseline of 22.8 correct answers control reached 23.7 and experimental 25.5, of a maximum of 41. Therefore, a battery of 180 messages achieved less than two more correct answers than the usual flow of information that the control arm had access to. For more than one third of the questions (($41 - 15.5)/41$) on average it failed to teach the knowledge for answering correctly. This clearly raises several question. One is about a reasonable effort – effect relation. Therefore, we subsequently look at means to keep the effort at a reasonable level. It also raises the question of interest and attention: If subjects did not feel affected by the topic they were not motivated to memorize the message content, as we can also see in the quiz described in Sect. 10.2.1. Third, SMS is too inferior to all kinds of graphical or animated material to illustrate such knowledge.

In a RCT for the potential of SMS to motivate HIV-positive individuals in Kenya [19] to ART adherence compare a control arm to two times two SMS sending schemes: short or long, and daily or weekly, for a period of 48 weeks. Short is not just short; it is the harsh reminder "This is your reminder". Long is not just longer but purposefully motivational ("... we care about you"). Here the content and style turns out not to be the strongest factor but in other investigations format does matter [4].

ART adherence was measured through servings taken from a Medical Event Monitoring System (MEMS) that registers every opening of a dispenser bottle and that was read out at monthly checks at the rural health center conducting the trial where also control arm patients were requested to go.

Targeted outcomes were the binary variables >90 % adherence and no 48 hours interval without doses throughout 48 weeks. The weekly reminder arms when lumped together were significantly superior to control regarding both outcomes. This is the more noteworthy because the control group was not just usual care: the monthly checkups where MEMS readings were taken may have had both a reminder and a social desirability effect such that the true size of the effect of the weekly reminders is even larger. More important, however, is the significant inferiority of control against the merged two weekly message arms. To remind of medications to be administered daily, this suggests, weekly messages achieve more than daily messages.

Two other aspects should be mentioned. Participants could select between English and two local languages for their messages. When showing for a checkup appointment participants in the control arm and all experimental arms received fresh airtime worth 1 US$ as an incentive. Here the monetary stimulus is offered all participants equally. In Sect. 10.3.1 we see that different incentives may lead to different outcomes.

In a secondary evaluation of data collected from IVR based interventions in the fields of diabetes and depression Piette and coworkers [18, 23] show that "the technical feasibility of gathering high frequency health data ... in some instances exceeds the clinical benefit" [23, p. 2]. Drawing on thousands of completed IVR recordings they address questions about the predictability of item values from other item values.

(1) Within one IVR call: Can the answer to some item be predicted from answers to other items?
(2) Across weekly IVR calls: Can the answer for an item at the sixth week be predicted from answers in the immediately preceding 5 weeks?
(3) Across less frequent IVR calls (2-weekly, 3-or-4-weekly): How much does the prediction accuracy decrease compared to weekly?

A large number of individual findings indicate that indeed high accuracy prediction is possible and consequently some items need not be asked at short intervals or not even asked at all. While correlation between different items as in (1) is moderate, prediction from earlier values of the same item is nearly equally good in (2) and (3) for some and moderate for some other items. Statistical procedures the details of which go beyond the scope of this volume suggest the following approach and conclusions.

From longitudinal data individual likelihoods for the problem areas are calculated. Where these are low (here set to $\leq 5\%$) the prediction accuracy from weekly and less frequent prior data is calculated. For diabetes and depression it turns out that for some items 85% or more of upcoming problems can be detected while reducing IVR call frequency to between 60% and 90%. This typically holds for broad general items such as general health (depression and diabetes) and for habits such as medication adherence. In the case of diabetes hyperglycemic symptoms and foot checking adherence can also be predicted, as can be depressive feelings in depression. Predictive power is less for days in bed (both conditions), hypoglycemic events and hypo- or hyperglycemic glucose self measurement readings. Explanations can be sought why some items are better versus less predictable. One may suspect that such incisive events as hypoglycemias will not be forgotten and their variation maps into unpredictability while items pertaining to the unspectacular daily chores are subjectively felt the same throughout. More important than such speculation, however, is that with some amount of data, some effort and analytic sophistication patients can be assigned their personal likelihoods for problem areas and IVR call

10.5 Expanding the Scope

intervals can be adapted to individual needs such that Consumer Health Informatics services "use patient contact time more efficiently for promoting behavior change or attending to comorbidities" [18, p. 517]. This is certainly worth the effort when services are meant to be offered for years. In the light of Chaps. 8 and 12 it finds its limits where items cover fast deteriorating, maybe life threatening problems.

In another outreach investigation [4] to motivate cell phone service subscribers in South Africa to seek HIV testing mixed effects of dosage and content seem to be present. In a RCT with 2533 citizens control arm participants were just enrolled and equally and synchronously as the experimental arm participants received one message encouraging to test and 3 weeks later a request to report whether they had or had not tested. Meanwhile the experimental arms received three messages in 9 days or ten messages in 4 weeks, informational or motivational of style. Ten motivational messages achieved the only significantly higher testing rate than control. The authors assume a sub-threshold effect size with three messages but also concede that the self reported "tested: yes/no" may be affected by a social desirability effect. But the sample is large enough, the setting naturalistic and anonymous enough and the likelihood of a false positive result so low ($p < 0.0036$) that content and dosage as factors must be taken into account. The stronger effect of motivational material is in accordance with results discussed in Sect. 3.2.2.

Take Home

The relation between amount and effect of SMS/IVR services shows a differentiated picture with no clear message.

- Long duration and high number of educational messages alone does not guarantee a learning effect.
- Reminders for a medication to be taken daily are more effective than no reminders and are more effective when delivered weekly than daily, irrespective of message format. Reminders for HIV testing, by contrast, are most effective in the arm with the highest number of individual messages.
- Services that collect patient inputs can in some cases be lowered in frequency and hence intrusion because the character of the disease allows to predict values highly reliably from recently collected values.

10.5 Expanding the Scope

10.5.1 Enhancing the Technology

We have seen fully automated services where the functionality was very limited and stereotypical (e.g. Sect. 10.2.2.1) but also very comprehensive services where nearly 70 % of the service was conveyed in person through phone calls (Sect. 10.4.2). We have also seen limitations of accuracy when services targeted behaviors and the only available resource to assess outcome was patient self-report (Sects. 10.4.2 or 10.2.3). We will now see one example of a service where SMS essentially remains the sole medium of exchange between provider and client but where personalized advice and encouragement is automatically supplied if the client sticks to a simple syntax in his answers. The second example combines SMS with automated recording of medications taken.

Ingersoll and coworkers [10] present the design and preliminary usability and usage data of a dialogue system to support HIV-positive clients with a history of substance abuse in managing their moods and their behaviors, mainly their ART. It typically runs a handful of dialogues per day with its clients, asking them about medication adherence and mood, plus in an intuitively coded and hopefully not exposing form ("How were the skies ...?") about the use of substances, with answers "cloudy" for marijuana and alike, also coded. For mood questions clients should openly reply "mood <cipher>", for medications yes or no. In the favorable case the client answers in correct syntax in a dialogue initiated by the service and then gets a personalized feedback message. Personalized means reinforcing if the client's answer code is for "good" behavior and encouraging for negative answers. Each client could design his individual texts for all answering options available.

Data from more than 16,000 messages exchanged with 31 patients enrolled at the University of Virginia in 10 months demonstrated high response rates. Clients answered between 64 % and 69 % of received questions in correct syntax and consequently received a reinforcing or encouraging message. Regarding the demographics, diagnoses and behaviours of the study population (more than 40 % each high school as highest education, African American, harmful drinking, substance abuse, major depression, generalized anxiety) the answering rate appears amazingly high. Their was no incentive except the SMS text each client had chosen for him personally for every answer he gave. Data whether this intervention improved behaviors and maybe viral load are still due. The high response rates may be in accordance with the observation that for all questions positive answers (medication yes, skies clear etc.) were given much more often. We may be seeing the clients struggle for a positive self image, an inclination to enact themselves socially desirable. In this situation this may be part of their cure and we need not dismiss it as a bias because positive and negative self reports are not used to measure outcomes.

In the next technical enhancement accurately measured medication behavior is fed back to control the sending of SMS. Diabetic patients in the Netherlands, whose sub optimal medication adherence was known because they had refilled less than 80 % of the prescribed drugs in the past were randomized to control or to RTMM or to RTMM with SMS reminders. RTMM or Real Time Medication Monitoring is a medication dispenser device which connects through mobile data communication with central servers and registers synchronously with the patient's identification each event of taking the contained medication. The transmission of the data works wherever SMS works.

The target of the investigations was the added value of SMS reminders whenever the RTMM had not registered a due medication. I.e. compared to services described

10.5 Expanding the Scope

in Sect. 10.4.3 SMS are only sent upon need. In a RCT with 104 patients monitored for 6 months completeness of taking medications within a 1 hour window or 4 hour window were both significantly higher in the RTMM with SMS arm. It should be noted that RTMM alone also is an experimental rather than a control condition where adherence is presumably higher through a Hawthorne effect (Sect. 15.2.3.3.1) and a true reminding character of the RTMM device. Therefore, the true effect size between usual care and RTMM and SMS is likely even higher. The intervention mainly improves accurate timing, though, while full days without medication did not differ significantly between RTMM alone and RTMM with SMS. But timing of course is important due to the variation of the blood glucose concentration during the day. Depending on the price of RTMM devices the combination tested here is certainly worth a consideration because it avoids mass transmissions of reminders to clients who need not be reminded and hence reduces what is known as alert fatigue in clinical medicine.

Take Home

While still operating mostly automatically SMS based Consumer Health Informatics services can be more personalized and achieve encouraging responses.

- HIV patients with severe behavioral comorbidities use the opportunity to communicate about their medical situation and moods through tailored SMS intensely. In preparation of the service they deliver their own personalized enforcing or encouraging messages which they will receive in response to their codified status reports.
- Diabetics with a history of low medication adherence achieve a better timed medication behavior when they are supported through a fed back medication monitoring (RTMM) and SMS system: Clients receive messages exclusively when the RTMM indicates a missed administration of a drug.

10.5.2 Involving Clients' Peers

The technology underlying SMS and IVR makes it easy to include human helpers for the client, be it in his physical environment or in virtual space. Whenever a client and a second person willing and appropriate to help are registered as a bundle with their phone numbers, stereotypical as well as deeply personalized services can be deployed to the client and his relation. Depending on the role that the second person plays, "treatment partner", "informal caregiver" or "buddy" are commonly used terms.

In investigations in Thailand which is among the countries with highest prevalence and incidence of tuberculosis, different combinations of treatment partner and phone or SMS message service were tested as to their efficiency and cost effectiveness both for the easier to treat non-MDR-TB (non-Multi-drug resistant tuberculosis) and the harder to treat MDR-TB. A WHO recommendation has it that infected persons should have a trusted person in their environment, the "treatment partner", eyewitness the daily taking of the medicine. This is part of a five step procedure DOTS, i.e. "Directly Observed Treatment, Short-course". Sputum conversion, i.e. the fact that from a patient's sputum a cell culture can no longer be infected is an easily available criterion that is taken as an indicator of achieved cure or very good prognosis of cure in the near future; a convenient as well as rather accurate outcome measurement. On a small scale with 38 MDR-TB and 60 non-MDR-TB patients randomized to either just family member provided DOTS or such DOTS plus daily phone calls [11] sputum conversions were taken for 6 resp. 18 months for non-MDR-TB resp MDR-TB patients. The phone calls achieved higher conversion rates under various circumstances, with a very strong "novelty" effect in the critical MDR-TB arm: 90 % were sputum converted after 1 month, versus only 20 % without phone calls. The long term cure (6 resp 18 months) with phone calls was 100 %, highly significantly superior for the critical MDR-TB group where DOTS alone achieved 73.7 % only.

Kunawararak et al.[11] report some more results but the ones presented here take us to the next consideration. One may have wondered whether in person calls are worth the effort, however, for the small percentage of MTB-TB it may be the case. Furthermore, automatically generated calls or some sophistication of IVR may do the job as well. We regard these considerations from a cost effectiveness review of various DOTS versus phone calls versus control (self-administered treatment) experiments to curb tuberculosis in Thailand. Hunchangsith et al. [6] calculate DALYs (Disability-Adjusted Life Years) that can be achieved with an effort made. From a large number of aggregated figures the following stand out from the perspective of Consumer Health Informatics. DOT provided by a family member alone, the control condition of the study above, lies in the middle field in therapy success and DALYs gained. At the same time it is the cheapest in government spending and middle ground in patient cost. Mobile phone alone, whose cost is in the middle ground too, is inferior to all DOT variants but superior to control. An apparently easy conclusion is that the combined evidence from the two investigations suggests a strong positive interaction because two treatments when offered in isolation achieve mediocre results whereas together they are stunning. However, phone does not equal phone. In the small investigation by [11] phone calls were high quality health professional provided with certainly some observer expectancy going on: The caller knows the study and wants the success, and that determines how he behaves. In the study cited in [6] callers were volunteers who had recently been cured of tuberculosis. They may have been enthusiastic about there new role upfront but if their enthusiasm faded and first line therapy adherence of the patients faded at similar rates, the high incidence of MDR-TB finds a natural explanation. These are possible but not compelling explanations. But they raise doubt that will be materialized soon that volunteer buddies are not always the helpers of choice.

An attempt is reported by [24] to adapt a group counseling service for African Americans to prevent diabetes mellitus 2 and its complications to a service for women in a Capetown township, with partly group counseling and partly SMS. The US Power to Prevent http://www.ndep.nih.gov/media/power-to-prevent-508.pdf?redirect=true is a program of twelve lessons from a "DPP" ("Diabetes Prevention Program") that has some history in the USA where motivational, medical, environmental, and coping elements are assembled. The US original has two of the twelve lessons devoted to "Physical Activity for Families" and "Get Your Family and Friends Involved".

The Cape Town replication has about half the lessons similar and while the other half was tried to adapt purposefully. The adaptation replaces the family physical activity related lesson through "Being a social support buddy, using the mobile phone". Concretely, participants were randomly assigned a buddy within the group hoping that the respective bonding would lead to mutual encouragement to exercise. Another Consumer Health Informatics element was automated SMS probes from the provider, one question from a list of 15 per day, about that day's health, expected to be answered by the participants. Various physical and mental health and well being indicators were taken at baseline, at 3 and at 6 months.

Adherence to the group session part was very satisfactory. The 22 participants responded to probes 83 times and sent 123 messages among buddies as a weekly average of the whole group. This appears as an appropriate adherence level, but outcomes are dire. BMI, blood pressure an blood glucose worsened on average. Mental health and well being indicators did not change except a *decrease* in spiritual hope. So what happened here?

Two interpretations suggest themselves, supported through some other data. First, when splitting the participants at the median into "high" and "low" texters (averages of 1002 vs. 754 texts throughout the study) the high texter cohort had and kept higher BMI and their step count decreased by 40 % from baseline to 6 months. "High-texting women appear ... (to have) used texting to replace walking." [24, p. 362]. The service added a new addiction on top of an existing one. The second is more subtle and draws on baseline assessments of attitudes and beliefs which included that all women were seeking explanations why they had diabetes, many were religious and prayed often and also believed in witchcraft and retribution of sins. With the experimental Consumer Health Informatics service imposed on them their whole view of the world was shaken and nothing new and sound was offered through the mechanics of caloric uptake and consumption underlying the educational concept of Power to Prevent.

Two major lessons can be learnt for Consumer Health Informatics. First replacing a therapy element that presumably helps in the real situation of a family exercising together through an apparently equivalent virtual one – SMS buddies encouraging each other to exercise – may have no or even reverse effects. Second, the whole mindset of a new target group must be taken into account when transferring a service approved for one target group.

Buddies may be a risk when the whole approach lacks a sound foundation. Buddies, in the following concept called "informal caregiver", can be instrumental to an improved Consumer Health Informatics service when their contribution has a designated place and role and they are actively informed and encouraged to embrace that role. In a preliminary investigation much alike the ones described in Sect. 10.4.3 Piette and coworkers [20] report about an experiment to bring IVR coaching to a diabetics population with one quarter illiterate in semi-rural Honduras. Here we concentrate on informal caregivers, mostly patient's family, who "received structured IVR call ... that included feedback and suggestions ... to support the patient ... self care." [20, p. 3]. Patients who had chosen support by an informal caregiver improved more at HbA1c, one of the crucial indicators of future complications of diabetes mellitus 2 although this group scored worse on an important predictive factor, depression. In other investigations (e.g. with heart failure patients) Piette's group finds high emotional approval of involving an informal caregiver which dwarfs feelings of confidentiality breeches, pretty well in accordance with observations in Sect. 11.3.

Take Home

Involving family and peers in the care of a chronically ill person can be beneficial when appropriately integrated into the flow of information and action of the Consumer Health Informatics service but can as well create new risks if left to chance.

- To achieve therapy adherence in tuberculosis WHO recommends health worker supervised medication administration. Combinations of reminder phone calls and family supervision achieve similar success rates as the resource intensive health worker supervision, however, cost effectiveness and whether personal calls can replace in-person calls remains open.
- Involving family in an IVR support of patients of chronic diseases many of whom are illiterate improves clinical outcomes.
- Trying to replicate a successful service where severely overweight clients are supported through real family living together with the client through randomly assigned SMS buddies, fails for many: Rather than exercising the clients text.

References

1. Cohen-Cline H, Wernli KJ, Bradford SC, Boles-Hall M, Grossman DC. Use of interactive voice response to improve colorectal cancer screening. Med. Care. 2014;52:496–9.
2. de Lepper AM, Eijkemans MJC, van Beijma H, Loggers JW, Tuijn CJ, Oskam L. Response patterns to interactive SMS health education quizzes at two sites in Uganda: a cohort study. Trop Med Int Health. 2013;18(4):516–21. doi: 10.1111/tmi.12059.
3. D'Arcy S, Rapcan V, Gali A, Burke N, Crispino O'Connell G, Robertson IH, Reilly RB. A study in into the automation of cognitive assessment tasks for delivery via the telephone: lessons for developing remote monitoring applications for the elderly. Technol Health Care. 2013;21:387–96. doi: 10.3233/THC-130740.
4. de Tolla K, Skinner D, Nembaware V, Benjamin P. Investigation into the use of short message services to expand uptake of human immunodeficiency virus testing, and whether content and dosage have impact. Telemed E Health. 2012;18(1):18–23. doi: 10.1089/tmj.2011.0058.

5. Giorgio MM, Kantor LM, Levine DS, Arons W. Using chat and text technologies to answer sexual and reproductive health questions: planned Parenthood pilot study. JMIR. 2013;15(9):e203. doi: 10.2196/jmir.2619.
6. Hunchangsith P, Barendregt JJ, Vos T, Bertram M. Cost-effectiveness of various tuberculosis control strategies in Thailand. Value Health. 2012;15:S50–5. doi: 10.1016/j.jval.2011.11.006.
7. Huang H-L, Li Y-CJ, Chou Y-C, Hsieh Y-W, Kuo F, Tsai W-C, Chai SD, Lin BY-J, Kung P-T, Chuang C-J. Effects of and satisfaction with short message service reminders for patient medication adherence: a randomized controlled study. BMC Med Inform Decis Mak. 2013;13:127. doi: 10.1186/1472-6947-13-127.
8. Hartzler A, Wetter T. Engaging patients through mobile phones: demonstrator services, success factors, and opportunities in low and middle-income countries. Yearb Med Inform. 2014;182–94. doi: 10.15265/IY-2014-0022.
9. Hall KS, Westhoff CL, Castaño PM. The impact of an educational text message intervention on young urban women's knowledge of oral contraception. Contraception. 2013;87:449–54. doi: 10.1016/j.contraception.2012.09.004.
10. Ingersoll K, Dillingham R, Reynolds G, Hettema J, Freeman J, Hosseinbor S, Winstead-Derlega C. Development of a personalized bidirectional text messaging tool for HIV adherence assessment and intervention among substance abusers. J Subst Abus Treat. 2014;46:66–73. doi: 10.1016/j.jsat.2013.08.002.
11. Kunawararak P, Pongpanich S, Chantawong S, Pokaew P, Traisathit P, Srithanaviboonchai K, Plipat T. Tuberculosis treatment with mobile-phone medication reminders in Northern Thailand. Southeast Asian J Trop Med Public Health. 2011;42(6):1444–51.
12. Kempe KL, Shetterly SM, France EK, Levin TR. Automated phone and mail population outreach to promote colorectal cancer screening. Am J Manag Care. 2012;18(7):370–8.
13. Lund S, Hemed M, Nielsen BB, Said A, Said K, Makungu MH, Rasch V. Mobile phones as a health communication tool to improve skilled attendance at delivery in Zanzibar: a cluster-randomised controlled trial. BJOG. 2012;119:1256–64. doi: 10.1111/j.1471-0528.2012.03413.x.
14. Martin L, Knight V, Read PJ, McNulty A. Clients' preferred methods of obtaining sexually transmissible infections or HIV results from Sydney Health Centre. Sex Health. 2013;10:91–2. doi: 10.1071/SH12062.
15. Mehran L, Nazeri P, Delshad H, Mirmiran P, Mehrabi Y, Azizi F. Does a text messaging intervention improve knowledge, attitudes and practice regarding iodine deficiency and iodized salt consumption? Public Health Nutr. 2012;15(12):2320–5. doi: 10.1017/S1368980012000869.
16. Nazeri P, Mirmiran P, Asghari G, Shiva N, Mehrabi Y, Azizi F. Mothers' behaviour contributes to suboptimal iodine status of family members: findings from an iodine-sufficient area. Public Health Nutr. 2015;18(4):686–94. doi: 10.1017/S1368980014000743.
17. Odeny TA, Bailey RC, Bukusi EA, Simoni JM, Tapia KA, Yuhas K, Holmes KK, Scott McClelland R. Effect of text messaging to deter early resumption of sexual activity after male circumcision for hiv prevention: a randomized controlled trial. J Acquir Immune Defic Syndr. 2014;65(2):e50–7.
18. Piette JD, Aikens JE, Rosland AM, Sussman JB. Rethinking the frequency of between-visit monitoring for patients with diabetes. Med Care. 2014;52:511–8.
19. Pop-Eleches C, Thirumurthy H, Habyarimana JP, Zivin JG, Goldstein MP, de Walqe D, MacKeen L, Haberer J, Kimaiyo S, Sidle J, Ngare D, Bangsberg DR. Mobile phone technologies improve adherence to antiretroviral treatment in a resource-limited setting: a randomized controlled trial of text message reminders. AIDS. 2011;25(6). doi: 10.1097/QAD.0b013e32834380c1.
20. Piette JD, Mendoza-Avelares MO, Ganser M, Mohamed M, Marinec N, Krishnan S. A preliminary study of a cloud-computing model for chronic illness self-care support in an underdeveloped country. Am J Prev Med. 2011;40(6). doi: 10.1016/j.amepre.2011.02.014.

21. Junod Perron N, Dominicé Dao M, Camparini Righini N, Humair J-P, Broers B, Narring F, Haller DM, Gaspoz, J-M. Text-messaging versus telephone reminders to reduce missed appointments in an academic primary care clinic: a randomized controlled trial. BMC Health Serv Res. 2013;13:125. doi: 10.1186/1472-6963-13-125.
22. Piette JD, Marinec N, Gallegos-Cabriales EC, Gutierrez-Valverde JM, Rodriguez-Saldaña J, Mendoz-Alevares M, Silveira MJ. Spanish-speaking patients' engagement in Interactive Voice Response (IVR) chronic disease self-management support calls: analyses of data from three countries. J Telemed Telecare. 2013;19(2):89–94. doi: 10:1177/1357633X13476234.
23. Piette JD, Sussman JB, Pfeiffer PN, Silveira MJ, Singh S, Lavieri MS. Maximizing the value of mobile health monitoring by avoiding redundant patient reports: prediction of depression-related symptoms and adherence problems in automated health assessment services. JMIR. 2013;15(7):e118. doi: 10.2196/jmir.2582.
24. Rotheram-Borus MJ, Tomlinson M, Gwegwe M, Comulada WS, Kaufman N, Keim M. Diabetes buddies: peer support through a mobile phone buddy system. Diabetes Educ. 2012;38:357. doi: 10.1177/0145721712444617.
25. Stockwell MS, Kharbanda EO, Martinez RA, Vargas CY, Vawdrey DK, Camargo S. Effect of a text messaging intervention on influenza vaccination in an urban, low-income pediatric and adolescent population. JAMA. 2012;307(16):1702–8.
26. Sims H, Sanghara H, Hayes D, Wandiembe S, Finch M, Jakobsen H, Tsakanios E, Ify Okocha C, Kravariti E. Text message reminders of appointments: a pilot intervention at four community mental health clinics in London. Psychiatr Serv. 2012;63:161–8. doi: 10.1176/appi.ps.201100211.
27. Sherrard H, Struthers C, Kearns SA, Wells G, Chen L, Mesana T. Using technology to create a medication safety net for cardiac surgery patients: a nurse-led randomized control trial. Can J Cardiovasc Nurs. 2009;19(3):9–15.
28. Strandbygaard U, Thomsen SF, Backer V. A daily SMS reminder increases adherence to asthma treatment: a three-month follow-up study. Respir Med. 2010;104:166–71. doi: 10.1016/j.rmed.2009.10.003.
29. Vahdat HL, L'Engle KL, Plourde KF, Magaria L, Olawo A. There are some questions you may not ask in a clinic: providing contraception information to young people in Kenya using SMS. Int J Gynecol Obstet. 2013;123:e2–6.
30. Wakadha H, Chandir S, Were EV, Rubin A, Obor D, Levine OS, Gibson DG, Odhiambo F, Laserson KF, Feikin DR. The feasibility of using mobile-phone based SMS reminders and conditional cash transfers to improve timely immunization in rural Kenya. Vaccine. 2013;31:987–93. doi: 10.1016/j.vaccine.2012.11.093.
31. Ybarra M, Bağci Bosi AT, Korchmaros J, Emri S. A text messaging-based smoking cessation program for adult smokers: randomized controlled trial. JMIR. 2012;14(6):e172. doi: 10.2196/jmir.2231.
32. Zou H, Fairley CK, Guy R, Bilardi J, Bradshaw CS, Garland SM, Sze JK, Afrizal A, Chen MY. Automated, computer generated reminders and increased detection of gonorrhoea, chlamydia and syphilis in men who have sex with men. PLOS One. 2013;8(4):e61872. doi: 10.1371/journal.pone.0061972.

Chapter 11
Smart Homes: Empowering the Patient Till the End

George Demiris

11.1 Overview

The significant and continuous increase of the segment of the population globally 65 years of age or older (cf. Sect. 2.3 and Table 2.2) is calling for innovative solutions to supporting new models of aging. Technology can play an empowering role in allowing people to lead meaningful lives in the community while preserving quality of life and independence. With aging, people often try to cope with health related issues such as falls, sensory impairment, diminished mobility, isolation, diminished mobility, and in some cases the challenge of complex medication management. "Smart home" developments are being pursued worldwide in response to advancing technology, rising health care costs and the desire of older adults and individuals with disabilities to remain independent at the residence of their choice.

A "smart home" is a residential setting with embedded technological features that enable passive monitoring of the well-being and activities of their residents aiming to improve primarily overall quality of life, to detect or even prevent emergencies and ultimately increase independence for the involved residents. The technology is integrated into the infrastructure of the residence and, therefore, does not require training of or major operation by the resident, distinguishing thereby smart home applications from stand alone information technology (IT) systems that are operated by a user in a home setting (e.g., a videophone, a blood pressure cuff, a glucose meter etc.).

The number of research projects and commercial initiatives exploring the concept of smart homes has been growing worldwide. The Center for Future Health at the University of Rochester in the United States has developed a Smart Medical

---

G. Demiris
Department of Biomedical Informatics and Medical Education, University of Washington School of Medicine, Seattle, WA, USA

Home as a highly controlled environment including infrared sensors, biosensors, and video cameras [14]. The Aware Home at the Georgia Institute of Technology explores ubiquitous computing technologies that sense and identify potential crises, assist a senior adult's memory and track behavioral trends [13]. Researchers from five countries (the UK, Ireland, Finland, Lithuania and Norway) joined their efforts for the ENABLE project [3], which promotes the well-being of people with early dementia with several features such as a locator for lost objects, a temperature monitor and an automatic bedroom light. In Toulouse, France, the PROSAFE project is utilizing a set of infrared motion sensors to support automatic recognition of resident activity and possible falls [4].

The following Table 11.1 showcases some of the most cited smart home projects worldwide targeting specifically or broadly older adults . This list captures some of the diversity of technological approaches, geographic areas and overall design, and also includes some of the earlier pioneering efforts in this area, but is by no means a comprehensive list of smart home projects.

Table 11.1 World wide smart home projects

Project	Target audience	Technologies
Assisted Interactive Dwelling House [2] UK	Frail elderly and persons with disabilities	• Environmental control technologies (e.g., for windows, curtains, doors) • Sensor (e.g., bedside pressure pad, passive infra-red detectors, video door entry system) aiming to assess health, activity, and provide security monitoring and response
Aware Home [13] Georgia Institute of Technology, USA	Older adults and their families	• Health-related motion/activity monitoring technology (e.g., video cameras, "Smart Floor", pendant-based camera, ultrasonic sensors) for early detection and emergency response • Communication technology for enhancing social connection, including Digital Family Portrait which provides users and family members health, social, activity, and event information about each other, using icons framed in a dynamic, flat panel display • Memory aid technologies, including finding lost objects using radio frequency tags and Family Video Archive aimed at improving long-term memory
BESTA project [3], Norway	Persons with early dementia	• Environmental monitoring and control technologies (e.g., automatic lighting, stove monitors) • Activity monitoring (e.g., alert activated if user out of bed for over 30 min at night, door monitors to detect out-of-residence wandering)
comHOME [11], Sweden	Persons with cognitive disabilities	Video Mediated Communication technologies for everyday home activities

(continued)

11.1 Overview

Table 11.1 (continued)

Project	Target audience	Technologies
ENABLE Project [3], UK, Ireland, Finland, Lithuania, and Norway	Persons with early dementia	• Safety and assistive technologies for monitoring and controlling bath and wash basin water level, temperature and gas stove burners • Locating lost objects • Programming telephones with photos instead of numbers • Dispensing medications digitally
Gator Tech Smart House [9] Rehabilitation Engineering Research Center on Technology for Successful Aging at the University of Florida, USA	Older adults and persons with disabilities	• Environmental sensors for comfort and energy efficiency (e.g., smart thermostats), safety (e.g., smart stove, smart leak detector, smart bathroom that monitors water temperature), and security (e.g., home security monitors) • Activity/motion monitoring (e.g., smart bed that tracks sleep patterns; ultrasonic sensors and smart floor with pressure sensors that detect movement and location) • Fall detection system with emergency alert in development • Other smart devices and smart appliances (e.g., smart phone, smart mailbox, and development of smart microwave) • "Immersive" audio-video communication technology under development to be used for "social-distant dining" with relatives • Biometric technologies are under development for physiological monitoring (e.g., weight, temperature)
Gloucester Smart House [1], UK	Persons with dementia	• Sensor technologies that use voice messages to remind or alert residents, including sensors that monitor bath, stove, ambient temperature, and automatic lighting • Picture-phone and lost-item locator
Oatfield Estates [15] Oregon, USA	Older residents of an assisted living facility	• Sensor technologies for activities/movement (including locator badges or wristwatches) • Sensors for environment control (e.g., lighting, appliances) • Physiological monitoring (e.g., pulse, respiration, moisture level) • Other health-related monitoring technology (e.g., restlessness in bed) • Communication technology (including a portal that provides stakeholders, including family, web access to health and social information of residents)

(continued)

Table 11.1 (continued)

Project	Target audience	Technologies
PlaceLab [10] Part of House_n project of Massachusetts Institute of Technology, USA	General population	• Ubiquitous sensor technologies for activity and health monitoring, including wearable biometric technologies • Energy system monitoring and distribution (e.g., temperature, water, lighting, gas flow) • Development of technologies for learning, communication, commerce, entertainment, and work
PROSAFE [17] Toulouse, France	Persons with Alzheimer's	Infrared motion sensors to monitor activity and alert to possible falls
Smart Medical Home [14] Center for Future Health, University of Rochester, New York, USA	General population Strong focus on older adults through the Center's Aging Well Consortium	• Sensor technologies (including biosensors, infrared sensors, video cameras, microphones) for: • Physiological monitoring (e.g., blood pressure, pulse, respiration) • Motion/Activity monitoring (e.g., gait and behavior, sleep, and exercise patterns as compared to "normal" patterns for user) • Assistive technologies, such as: Personal Medical Advisor System, which includes a voice interaction system for medication compliance • Memory Assistance Aids, including object recognition system for frequently lost items such as keys
SmartBo and SmartLab [7] Swedish Handicap Institute, Sweden	Persons with visual, hearing, mobility, or cognitive disabilities	• Environmental control and safety technologies, such as for lighting, windows, doors, locks, water, electricity, and stove • Signaling devices, including a text enlargement program, speech synthesizer, and Braille display
Smartest Home of the Netherlands [18] Tilburg, The Netherlands	General population (Designed with input from older adults.)	Environmental technologies for safety, security, energy efficiency and comfort (e.g., automated security alarm; TV video of visitors at front door, activated by doorbell; automated lighting and heating)
Tiger Place [6] University of Missouri-Columbia, USA	Residents of assisted living facility	• Motion/activity sensors that monitor overall activity and location • Anonymized video sensor system for activity analysis. Pressure switch pads for activity monitoring and assistance such as automatic activation of lights • Bed sensor which monitors restlessness in bed and respiration and pulse parameters
Welfare Techno-House project [12], Japan	Older adults and persons with disabilities	• Sensors that monitor activity, environment • Development of biometric sensors that do not have to be attached to body (e.g., ECG measurement via electrodes attached to bath tub wall or to the foot and head of bed; and excretion or voiding measurement via load sensor on floor adjacent to toilet bowl • "secured lifelines" for natural disasters

11.2 Smart Home Functionalities

When examining the broad spectrum of technologies and the purpose they serve, smart home functionalities serve the following purposes:

- Physiological monitoring: Collection and processing of data pertaining to physiological measurements such as vital signs of pulse, respiration, temperature, bladder and bowel output, etc.
- Functional monitoring: Collection and processing of data pertaining to functional measurements such as general activity level, motion, gait, meal intake, and other activities-of-daily-living.
- Safety monitoring: Collection and processing of data pertaining to measurements that detect environmental hazards such as fire or gas leak. Safety assistance includes functions such as automatic turning on off bathroom lights when getting out of bed, facilitating safety by reducing trips and falls. Location technologies aimed at safety also fit into this type.
- Security monitoring and assistance: Measurements that detect human threats such as intruders. Assistance includes responses to identified threats.
- Social interaction monitoring and assistance: Collection and processing of data pertaining to social interactions such as phone calls, visitors, and participation in activities. Social interaction assistance includes technologies that facilitate social interaction, such as video-based components that support video-mediated communication with friends and loved ones, virtual participation in group activities etc.
- Cognitive and sensory assistance: Provision of automated or self-initiated reminders and other cognitive aids such as medication reminder and management tools, lost key locators, etc., for users with identified memory deficits. Cognitive assistance applications also include task instruction technologies, such as verbal instructions in using an appliance. Sensory assistance includes technologies that aid users with sensory deficits such as for sight, hearing, and touch.

While formal smart home initiatives targeting older adults date back to the late nineties, this is a relatively new and still emerging concept and research domain which calls for further examination of older adults' acceptance, ethical and practical considerations and the solidification of scientific evidence of the effectiveness of such systems.

11.3 Acceptance

The diffusion of smart homes and their adoption by the population ultimately depend on user acceptance of the concept. Introducing technologies in the residential infrastructure that support the ongoing passive monitoring of all inhabitants and visitors calls for the consideration of numerous factors. We believe that the concept of obtrusiveness, defined as "a summary evaluation by the user based on characteristics or effects associated with the technology that are perceived as undesirable and physically and/or psychologically prominent" [8], needs to be systematically examined in the context of smart homes. Obtrusiveness covers several underlying constructs and is meant as a summary evaluation, namely the cumulate effect of a number of characteristics or attributes that may be important or prominent to a user [8]. Obtrusiveness is also a subjective assessment (i.e., what one person perceives as obtrusive may not be perceived the same way by another). The user in this context is not only the patient or the older adult but also all other residents in the home. Given that perceived obtrusiveness is a subjective assessment, it is important to take the needs and expectations of the specific stakeholders in consideration. There is evidence that people will weigh their perceived need for such health care technology against potential privacy considerations [5].

11.4 Ethical Considerations

The research agenda for smart homes must include ethical considerations for their design and implementation. Implications, including those for social relationships and interaction, over-reliance, and privacy, must be fully considered. Moran [16] was one of the first to pose crucial questions about the social impact of smart technologies. She stated that

> The introduction of advanced technology into the home has the potential to change qualitative and quantitative aspects of relationships between household members, as well as the role and function of the home and its relationship with the wider environment.

As we design smart home features we are called to examine the possibility of such technologies removing choice and control from users as they learn to rely on automation. One may even hypothesize that smart homes would result in a reduction of social interaction, or may provide tools that substitute for personal forms of care and communication [20]. As we consider ways to implement smart home systems, we need to address the warning by Wylde and Valins [21] that we may be indeed creating "societies of high tech hermits".

An additional consideration is the extent to which smart homes may lessen the sense of personal responsibility on the part of residents or their formal or informal caregivers. Family caregivers, for example, may become less vigilant in monitoring health changes in their loved one and the residents themselves may become less vigilant in health self-monitoring and/or self-management as they rely on an automated process. This in turn introduces the question about the appropriate eligibility criteria or characteristics that make a smart home intervention appropriate for a population. Stip and Rialle point out [19] that the issues of individual freedom, personal autonomy, informed consent, and confidentiality have to be examined in the context of the target population. They provide an example of applications for residents with schizophrenia, a condition that causes distortion of reality in the form of delusions of persecution and psychosensorial phenomena, and highlight the likelihood that surveillance technologies may exacerbate such symptoms. Similarly, smart home systems may be of benefit to people with dementia as they facilitate monitoring and detection of emergencies; at the same time, it is hard to assess what the resident's true wishes may have been in terms of being monitored, if they themselves cannot provide consent for such an intervention and their participation is determined by a loved one who acts on their behalf. Such challenges raise the question how smart homes may affect or alter the relationship between a patient/resident and their family or other members of their social network.

Smart home systems create a large amount of new datasets. While data mining and advanced algorithms processing these data may result in the identification of abnormalities or trends that require immediate attention, questions are being raised who and how often should be monitoring such data sets. Health care providers are already struggling with limited time and may not easily integrate these new streams of data into their workflow. The challenge becomes in applying sophisticated data mining and pattern recognition tools to create meaningful information that can be used in a timely manner by health care providers, rather than overwhelming data that will be burdensome for clinicians to take into consideration and will raise questions of accountability and liability.

11.5 The Evidence for Smart Homes

Scientific literature is lacking evidence of the effects of smart homes on health outcomes, including earlier disease, illness, and injury detection and intervention. There is a lack of research studies addressing the effect of a smart home on acute episodes requiring emergency care or a possible delay or prevention of nursing home placement. Ultimately, such questions will necessitate large randomized and controlled studies, possible only with more widespread penetration of smart homes. Conducting such large experimental research studies, however, may prove to be challenging given the cost of implementing or retrofitting large number of residences and furthermore, observing other homes as a control group for long periods of time. Many argue that randomized clinical trials may not even be feasible in this domain. In order, however, for health systems to consider smart homes as tools that can play a role in the health care and well-being of older adults, and to introduce mechanisms for reimbursement of such systems or services, further evidence is needed. In order to assess the cost-effectiveness of smart homes, we need to have evidence of potential health care or quality of life related benefits. Currently, the evidence base consists of small pilot and feasibility studies and some larger studies that have followed cohorts of residents over a longer period of time. As initiatives continue to emerge, the body of scientific literature for smart homes will also continue to increase, and one would hope that the quality of scientific evidence would also improve (cf. Chap. 15).

11.6 Future Trends

The advancement of personal health records that allows the collection of management of health related information by the patients themselves can play a great role in the future of smart homes. The large amount of data generated by continuous passive monitoring can be processed to identify trends and patterns (for example, of overall mobility or sleep quality). Such information can be integrated into personal health records, allowing for a more comprehensive assessment and documentation of one's health and furthermore informing potential lifestyle changes that may be needed for disease prevention and management. The behavioral sensing component that is enabled by smart home technology can be integrated into personal records to provide a comprehensive view of one's status; such aggregate information can then be shared with health care providers and informal caregivers to facilitate shared decision making. One such example would be for decisions pertaining to transitions of care; often older adults themselves and their families have to make decisions about transitioning to a different setting with a higher level of institutionalized care, based on subjective or incomplete information. Health care providers in this case may only have episodic fragmented snapshots of one's overall wellness without information on the actual health related trajectory. A personal health record that integrates smart home data could in such a case become a meaningful tool to facilitate decision making and improve communication between the stakeholders.

Smart homes in the future and as a direct result of the rapid technological advances will strengthen their three attributes of *invisibility, ubiquity and adaptivity*. As technologies integrate into the architecture, furnishings, appliances and clothing, they become effectively invisible to residents and visitors. Moreover, they are located in multiple rooms, making them ubiquitous in the home and some support monitoring and data collection outside the home as well. Smart home systems often include artificial intelligence (AI) features, allowing them to learn and adapt to the particular patterns of residents.

The field of smart homes demonstrates the potential of information technology to support aging. As technological advances enable more sophisticated and tailored home-based solutions, we face the challenge to ensure that the design and implementation of informatics applications for older adults are not determined simply by technological advances but by the actual needs of older adults and their families.

References

1. Adlama T, Gibbs C, Orpwood R. The gloucester smart house bath monitor for people with dementia. Phys Med. 2001;17(3):189.
2. Bonner S. Assisted interactive dwelling house. In: Proceedings 3rd TIDE congress: technology for inclusive design and equality improving the quality of life for the European citizen, Helsinki, 23–25 June 1998.

References

3. Cash M. Assistive technology and people with dementia. Rev Clin Gerontol. 2003;13(4): 313–9. doi: 10.1017/S0959259804001169.
4. Chan M, Bocquet H, Campo E, Val T, Pous J. Alarm communication network to help carers of the elderly for safety purposes: a survey of a project. Int J Rehabil Res. 1999;22(2):131–6.
5. Courtney KL, Demiris G, Rantz M, Skubic M. Needing smart home technologies: the perspectives of older adults in residential care communities. Inform Prim Care. 2008;16(3):195–201.
6. Demiris G, Skubic M, Keller J, Rantz MJ, Oliver DP, Aud MA, Lee J, Burks K, Green N. Nurse participation in the design of user interfaces for a smart home system. In: Nugent C, August JC editors. Smart homes and beyond. Amsterdam: IOS; 2006. pp. 66–73.
7. Elger G, Furugren B. SmartBo – an ICT and computer based demonstration home for disabled people. In: Proceedings 3rd TIDE congress: technology for inclusive design and equality improving the quality of life for the European citizen, Helsinki. IOS; 23–25 June 1998.
8. Hensel BK, Demiris G, Courtney KL. Defining obtrusiveness in home telehealth technologies: a conceptual framework. J Am Med Inform Assoc. 2006;13(4):428–31. doi: 10.1197/jamia.M2026.
9. Helal A, Mann W, Elzabadani H, King J, Kaddoura Y, Jansen E. Gator tech smart house: a programmable pervasive space. IEEE Comput Mag. 2005;38(3):50–60. doi: 10.1109/MC.2005.107.
10. Intille SS, Larson K, Tapia E, Beaudin J, Kaushik P, Nawyn J, Rockinson R. Using a live-in laboratory for ubiquitous computing research. In: Proceedings of PERVASIVE, Number 3968 in LNCS. Springer; 2006. pp. 349–65. doi: 10.1007/11748625_22.
11. Junestrand S, Keijer U, Molin G, Tollmar K. User study of video mediated communication in the domestic environment with intellectually disabled persons. Int J Hum Comput Interact. 2003;15(1):87–103. doi: 10.1207/S15327590IJHC1501_07.
12. Kawarada A, Nambu M, Tamura T, Ishijima M, Yamakoshi K, Togawa T. Fully automated monitoring system of health status in daily life. In: Engineering in medicine and biology society. Proceedings of the 22nd annual international conference of the IEEE, volume 1; 2000. pp 23–8. doi: 10.1109/IEMBS.2000.900794.
13. Kidd CD, Orr R, Abowd GD, Atkeson CG, Essa IA, MacIntyre B, Mynatt ED, Starner TE, Newstetter W. The aware home: a living laboratory for ubiquitous computing research. In: Proceedings of CoBuild'99. Position paper, Oct 1999. pp. 191–8. doi: 10.1007/10705432_17.
14. Marsh J. House calls. Rochester Rev. 2002;64(3):22–6.
15. Mulvenna MD, Nugent CD, editors. Supporting people with Dementia using pervasive health technologies. 7th ed. London/New York: Springer; 2010.
16. Moran R. The electronic home: social and spatial aspects. Dublin: European Foundation for the Improvement of Living and Working Conditions; 1993.
17. Rialle V, Rumeau P, Ollivet C, Herve C. Smart homes. In: Wootton R, Dimmick SL, Kvedar JC, editors. Home telehealth: connecting care within the community. London/Ashland: RSM Press; 2006.
18. Shuai Z, McClean S, Scotney B, Xin H, Nugent C, Mulvenna M. Decision support for Alzheimer's patients in smart homes. In: Proceedings 21st IEEE international symposium on computer-based medical systems CBMS '08. Los Alamitos: IEEE Computer Society; 2008. pp. 236–41.
19. Stip E, Rialle V. Environmental cognitive remediation in schizophrenia: ethical implications of "Smart Home" technology. Can J Psychiatry. 2005;50(5):281–91.
20. Tetley J, Hanson E, Clarke A. Older people, telematics and care. In: Warnes AM, Warren L, Nolan M, editors. Care services for later life: transformations and critiques. London: Jessica Kingsley Publications; 2001. pp. 243–58.
21. Wylde M, Valins MS. The impact of technology. Oxford: Blackwell Science; 1996. pp. 15–24.

Chapter 12
Partial Solutions for Patient Safety

12.1 Introduction

In Chap. 8 we outlined various risk dimensions and made claims for safeguards to be erected in protection of a Consumer Health Informatics client. In this chapter we report on some safeguards already in use in Consumer Health Informatics and address some others from other fields that suggest themselves to be considered for certain Consumer Health Informatics services.

12.2 Medical Risk

12.2.1 Medical State and History

12.2.1.1 Methods in Use

We analyse three Consumer Health Informatics services that combine form filling and numeric scales with measurement of physical signals to assess the medical risk dimension (cf. Sect. 8.4.1). Before going into detail, however, we consider the risks specifically lurking for the given conditions with subjective self assessment and forms filling.

In't Veen and coworkers provide experimental evidence that indeed subjective assessment and staging of bodily complaints can be flawed in a way that puts a patient at severe if not fatal risk [8]. They compare how well subjective assessments of breathing capacity match actual breathing capacity as measured through FEV_1 in a methacholine provocation test which induces stepwise broncho-constriction. Subjective assessments are the Borg scale and a visual analog scale which had both been proved to be in good accordance with 1 min ventilation capacity when tested with healthy subjects under physical exercise conditions.

For severe and brittle asthma patients the authors, however, find that the slopes of the curves for both, Borg and visual analog scale over reduction in breathing capacity (FEV_1) are much flatter than for patients with mild steroid-naïve asthma. This compares to earlier studies where near fatal asthma attacks were associated with much lesser perception of hypoxia than objective measurements revealed. The subjective perception of hypoxia in terms of Borg and VSA scale values is the lowest in the group with frequent exacerbations. The patients with highest need for personalized and timely interventions are just those who can contribute the least through accurately reporting their level of breathing impairment. In their experimental setting with availability of all pertinent clinical and lab resources in't Veen and coworkers could show that eosinophil granulocytes may provide an explanation for the reduced sensitivity to hypoxia because their sputum concentration correlates positively with reduction in breathing capacity in mild asthma while it inversely correlates in severe asthma. But eosinophils certainly do not suggest themselves for routine home staging of the level of asthma activity in a Consumer Health Informatics service.

Just to add one level of complexity until we move on to humble attempts of staging asthma through a combination of assessment methods: When it is not clear whether a patient has asthma or COPD, face-to-face medical expertise is even more necessary. So in the sequel we regard cases where the differential diagnoses between asthma and COPD is definite.

In Sect. 5.2.3.2 we see a strategy that does not rely on subjective self-assessments alone. In an app based Consumer Health Informatics service Liu and coworkers [11] let the patient every day report PEFR (a short term breathing capacity indicator), a few subjective four level self staged complaints and the objective observation whether rescue medication was used in the past 24 hours. Behavioral recommendations are based on a score where notable PEFR signs and the need for rescue medication each contribute 1 full point to an overall score. The score stages clients as "partially controlled" between 1 and 3 and "uncontrolled" with 4 or more. Notable PEFR signs for bad control essentially are strong decline compared to the day before and high 7 day variation. This points to the fact that Liu and coworkers establish and actively use a service specific partial ER (cf. Sect. 8.4.1.2.2) to capture the medical history.

Anhøj and Nielsen [3] proceed similarly in their Internet based service LinkMedica. Instead of PEFR they use daily FEV_1 combined with few observation that clients enter into their electronic "asthma diary". These are number of rescue medications and presence of asthma symptoms in the past night. LinkMedica suggest steroid aerosol dose increase when a score which also includes comparison with past data exceeds a threshold. It should be mentioned that the service has various convenience functions. One addresses the challenges outlined in Sect. 8.4.3.1 of addressing different education levels of their clients: selected articles are made available in "'In summary,' a user-friendly summary ... in consumer language ... and 'In detail.' fuller version ... link to ... paper abstract [3]".

In van der Heijden and coworkers' ([18], cf. Sect. 4.5.2) app based Consumer Health Informatics service AERIAL for COPD patients the approach is also similar

12.2 Medical Risk

but takes into account the less volatile nature of obstructive airways disease. While asthma severity can change within short time through whatsoever stimuli, COPD develops more steadily most of the time such that weekly FEV_1 and measurement values plus eight self assessed symptoms (present/not present) are regarded sufficient for a client in good control of his disease. AERIAL suggests more frequent data capture when symptoms suggest a beginning exacerbation. They add a safeguard against the risk that the user fails to manually enter measurement values by having the FEV_1 and oximetry reading sent to the cell phone though a specialized Bluetooth® protocol. Besides monitoring the medical severity they also reduce the risks of technological failure, as requested in Sect. 7.5 by providing the decision support locally on the smart phone.

All three are instances that satisfy the request in Sect. 8.4.1 to back self reported subjective symptom levels (cf. Sect. 8.4.1.1.1) up through objective measurements (cf. Sect. 8.4.1.1.3) and reference to a service specific partial ER (cf. Sect. 8.4.1.2.2).

Take Home

For asthma and COPD different Consumer Health Informatics services successfully combine patient self-assessment and self-report through forms and scales with physical measurements for a valid staging and heading towards automated dose adaption advice.

Since subjective self assessment does not validly estimate true breathing capacity a service without physical measurement would be reckless.

One service [3] offers advice in different forms targeted at different levels of health literacy.

12.2.1.2 Options for Future Use

Some investigations attempt to migrate paper questionnaires approved for diagnosis and staging of another type of medical risk, mental disorders such as depression, to digital forms and the Internet. We analyze two of them as to their methodological soundness and feasibility for routine use.

Evidence reported in [5] suggests that a questionnaire that has been thoroughly developed and migrated to online presentation can be used for Level 2 type diagnosis of depression in youths. Cawthorpe compared the results for 122 (38 males) psychiatric patients aged 11–17 – 75 of them depressive according to the attending psychiatrist's judgment – through various diagnostic procedures and against the diagnosis of the psychiatrist.

A computerized version of an originally face-to-face standardized diagnostic interview for child and adolescent disorders forms the core diagnostic method. Patients fill the Computer-Based Diagnostic Inventory Schedule for Children – Revised (CDISC-R) plus three other questionnaires that explore different factors of depression: the 20 item true/false Beck Hopelessness Scale (bhs) which features negative beliefs, the 10 item Rosenberg Self-Esteem (Likert) Scale (rose) and the 27 Likert item Child Depression Inventory (cdi).

Physician and CDISC-R diagnosis match in 76.2 % of the cases. For males and females concordance differs slightly. Leaving this small variation aside deviations were as follows: False positives (only CDISC-R-score: depressive) outweigh false negatives (only physician-judgment: depressive) by 21 to 8. In other words: The risk that CDISC-R scores "depressive" for healthy clients is notably higher than that it misses a depressed youth. So medically, the presented CDISC-R form is on the safe side. Its decision is mostly supported by the three factor related scores bhs, rose and cdi: in the female subgroup all three are higher in those subjects classified depressed through CDISC-R-score than in those classified depressed according to psychiatrist-judgment. Existing respective trends in the male subgroup are too few to allow conclusions.

In a similar investigation Donker and coworkers [7] migrate two paper questionnaires that are in use for diagnosis of depression in adults to an Internet-based online form. A structured extended telephone interview serves as gold standard against which online CES-D and K10 scores are compared, concretely, whether they exceed thresholds. Sensitivity resp. specificity are 0.94 resp. 0.64 for CES-D and 0.69–0.81 resp. 0.79–0.67, depending on the threshold chosen.

Equally appropriate, it appears. All three instruments have a history of successful face-to-face presentation. All prefer sensitivity over specificity i.e. have a safety margin of more false positives than false negatives.

However, concerns remain. In the [5] investigation the sample used for testing the discriminatory power is not representative of a normal population but consists of psychiatric patients. The sample is not large, especially the male sub-sample. Also the effort of filling CDISC-R, the person-to-person version of which takes up to 2 hours, may be too high for routine use, especially in case of fragile personality.

Donker et al. [7] also has sampling problems. Recruiting happened through banner ads on psychiatric service sites plus a small part of student services of a university psychology department. Internet savvy persons are likely overrepresented. Furthermore a drop out rate of 355 of the 502 showing initial interest indicates a second selection bias of unknown provenience on top of the Internet affinity related one.

Finally, the inclination of all instruments to over-diagnose does not only have advantages. The major advantage in the sense of safeguards requested in Sect. 8.4.1 is the high likelihood to not miss sick clients and hence to offer treatment before the disease has fatal consequences. However, the exposure of an intriguing diagnosis, even if the information actually is false, may also cause harm. As outlined in Chap. 13 such instruments should not be offered freely in open networks, since clients may be traced and identified, together with their scores. We must also be aware of risks of false positive bad news conveyed to individuals some of whom are already emotionally fragile. In a face-to-face setting human beings can sense a respective emotionality. In a virtual only Level 2 setting the client is on his own (cf. Sects. 8.4.2.1 and 12.3) unless personality inventories as discussed in Sect. 12.3.1.1 are a "gatekeeper" part of a service, before access to potentially frightening information is granted. Finally, in countries or populations where depression is tabooed, even the correct diagnosis conveyed to a person who successfully "passed the gate" may be irresponsible.

> **Take Home**
> A research process of making online depression screening or diagnosis tools available is under way.
> Samples and results are not compelling yet.
> Although the general tendency to prefer false positive over false negative appears rational and responsible at first sight, negative implications of online communication of false positive and of true positive diagnoses should be thoroughly considered.

12.2.2 Identification of Familial Risk

As opposed to an active disease such as asthma or depression a genetic disposition mostly does not require immediate action but considerate management. The follow up of a positive finding can reasonably reach from fully ignoring to immediate clinical review. Therefore, this section has two points of emphasis: Consumer Health Informatics services to identify a risk and services to manage the consequences of an identified risk.

12.2.2.1 Family Tree Services

Peace and coworkers [16] summarize experiences with collecting genetic, better to say familial health excess risk through various channels including face-to-face and Internet forms such as http://familyhistory.hhs.gov/ and http://www.familyhealthware.com/. Those face-to-face investigations where gold standard correct family relation and diagnosis could be established through independent methods accuracy of the client provided information was found to be between 56 % (asthma of spouses, parents, or siblings) and 95 % (breast cancer of 1st degree relatives). Accuracies of prominently showing diseases such as breast cancer clearly outweigh those of more embarrassing silent ones such as prostate cancer and less spectacular ones such as diabetes. Accuracy also decreases with farther distant relation or farther distant past, as would be expected.

http://familyhistory.hhs.gov/ applies quite some care to assist in exploring familial conditions. It exists in English, Español, Português and Italiano. Clients can start anonymously and refrain from providing identifying information, but unless they cheat on data such as date of birth and some other, re-identification remains a risk. Clients can also choose to have their Microsoft® Health Vault™ ER data uploaded and receive a warning that they are "taken to a non-federal website"; in other words contents and confidentiality are as good as Microsoft offers them, cf. risks described in Chap. 13. The own and family members' medical history are asked in somewhat lay language, well designed dialogues, where a more detailed description is solicited when the client has entered a broad diagnosis for himself or family members.[1] Instructions encourage to concentrate on genetic family (not adopted, step, ...). However, it takes quite a while with an extended family and multiple diagnoses to fill the forms. The delivered result is not more and not less than a well laid out display in various graphical (tree), tabular and computational (xml) forms. Client attention is drawn to aggregations of similar presumably meaningful risks in a naturally appealing way. The graphical displays are well suited to seek professional assistance while the xml report form is well suited to be used by other services. http://familyhistory.hhs.gov/ does not encourage actively to follow up on findings. However, when used as embedded resource by a Consumer Health Informatics service provider that handles heritable diseases, it would be instrumental to a better pre-assessment of a client's excess risks for certain diseases.

http://www.familyhealthware.com/, originally from CDC , now from Sanitas and showing a strange disclaimer[2] does not give access immediately but requests an e-mail address for a registration. It addresses client's behavior (smoking, exercise, ...) plus diagnoses, as well as diagnoses of family members. In contrast to http://familyhistory.hhs.gov/ it is less detailed and does not go into the depth of a broad diagnosis such as cancer. However, in addition to a family tree it delivers the client's "Family Healthware Health Score" as x/100, together with personal risk factors, suggested lifestyle changes, and suggested tests. The latter do not encourage to over-utilize or to seek intrusive diagnostics. Lifestyle changes and options for personalized screening schedules dominate. Therefore, http://www.familyhealthware.com/'s purpose is a more conscientious management of one's personal health related behaviors, like an open ended self contained Level 2 service. In a large study with 3785 users of the service O'Neill and coworkers show that an essential percentage (between 4 % and 34 %) actually have notable excess risks for one of the included diseases [15].

Both services appropriately cover adjacent purposes of incorporating familial risks in health care and health management as long as underlying assumptions are warranted. These include that familial risks essentially are genetic risks and that clients exclusively and correctly report their genetically related family. Neither is fully true, however, as [16] reports. Some of their subjects feel inclined to include individuals that are perceived as family although the subject knows that biologically

---

[1] E.g. a pull down menu with many concrete cancers when the client has entered "cancer".

[2] "CDC does not directly or indirectly endorse Family Healthware or services provided by this tool".

they are not. If meant for persons living in the same household this is not without reason, e.g. when a subject reports about a quasi-family person that he smokes a lot; common sense may tell the subject that his role of a passive smoker in the vicinity of that quasi family increases his risk of cancers or respiratory diseases. Similar arguments apply to unhealthy behaviors of the metabolic syndrome type that are learnt from household members perceived as family.

Two more types of uncertainty and risks for the validity of inferences and recommendations showed with the 21 subjects. Firstly, it turned out to be not always clear who truly is family and who is in-law, mainly in far distant branches of a family, not to speak of misbegotten individuals whose true fathers remain out of consideration forever. Secondly precise diagnoses were not always known.

Additionally, the 21 subjects, whose reporting of familiality of health problems and handling of and satisfaction with online family health services was investigated in depth show typical sampling biases outlined in [17]: Like the "psychology sophomores" which gave the name to a psychology sophomore phenomenon that most psychological theories have been experimentally tested against samples of younger psychology students, the familiality of health problems services have been tested with 21 students, 18 female, who visited a university health clinic and were not at "significant or psychological distress". The assumption that they were not emotionally involved and their participation was a totally transient peripheral experience – in other words that they did not actually care – is underlined through the fact that 20 of the subjects were not interested to receive their printed pedigrees after they had volunteered their data.

12.2.2.2 Gene and Tumor Marker Scan

In Sect. 3.3.2.2 we analyze the risks emanating from clients finding lab services and giving in to the temptation to mail a sample and to receive a report: that without interpretation and professional assessment the first step likely entails the second: to undergo clinical, maybe intrusive procedures to clarify.

Lovett and coworkers [12] rightly criticize such services because of their subtle yet compelling advertizing. Given an appropriate role, however, they may be beneficial. As for http://familyhistory.hhs.gov/, when some Consumer Health Informatics service reports a tentative diagnosis for a client and a lab service exists that provides the client's individual risk for that diagnosis why not include that auxiliary information, by subcontracting the lab service, and resume with interpretation of the results and considerate management of the overall risk rather than suggesting intrusive procedures immediately?

> **Take Home**
> Diverse Consumer Health Informatics services offer their clients an assessment of their excess medical risks based on personal behaviors and inherited diseases.
> When volunteering accuracy and time when filling forms about own and familial diseases (family trees) clients can receive a fair and well organized account of their individual risks.
> Accuracy of data that clients provide is deficient concerning precise identification of diagnoses and familial relations.
> The presented Consumer Health Informatics service encourage a considerate follow-up on findings, neither encouraging negligence nor over-utilization of diagnostic resources.
> By contrast, Consumer Health Informatics services that solicit mail in of specimens for gene, gene expression or tumor marketing scans tend to encourage over-utilization even on marginal findings.

12.2.2.3 Managing Genetic Risks

We use the example of breast cancer to analyze considerate incorporation of presumable genetic risks as part of the medical risk assessment requested in Sect. 8.4.1. Knowing that the genes BRCA1 and BRCA2 and therefore a hereditary factor of breast cancer has been found in the late 1990s, any Consumer Health Informatics service that covers breast cancer should by itself address the genetic risk and whether it may be in excess. This is not or only marginally the case in the services presented in this volume. Search for scholarly articles using (``Hereditary Breast and Ovarian Cancer Syndrome'' [Majr]) AND ``Consumer Health Information'' [Majr] against PubMed delivers various articles that confirm the importance of client awareness, but the only project where it is incorporated in an information package is about a paper brochure [6]. The authors in the sequel studied effects in a community setting rather than upgrading to an online Consumer Health Informatics service.

A health kiosk approach by Kreuter and coworkers [9] addresses indication for mammography screening and provides printed journals to clients who answer a questionnaire of between 11 and 24 questions, depending on the client's findings. Questions do not cover familial risks. Knowing, however, that filling the family tree data for an extended family takes hours rather than minutes familiality may be out of scope of a public kiosk setting.

The cancer survivor service http://www.oncolink.com/oncolife/ presented in Sect. 5.2.3.3 takes a different approach. Rather than helping the client to find out herself it asks whether others have. Among the questions is: "Have you been told you have a genetic abnormality or syndrome?" If the answer is yes the plan explains the character of a genetic risk and then advises that "if you are concerned (for yourself or family; the author)... consult with a genetic counselor... will also help to outline a plan for cancer screening that is tailored to your level of risk."

Those clients who actively use related topics as search terms and venture into search engines such as Google™ may also succeed but all concerns about the indeterminacy and risk raised in Sect. 3.3.1.2 apply. There are good services, though, e.g. http://www.cancer.gov/cancertopics/factsheet/detection/mammograms provided by the NCI which is Google™'s first hit[3] when tentatively searching `breast cancer mammography schedule`. It mentions the excess risks in a subsection of "What are NCI's recommendations for screening mammograms BRCA ", suggesting that "Women ... with family history ... or known mutation on ... BRCA1 or BRCA2 ... should talk with their health care providers whether ... mammograms before age 40 and how often ...". Those who happen to search Google™ for `breast cancer genes screening` first find[3] http://www.breastcancergenescreen.org by the Georgia Breast Center which also asks various detailed questions and, if those pointing to a genetic risk are answered positively, prominently presents a summary that includes that "Your risk for breast and/or ovarian cancer may be greatly increased over the general population. Cancer Genetic Counseling is recommended ... review family history ... assess risks ... discuss benefits and limitations of genetic testing". Hyperlinks lead to Information broker (Sect. 5.2.5.1) and Logistics support (Sect. 5.2.5.2) type service.

Take Home

Although the importance of the genetic risk is undisputed in diagnoses such as breast cancer, it is disregarded by some Consumer Health Informatics services, appropriately incorporated by some, but also overemphasized by others.

The http://www.oncolink.com/oncolife/ service stands out in assisting cancer survivors in pulling together personalized data and information and mildly rather than dramatically encouraging for vigilance and healthy lifestyle.

12.3 Personality

According to the intention of this volume on Consumer Health Informatics to enable the client to safely play a more active role, attending to his capacity or limitations to actually contribute is an important prerequisite. We analyze two partially overlapping categories of identifying limitations in a client to being an active "compliant" partner: personality traits and mental conditions.

---

[3] Searched in September 2013.

12.3.1 Personality Traits

Absolutely healthy persons still vary dramatically as to their perseverance, tolerance for adversity, stability under stress, self-efficacy and many more. Consumer Health Informatics services may necessitate well developed capacities in one or the other dimension of these dimensions and should then check before enrolling a client.

12.3.1.1 Personality Inventories

Among numerous personality theories and respective diagnostic tools we analyze two that suggest themselves for use in conjunction with Consumer Health Informatics services.

Wilson and coworkers [20] address the question whether youths' and young adults' risk of addictive behavior in online resources such as social networks can be assessed through general-purpose personality inventory instruments. They apply the NEO Five-Sector Personality Inventory and the Coopersmith Self-Esteem Inventory in a sample of 201 students (46 males) together with self-reported estimates on amount of time spent in social network and behaviors that indicate addictive tendencies such as the feeling of deprivation when having no access. Student inclusion criteria included being owner of a personal page in a social network system. The inventories cover dimensions neuroticism, extroversion, openness, agreeableness, and conscientiousness. Self-esteem is inquired about domains academic, social, family, and personal experience.

Not surprisingly the authors find that subjects who score high on extroversion and low on conscientiousness are at higher risk of extensive use and addiction to social network services. What appears as a truism when regarded out of context may be very helpful in the following context: a provider of whatsoever Consumer Health Informatics service for youths and young adults knows that for the service to be effective the clients have to visit pretty regularly and for extended periods of time. The provider then has the responsibility to not enroll clients who already are on the verge of or fully developed social network addicts. If the service is Level 2, with no opportunity to meet with prospective clients and get a sense of their control of social network habits, the two instruments and mainly the NEO Five-Sector Personality Inventory suggest themselves to identify individuals that require double checking before enrolling.

Ashton and coworkers [1] and [2] investigate various aspects of understanding personality and identifying individuals on the verge of psychiatric diagnoses. With samples of several hundred Dutch and Canadian students they have substantiated a six dimensional theory of personality and a related questionnaire HECAXO (with the short form HEXACO-60), plus a specific seventh dimension meant to cover schizotypy/dissociation in a questionnaire (Curious Experiences Scale). HEXACO dimensions are honesty-humility, emotionality, extroversion, agreeableness versus anger, conscientiousness, openness to experience. For the time being these instruments have not been applied in a concrete diagnostic context, let alone Consumer Health Informatics service. However, in personal communication [4] the lead author agreed that it would make sense to use certain axes for preliminary screening of clients before enrolling to certain types of Consumer Health Informatics services. For instance could individuals scoring high on emotionality and low on conscientiousness or agreeableness be at risk to overreact on intimidating findings. Conversely, prospective clients with high conscientiousness would likely adhere well to programs or diet or exercise or medication.

HEXACO can also be related to the widely used PID-5, the Personality Inventory for the five factor personality model DSM-5. Since maladaptivity is a risk for predictable "compliant" behavior, characterizing maladapted individuals through general-purpose instruments such as HEXACO would help a lot. Indeed do most dimensions of HEXACO correlate well with dimensions of PID-5. Another approved model of personality, the Five-Factor Model, together with PID-5 also brought forth the six HEXACO factors plus a factor for schizotypy/dissociation.

12.3.2 Mental Healthiness

Mental healthiness is closely related to absence of personality disorders. Therefore, basically dedicated dimensions of personality or psycho-diagnostic instruments can be considered. In Sect. 12.2.1.2 we saw instruments for depression screening where depression was meant as the target of a service. Depression may also be a prognostic factor before enrolling to a weight reduction, cancer prevention or other Consumer Health Informatics service. Then instruments such as CES-D can be used here as well. Similarly, addictive tendencies can be identified through subscales of NEO Five-Sector Personality Inventory but also of scales used in [13] for addictive patterns of alcohol use. Some clients may escape all such effort because they pathologically distrust care, be it conveyed in person or as a Consumer Health Informatics service [14].

> **Take Home**
> Empirical results on personality and mental health instruments show promise for pointing to clients' individual risks that matter for a service.
> They do not achieve off-the-shelf safe universal personality clearance for Consumer Health Informatics services.
> Rather should they encourage the effort to identify existing or to develop new instruments for personality traits required or to be avoided in a planned service.

12.3.3 Interfering Attitudes

Most Consumer Health Informatics services of Level 1 and Level 2 have sophisticated informed consent procedures. However, the sophistication lies in law or in research ethics. Typical commercial online pharmacy (Sect. 5.2.4) or virtual service (Sect. 5.2.5.4) offerings request consent that the client waives all rights to legally sue the provider in case of adverse effects. Typical scientific investigations about effectiveness or cost effectiveness of a Consumer Health Informatics service present consent forms that withstand the scrutiny of IRBs, Ethikkomissionen etc. Emphasis in both cases is that the client is aware of the balance of risks and opportunities and not to what extent he may be willing to cooperate with the Consumer Health Informatics service provider.

Learnt and willingly maintained attitudes against trustful cooperation are probably harder to test than innate or unconsciously acquired personality traits. An example of perfectly faked cooperation is provided by Lenny and Dear [10]. They show that when so instructed subjects are capable to answer to an instrument that is in wide use in custody evaluations (MCMI – Millon Clinical Multiaxial Inventory) in such a way that they come out as "good parents" irrespective of what they actually are and can even simulate different types of "goodness" such as administrative, clinical. We should, therefore, be warned about the validity of instruments meant to explore learnt or community approved attitudes: If the client wants to conceal he likely can.

> **Take Home**
> While consent forms principally are appropriate to inquire willingness of a client to cooperate and Consumer Health Informatics service providers should be aware of far ranging human capabilities to cheat on respective instruments.

12.4 Cognition

In Sect. 8.4.3 we have explored the meaning of health literacy and reading level including various methods to measure and adapt. Here we analyze an example of a medical condition and a target population that call for material adapted to their comprehension and where this has been addressed in a low profile Level 1 Consumer Health Informatics service.

Vargas and coworkers [19] developed dedicated educational material and evaluated client capabilities and comprehension of the material under several aspects. A mobile unit tours under-served communities of Phoenix, AZ, for free of charge services for parents of children with asthma. While trying to provide evidence that video and touch screen educational material informs clients better than paper and pencil material of equal contents the authors also record several co-factors under consideration as modifiers of the capability to comprehend medical contents. To answer the key question they let randomized subgroups of their sample of 48 parents either learn from the video or the paper and pencil. In both the video and the paper and pencil condition questions are embedded between instructions, with all desired freedom for the clients to move forward and backward and to change answers. Final answers are taken for further evaluation. In subsequent extended structured interviews with all subjects nurses identified their actual states of knowledge to be used as gold standard. Correlation of this gold standard with final answers was significantly higher in the video arm than in the paper and pencil arm (.68 vs. .54, $p < .01$). Therefore, the presumably easier to comprehend video material indeed achieves a higher level of understanding.

A closer look delivers interesting other predictors of the concordance between final answers and interview gold standard. Clients could choose to use an English or Spanish version of their educational material. All also underwent the STOFHLA test of functional health literacy in the chosen language, and age and years of formal training were recorded. All but one English client had adequate medical literacy skills, while 22 % of the Spanish speaking sub-population had marginal skills only and 11 % had inadequate skills. In this sample of nearly equal young age (median 32 years) subjects STOFHLA also correlated with years of education.

Among all factors analyzed as to their effect to the level of knowledge demonstrated in the interview, the strongest were experimental arm (video over paper), age of the client and years of education. Despite the general skepticism towards formal education of Sect. 8.4.3.2.3 as indicator for health literacy the circumstances given here of equally limited quality in minority neighborhood high schools lets the years in school count.

> **Take Home**
> While years of education is a poor predictor of health literacy across whole nations it contributes positively in homogeneous local environments, together with age.

12.5 Identify and Authentication

Identification and authentication in Consumer Health Informatics is as work in progress as it is for other services. Some services do not request client identification, some for good reason e.g. general counseling for embarrassing conditions (cf. Sect. 5.2.3.1). Methods for providers to identify themselves as trustworthy towards lay persons are outlined in Sect. 3.4.

We outline in Chap. 13 what can and should be done when Consumer Health Informatics moves center-stage and services persist over extended periods of time and a persistent true identity becomes a must. Secure methods tend to rely on encryption and on two factors that the client commands independently and which are never available to an intruder simultaneously, such as a password and a physical token or biometric pattern. Biometric patterns require higher protection against intruders than any kind of artificially assigned identifier, as outlined in Sect. 8.4.4.2.3. This may pose new challenges when physiological signals "innocently" collected in smart home services as just data turn out as being so individual, so much signature of a person, that they allow re-identification of their producers (Sect. 11.2).

To summarize: While functionality and medical range of Consumer Health Informatics grows as we speak identification and authentication are laggards which may hit the field in the face, especially in times where Assange,[4] Snowden,[5] and the likes inform the public intensively about leakage of information that was not meant to leak out.

> **Take Home**
> Regarding the obvious threats for sensitive health data to be become publicly exposed Consumer Health Informatics services must apply state of the art methods to secure privacy of entrusted data.
> Methods are outlined in Sects. 13.3 through 13.5. They rely on encryption and two factor authentication, among others.

References

1. Ashton MC, Lee K. The HEXACO-60: a short measure of the major dimensions of personality. J Pers Assess. 2009;91(4):340–5. doi: 10.1080/00223890902935878.
2. Ashton MC, Lee K, de Vries RE, Hendrickse J, Born MP. The maladaptive personality traits of the personality inventory for DSM-5 (PID-5) in relation to the HEXACO personality factors and schizotypy/dissociation. J Pers Disord. 2012;26(5):641–59.
3. Anhøj J, Nielsen L. Quantitative and qualitative usage data of an internet-based asthma monitoring tool. J Med Internet Res. 2004;6(3):e33. doi: 10.2196/jmir.6.3.e23.
4. Ashton MC. On medical and psychiatric use of psychological tests. Personal communication Sept. 2013, 2013.
5. Cawthorpe D. An evaluation of a computer-based psychiatric assessment: evidence for expanded use. Cyberpsychol Behav. 2001;4(4):503–10.
6. Cohn WF, Jones SM, Miesfeldt S. Are you at risk for hereditary breast cancer? Development of a personal risk assessment tool for hereditary breast and ovarian cancer. J Genet Couns. 2008;17(1):64–78. doi: 10.1007/s10879-007-9125-0.

---

[4]Julian Assange, one of the founders and best known protagonist of the whistleblower platform WikiLeaks, http://wikileaks.org, whose aim it is to provide to the public information that the WikiLeak organizers believe should be known to the public but is kept secret by the holders; source Wikipedia and WikiLeaks.

[5]Edward Snowden, former CIA and CIA subcontractor employee who revealed privacy breaches routinely committed by the US secret service NSA; source: Wikipedia.

7. Donker T, van Straten A, Marks I, Cuijpers P. Brief self-rated screening for depression on the internet. J Affect Disord. 2010;122:253–9. doi: 10.1016/j.jad.2009.07.013.
8. JCCM in't Veen, Smits HH, Ravensberg AJJ, Hiemstra PS, Sterk PJ, Bel EH. Impaired perception of dyspnea in patients with severe ashtma – relation to sputum eosinophils. Am J Respir Crit Care Med. 1999;158:1134–41.
9. Kreuter MW, Black WJ, Friend L, Booker AC, Klump P, Bobra S, Holt CL. Use of computer kiosks for breast cancer education in five community settings. Health Educ Behav. 2006;33:624–42. doi: 10.1177/1090198106290795.
10. Lenny P, Dear GE. Faking good on the MCMI-III: implications for child custody evaluations. J Pers Assess. 2009;91(6). doi: 10.1080/00223890903228505.
11. Liu W-T, Huang C-D, Wang C-H, Lee K-Y, Lin S-M, Kuo H-P. A mobile telephone-based interactive selfcare system improves asthma control. Eur Respir J. 2011;37:310–7. doi: 10.1183/09031936.00000810.
12. Lovett KM, Liang BA, Mackey TK. Risks of online direct-to-consumer tumor markers for cancer screening. J Clin Oncol. 2012;30(13):1411–4. doi: 10.1200/JCO.2011.37.8984.
13. Murray E, McCambridge J, Khadjesari Z, White IR, Thompson SG, Godfrey C, Linke S, Wallace P. The DYD-RCT protocol: an on-line randomised controlled trial of an interactive computer-based intervention compared with a standard information website to reduce alcohol consumption among hazardous drinkers. BMC Public Health. 2007;7:306. doi: 10.1186/1471-2458-7-306.
14. Maguire PA, Reay RE, Looi JCL, Cubis J, Byrne GJ, Raphael B. Neither the internist nor the internet: use of and trust in health information sources by people with schizophrenia. Aust N Z J Psychiatry. 2011;45:489–97. doi: 10.3109/00048674.2011.570308.
15. O'Neill SM, Rubinstein WS, Wang C, Yoon PW, Acheson LS, Rothrock N, Starzyk EJ, Beaumont JL, Galliher JM, Ruffin MT, for the Family Healthware™ Impact Trial Group. Familial risk for common diseases in primary care The Family Healthware™ impact trial. Am J Prev Med. 2009;36(6). doi: 10.1016/j.amepre.2009.03.002.
16. Peace J, Valdez RS, Lutz KF. Data-based considerations for electronic family health history applications. Comput Inform Nurs. 2012;30(1):37–45. doi: 10.1097/NCN.0b013e31822b865b.
17. Rosenthal R, Rosnow RL. The volunteer subject, chapter 3. In: Rosenthal R, Rosnow RL, editors. Artifact in behavioral research. New York: Academic; 1969. pp. 59–118.
18. van der Heijden M, Lucas PJF, Lijnse B, Heijdra YF, Schermer TRJ. An autonomous mobile system for the management of COPD. J Biomed Inform. 2013;46:458–69. doi: 10.1016/j.jbi.2013.03.003.
19. Vargas PA, Robles E, Harris J, Radford P. Using information technology to reduce asthma disparities in underserved populations: a pilot study. J Asthma. 2010;47(8):889–94. doi: 10.3109/02770903.2010.497887.
20. Wilson K, Fornasier S, White KM. Psychological predictors of young adults' use of social networking sites. Cyberpsychol Behav Social Netw. 2010;13(2):173–7. doi: 10.1089/cyber.2009.0094.

Part III
Additional Methodology

Chapter 13
Privacy and Data Protection: Mission Impossible?

Georgios Raptis

13.1 Protection of Your Data: Why?

Medical data are sensitive data in terms of confidentiality. Professional discretion in medicine has a great tradition of over 2500 years. Hippocrates defined in his oath that physicians shall keep information about their patients secret.

Modern information technology and ubiquitous interconnected networks around the world pose big challenges in protecting medical data. Consumer Health Informatics implies that medical data will be accessed, transferred and stored in public networks and services. We need to ask, if effective data and privacy protection is possible and feasible at a reasonable cost and effort.

13.2 What Data Should Be Protected?

In a discussion about protection of medical data most people have medical records written by a physician in mind. They include the diagnoses of the patient, the medication, care, medical history, laboratory results and some other relevant conditions such as pregnancy or lactation. It is clear, that this data needs protection, as most patients do not want to make them public.

But there are also other data that must also be considered as sensitive medical data, although they do not fall into the categories mentioned above.

Just think of a patient sending and receiving e-mails or making a video conference once a month with a cardiologist. Someone knowing this will suppose

---

G. Raptis
German Medical Association, Berlin, Germany

TH Mittelhessen University of Applied Sciences, Faculty of Health Sciences, Giessen, Germany that this patient could have a medical issue with his heart. Connection data can reveal a doctor-patient relationship. They must also be considered as medical data that needs protection.

The address book of a physician is a good source of information about his/her patients. Normally in "real life" no one would publish his address book in the newspapers or give it to a little known company abroad. Current apps in modern smart phones and tablet computers have in many cases unlimited access to the address book of the owner and regularly sent its entries to the server of the app producer. If thereby the relationships of a doctor to his patients are revealed, then this is quite problematic. Address books can contain sensitive medical data.

What about search queries (cf. Sect. 3.2.1)? Consider some person asking Bing®, Yahoo!™ or Google™ about myasthenia gravis and searching for information. Or she/he retrieves information from the homepage of a specific myasthenia gravis support group. Of course there is a chance that this person has just an academic interest in myasthenia gravis or searches on request of a friend. But someone observing the search queries and web browsing interests may consider that there is some risk for this person having myasthenia gravis. If this is your bank and you are asking for a long-term loan, then you may have a problem.

The following consumer health informatics related data can give information about medical conditions of patients and therefore should be protected:

- All electronic health records (EHR), e.g. diagnoses, care, medication, medical history, laboratory test results, medical images, conditions etc.
- Personal health records (PHR) [9] including information and observations with health content written by the patient, cf. Chap. 14
- All professional communication of a physician in any network
- Connection data of Consumer Health Informatics services or of communications between patients and physicians
- Search queries about medical conditions, diagnoses, medication, procedures etc.
- Information about visited web pages with medical content

13.3 What Kind of Protection Do We Need? How Can Protection Be Achieved?

It is obvious that confidentiality is a major goal in protecting health data. In Consumer Health Informatics this is of great importance because protecting confidentiality has become difficult in networks and the Internet. The Internet does not forget and you cannot erase information once published. Medical data is no exception from this rule. Once medical data had been revealed and become searchable, secrecy generally cannot be restored any more.

But confidentiality is not the only security objective applicable to health data. Consider a consultation with your doctor over a Level 1 service about your type 1 diabetes mellitus. Suppose that confidentiality of data is effectively protected because the service uses a virtual private network [14], which encrypts [11] all transferred data. Your doctor sends you a message and he recommends that you increase the insulin dosis by 2 IE in the morning. Unfortunately when you receive the message it says that you should increase the morning insulin dosis by 20 IE. The message has been somehow altered and next morning you will have a serious problem (cf. Sect. 5.3.4.4). Integrity is an important security objective not only for messages but for any medical content. Breach of integrity of health data can be life threatening. So we should protect the integrity of data and services in Consumer Health Informatics services so that you can be sure that health data has not been altered.

Are you actually sure that a message has been sent from your doctor? Or that the information about a new drug on a Level 0 service is from a trustworthy source? What if this is not the case? Most people receive lots of e-mails every day supposedly from big companies, banks or lotteries saying that they have won millions of dollars. This is a very common problem and some people really believe some of those messages. Such fake messages are not sent from the supposed senders, even when they say so. Maybe it is a good idea to protect not only confidentiality and integrity but also the authenticity of health data and services.

Suppose you receive this message saying that you should increase your morning dosis by 20 IE and the integrity and authenticity of the message is protected. That means, you are sure, the message is from your doctor and it is not altered. You suffer a major hypoglycemic episode while driving to work but your doctor insists that he did not send this message at all. You may choose to sue your doctor but how can you convince the judge that it was your doctor sending exactly this message? We need some mechanism providing evidence for the actions of each user and the information sent ("non-repudiation"). All this applies not only to health data but also to health services. Just think of a hacked service providing false medical information or manipulating patient records. This can also be life threatening.

> **Take Home**
> At least as important as confidentiality are integrity and authenticity of medical data and health services. Their breach can potentially lead to life threatening situations.

13.4 How Health Data and Services Should Be Protected?

This volume is about Consumer Health Informatics and not about computer security and cryptography. Furthermore consumers and patients are not computer security experts and cannot assess the security mechanisms of a service. We must assume that reputable companies operating health services use state of the art security mechanisms. However, security is a cost factor (cf. [8]) and adds complexity sometimes making handling and user experience difficult. So maybe data and systems security is not on the focus of any Consumer Health Informatics service. Therefore we give here an exemplary rough overview of some typical security mechanisms.

Confidentiality can be protected by many means. Data transferred in networks are typically protected by using cryptography [2], e.g. with the TLS (cf. [13]) protocol. It is important that secure algorithms (such as RSA^{TM} or AES) with long keys (like 2048 bit for RSA and 256 bit for AES) [6] and protocol parameters (like Perfect Forward Secrecy, cf. [1, 12]) are used and cryptographic keys are securely created and erased after use.

Stored data are usually protected by implementing access control mechanisms. This means, a user must first authenticate himself to the server and not until then he gets access to his/her data. The problem is that access controls can be overridden by attacks commonly known as "hacking". Usually someone exploits a vulnerability of the operating system or database engine of the server and gets unauthorized access to the data. As vulnerabilities in software cannot be fully excluded, access controls cannot guarantee a 100 % protection of the data. So it is a good idea to additionally apply a cryptographic protection to the data. It is virtually impossible to break a correctly implemented encryption if the decryption key is kept secret. The goal is that an attacker who manages to hack the service can get non-readable data only. However it is not always possible to encrypt medical data as management and processing of encrypted data can be very difficult.

Data integrity is usually protected by implementing access controls so that only authorized users (e.g. the doctor or the patient) can alter data. Use of cryptographic tools such as secure hash functions or electronic signatures is even better but not yet widely used.

Authenticity is achieved in many cases by using (only) passwords. Passwords are prone to attacks widely known as "identity theft", so if authenticity is a major issue at least a two factor authentication should be used. This means that a user must use two independent factors in order to prove his/her identity. For an attacker it is much more difficult to steal and use both factors. Examples are a password (something I know) and a PIN sent to my mobile phone (something I possess), or a chip card and a PIN (cf. Sect. 12.5). Even more secure is a two factor authentication if it is combined with cryptographic methods and protocols like electronic signatures (e.g. in TLS client certificate authentication) or zero knowledge protocols, [2, Chap. 14.3.3], [15].

Non-repudiation is usually supported by a health system by keeping track of the actions of the users and logging this information. For messages non-repudiation implies the usage of electronic signatures. In many jurisdictions there are laws regulating legally binding electronic signatures and defining specific technical and organizational requirements about them [5]. Electronic signatures are not yet widely used in health services.

> **Take Home**
> Use more cryptography! You can usually rely on mathematics, more than on software security and access control mechanisms.
> (Just) passwords are too weak to ensure authenticity. A two factor authentication mechanism or some suitable cryptographic protocol should instead be used.

13.5 The Bottom Line for Companies Running Health Services

- If you store medical records, use more cryptography! If you can reach your goal either by implementing access control mechanisms or by encrypting the data, encryption is the more confident way. You can still implement additional access control mechanisms. Sure, there are workflows where encryption does not work and key management can be very complicated, especially if you must share data between the patient and his doctors. But you can still use encryption where applicable, to the maximum possible extent.
- Establish an information security management system [3] and implement appropriate security measures! There is an established methodology for that [4] and a great variety of security tools like firewalls, intrusion detection systems, VPN-devices, hardware security modules or security appliances you can use in the scope of your security management. Computer security needs specialized know-how, so you must hire experts or charge a specialized company for this job.
- Prove the security of your service! You can charge a specialized reputable company with a security audit and get a security certification. Ideally your security architecture should be strong enough to even publish it, as this will create more confidence.

13.6 Know Your Enemy

Who is interested in breaching the confidentiality of patients' records? And why should someone hack a health service and pose the life and health of patients at risk? The most simple and cynical answer is, because she/he can do this. Many attacks to web services today are not specifically targeted. If a system is somehow vulnerable then someone who finds out may attack this system, either just for fun or to sell the stolen data, infect the server with a botnet malware and earn some money. The tools for most attacks are (mostly) freely available to the public. In fact, in many cases an attacker will not specifically seek health services or data. However, it is only the result that counts. Once your medical records are public they can be maliciously used by other people.

Medical records can be valuable information for many reasons. A bank may choose to not grant a loan if the customer has certain medical conditions and there is a risk of becoming ill. A potential employer would possibly choose a healthier applicant for a certain job. Of course banks and companies do not hack into health services in order to get information about their customers (and if some do that, you better do not want to do business with them). But what if the relevant data are already public? In many jurisdictions it is illegal to hack into computer systems but it is not illegal to search the Internet for publicly available information about customers or potential employees. Besides "information vandals" or criminals hacking into computer systems for fun or for money, they are also various authorities around the world, which may cause trouble to health services. Well, it is controversially discussed if governmental authorities should hack into computer systems and for most people it is unlikely that an intelligence agency is interested in their medical records. However, there is evidence that some standard software products, security hardware and software and even cryptography standards can be influenced by such authorities and may contain vulnerabilities [7, 10]. The problem is that such vulnerabilities are accessible not only to these authorities but can also be discovered and exploited by common hackers and criminals. Computer security and especially cryptography needs trust anchors like secure keys and algorithms. If the trust anchors cannot be trusted anymore, people will not have confidence to health services and will not use them.

13.7 Protection of Your Data: Can I Trust Health Services?

This is a very difficult question. And this question is even more complicated if you consider data protection not only in Consumer Health Informatics services but also in comparison to the data security of a doctor's office or hospital. Most doctors and hospitals use information technology to handle the records of their patients and they are usually very cautious taking data protection very seriously. But no one is immune against all cyber-attacks. Doctors are no exception of this rule. Because of this there are in some countries (e.g. Germany) recommendations from their professional organisations to avoid connecting computer systems with health records to the Internet.

A common statement is that there is no 100 % security. But the following statement is also true: you can usually trust in mathematics. The prime factorization problem, which is the foundation of the RSA encryption algorithm, has not been effectively solved since the days of Euclid of Alexandria 2300 years ago. But on the other hand, mathematics and cryptography provide effective security only if trust anchors like secure key generation and implementation of the algorithms are guaranteed. And for some algorithms it is possible albeit unlikely to experience "crypto-accidents" in the near future like a very good idea to solve a 2300 old mathematical problem or to build a really working large quantum computer. If security hardware, software and Consumer Health Informatics services are certified and monitored by independent and reputable third parties then consumers and patients may choose to trust them. In this context it is very important to have the right to choose, just because it is a matter of trust someone may or may not have in a specific health service, health informatics or generally in technology.

Consumers and patients normally cannot assess the security of a service, as this requires detailed information of the underlying security architecture and expert know-how. They have to trust the company running the service. Companies operating health services can generate trust if they are honest to the customers. It is a good idea not only to explain but also to prove why someone should entrust her/his data to a specific company. Certifications like ISO27001 are a good starting point as they demonstrate that security is taken seriously. A full security audit of the service by a widely recognized company or authority considering not only organizational but also all aspects of technical security would be even better as it creates confidence to the public.

Consumers and patients may also choose to trust health services in a more differentiated approach. One may not have a problem to trust a health service for diabetes or cancer management because all friends, relatives and colleagues anyway know about this. But some people may choose to be more cautious with specific medical records of greater personal importance. The criteria are very individual, starting for example from sexual or mental health and continuing with genetic analyses which can have implications to the following generations.

> **Take Home**
> A security audit or certification of a health service can be helpful to generate trust and acceptance.
> Please give patients the right to choose, whether they want to trust a health service.

References

1. Bernat V. SSL/TLS & perfect forward secrecy. http://vincent.bernat.im/en/blog/2011-ssl-perfect-forward-secrecy.html. Accessed 10 Oct 2013.
2. Buchmann J. Introduction to cryptography. 2nd ed. New York: Springer; 2004.
3. International Organization for Standardization. ISO/IEC27001. Information technology. Security techniques – information security management systems – requirements. Geneva. ISO/IEC.
4. International Organization for Standardization. ISO/IEC27002. Information technology – security techniques – code of practice for information security controls. Geneva: ISO/IEC; 2013.
5. Mason S, editor. Electronic signatures in law. Cambridge/New York: Cambridge University Press; 2012.

6. European Network of Excellence in Cryptology II. ECRYPT II yearly report on algorithms and keysizes. http://www.ecrypt.eu.org/ecrypt2/documents/D.SPA.20.pdf, Sept 2012. Accessed 10 July 2015.
7. Pelroth N, Larson J, Shane S. N.S.A. able to foil basic safeguards of privacy on web. The New York Times, http://www.nytimes.com/2013/09/06/us/nsa-foils-much-internet-encryption.html?smid=pl-share, Sept 2013. Accessed 10 Oct 2013.
8. Sonnenreich W, Albanese J, Stout B. Return on security investment (ROSI) – a practical quantitative model. JRPIT. 2006;38(1):45–56.
9. Tang PC, Ash JS, Bates DW, Overhage JM, Sands DZ. Personal health records: definitions, benefits, and strategies for overcoming barriers to adoption. J Am Med Inform Assoc. 2006;13(2):121–6. doi: 10.1197/jamia.M2025.
10. New York Times. Secret documents reveal N.S.A. campaign against encryption. The New York Times, http://www.nytimes.com/interactive/2013/09/05/us/documents-reveal-nsa-campaign-against-encryption.html?smid=pl-share, Sept 2013. Accessed 10 Oct 2013.
11. Wikipedia. Encryption. http://en.wikipedia.org/wiki/Encryption. Accessed 17 Oct 2013.
12. Wikipedia. Perfect forward secrecy. http://en.wikipedia.org/wiki/Perfect_forward_secrecy. Accessed 10 Oct 2013.
13. Wikipedia. Transport layer security. http://en.wikipedia.org/wiki/Secure_Sockets_Layer. Accessed 10 Oct 2013.
14. Wikipedia. Virtual private network. http://en.wikipedia.org/wiki/Virtual_private_network. Accessed 17 Oct 2013.
15. Wikipedia. Zero-knowledge proof. http://en.wikipedia.org/wiki/Zero-knowledge_proof. Accessed 17 Oct 2013.

Chapter 14
The Patient-Centered Electronic Health Record and Patient Portals

Lisa M. Vizer and Amanda K. Hall

Take Home

Terminology

- Electronic Health Record (EHR) – a health care provider's secure electronic record of patient information. Patients do not have direct access to the EHR, although a subset of information is usually viewable through the patient's Patient Portal.
- Personal Health Record (PHR) – an electronic application that allows a patient or patient proxy to maintain and manage his or her health information in a private, secure, and confidential manner. This record is owned by the patient and can contain information that is not included in a medical record.
- Patient Portal – a secure electronic application or website that gives a patient or proxy access to personal health information and medical records connected to his or her health care provider's EHR. Opportunities to interact electronically with the provider's office and provider are usually included.
- Meaningful Use (MU) – is a Centers for Medicare & Medicaid Services (CMS) program incentivizing the use of certified electronic health record (EHR) technology as a means by which doctors, patients, and family members can store and retrieve medical information to gain access to their medical records and to more completely engage in their care, to improve quality, safety, efficiency, and care coordination.

L.M. Vizer • A.K. Hall
Department of Biomedical Informatics and Medical Education, University of Washington School of Medicine, Seattle, WA, USA

14.1 Introduction

The health care industry touts the personal health record (PHR), and particularly the patient portal, as instrumental to the future of medical care and health management. Many experts see the patient portal as a powerful means to engage patients in their own care and empower them to manage their own health, especially for those with chronic health conditions. Studies also show that patients are enthusiastic about the idea of patient portals [15]. Specifically, one study [9] shows that patients are very interested in the self-management and administrative benefits of patient portals. However, recent studies [10, 14] also show insufficient evidence to claim improvement in health outcomes, cost measures, or health care utilization. Differing viewpoints make it difficult to understand the real impact of patient portals on patients' wellness and how the portals fit into patients' health care. This chapter will help disambiguate some of the claims.

This chapter will give an overview of the evolution of PHRs and patient portals, discuss the components of a PHR or patient portal, examine the political implications along with accessibility and usability factors, and consider the weaknesses of the system including liability and data issues.

14.1.1 Evolution of Patient-Centered Health Information Systems in the USA

In 1994, The Guardian Angel "Manifesto" Proposal envisioned the idea of patient-centered health information systems or electronic health records where the web could manage health care information and provide education and communication across the lifespan [20]. The dot.com era in the late 1990s and into the early 2000s and the widespread use of the Internet spurred the growth and availability of health and medical information on the web, which further prompted the development of PHRs and patient portals [3]. National surveys conducted in the early 2000s found that consumers were interested in receiving, viewing, and communicating health information from and with their health care providers online [23]. Survey findings led EHR developers to produce products (i.e., web interfaces) that linked health care providers and patients.

Patient portals allow patients to have access to a subset of the clinical record and from the provider's EHR. Columbia's PatCIS system and Beth Israel Deaconess's PatientSite were a few of the first patient portals developed in 1999 [5, 13]. Whereas, in 1999 Epic® systems, a widely utilized and established vendor of EHR systems, created a patient portal named MyChart® in collaboration with the Palo Alto Medical Foundation (PAMF) [13]. MyChart® launched in 2000 with great success and since then millions of patients in the USA are using the system, which is also used by Kaiser Permanente® and Group Health® Cooperative. MyChart® enables patients to review their medical record, such as diagnoses, test results, appointments, and allows patients to request appointments or prescription renewals as well as communicate with their health care providers.

Indivo, an open source subset of PHRs known as a Personally Controlled Health Record (PCHR), was developed in 2006. Indivo is based on a subscription model to integrate data from EHR systems across various hospitals. Indivo gives individuals control over who can access, write, and modify information in their records [13]. Indivo has not been successfully adopted by users, a fate also suffered by Google Health™. However, the future of Microsoft® HealthVault® remains to be determined. www.indivohealth.org/research outlines the relationship of PHR pioneers. Due to the relatively early developmental lifecycle of patient-centered health information systems and slow adoption, we look forward to more available research on their use and benefits [7].

14.2 PHR and Patient Portal Components

Personal Health Records are standalone records maintained entirely by the patient or patient proxy. Useful for managing family history and other personal health information, PHRs are especially important when the patient is engaged in acute disease or chronic illness management. Health tools often available through a PHR include vetted health information, disease management tools, and health education and promotion materials. These records are tied to the patient.

Unlike the PHR, patient portals are connected, or tethered, to a provider's specific EHR. Patients may need to access several patient portals to view their health information since it can be spread among several providers. Many commercial and private patient portals are in use. Popular commercial portals include Epic®'s MyChart®, Cerner®'s Patient Portal, and eClinicalWorks' Patient Portal. Health care delivery systems may also have their own patient portals, such as the US Veteran Administration's My HealtheVet.

For instance, My HealtheVet (MHV), the US Department of Veterans Affairs (VA) PHR system, was introduced in 2003 [17]. MHV (http://www.myhealth.va.gov) provides veterans with health education information, health management tools, and other useful resources. MHV includes health information entered by veterans and data from the VA's EHR system. MHV was designed to complement other services offered through the VA and provides access to health information so patients and their families can play a more active role in veterans' health care. MHV has three levels[1] of access, and functionality increases with each level (note, each level includes all the features and functionality of the previous level or levels) (refer to Table 14.1, page 284 for a list of levels of access and functionality of MHV). According to [17, p. S63],

---

[1]Levels here should not be mistaken for the Levels of Consumer Health Informatics services introduced in Chaps. 3, 4, 5, and 6.

Table 14.1 Levels of Access and Functionality of My HealtheVet (according to [17])

Level	Details
Level 1: Public access, available to anyone with an Internet connection	General information and resources (VA benefits, VA-related news), Research health (evidence-based health information, health screening tools), and My HealthVet Learning Center (online health courses)
Level 2: Veteran's online registration access	Get care (caregiver information, treatment locations, health insurance coverage), Health information card (print medical information on a wallet card), Personal health history, family health history, military health history, personal health summary, Health eLogs (track health measures such as blood pressure, weight etc.), Allergies, Immunizations, Tests, Medical events, Food and activity journals, health calendar, medications, and prescription refills
Level 3: Authenticated users (in-person identity verification)	VA prescription history, My complete medications, Wellness reminders, and Secure messaging (between patients and their health care team)

As of July 2009, MHV has been visited over 28 million times, more than 810,000 people have registered (16.3 % of veterans currently receiving VA health care services), and over 130,000 veterans have completed the in-person identity verification process.

The portal system available to a patient is chosen by the health care provider or health system, and is often dictated by the provider's choice of EHR. In this section we discuss the data accessible through and functions of PHRs and portals.

14.2.1 Data

As long as methods outlined in Chap. 13 to protect data against different forms of malevolent intrusion are carefully applied, PHRs provide a safe repository for health information; that data is inputted by the patient, either manually or through an import function. Patient portals provide access to a wide range of patient data that is pulled from the medical provider's EHR. We discuss types of data currently accessed through PHRs and portals and data that will soon be integrated.

14.2.1.1 Demographic Data

The personal information that users can input into a PHR or is displayed in the patient portal varies widely across vendors. Demographic information typically includes:

- Name
- Sex
- Date of birth
- Address

14.2 PHR and Patient Portal Components

- Phone number
- E-mail address

Additional information may include Social Security Number and emergency contact information.

PHRs allow the patient full control over personal data, but they require the patient to manage and curate that data. Portals, in contrast, pre-populate data, and allow patients to view their personal information, but only allow them to change a subset. This is to protect the patients and providers against unauthorized changes. For example, patients might be able to view name, date of birth, insurance information, and email address, but only be able to change their email address.

14.2.1.2 Clinical Data

Laboratory and other test results, such as those from radiology and pathology, are usually accessible to the patient through the patient portal and can be input into a PHR. Other common information is health history, allergies, immunizations, and medication and medical condition lists. Some patient portals also include physician notes on patient visits. The portal might also provide patients access to educational material about their medical conditions.

Some patients may have difficulty interpreting complex medical data and jargon [10, 14]. These issues might be addressed in part by patient education, but a more sustainable approach is to improve the way data is labeled and presented. For example, effective data visualization provides the user with an information display that allows clearer understanding of the data and use of lay language allows patients to understand information in their own words. These tools can reduce confusion about and misinterpretation of information, see, however, remaining limitations in Sects. 8.4.2 and 8.4.3.

14.2.1.3 Patient-Provided Data

Patients provide all of the data that is inputted to a PHR, but can also provide some of the information in a portal. This includes a subset of the data discussed above, but might also include data from personal devices and observations. Although not yet commonly available, consumers could upload health information from blood pressure monitors, blood glucose monitors, insulin pumps, sleep monitors, or notes on lifestyle and symptoms, such as sleep quality, mood, or headache. A PHR or portal system can use this information to produce visualizations, alerts to the patient or a clinician, reminders about healthy behaviors, or recommendations about behavioral changes, as outlined in many places in this volume.

14.2.2 Functionality

Anyone can create a PHR for herself or for someone under her care, but for a patient to use a patient portal the system or medical provider must verify her identity and she must register. Some providers require in-person verification for accessing the portal. Other methods include verification through email or postal mail. Authentication assures that unauthorized persons do not access sensitive health information.

However, registration and authentication are procedures that can cause a great deal of trouble for patients. For example, in a study of the US VA's My HealtheVet program [14], testing found that only 25 % of users successfully completed registration without problems. Participants were especially confused about password requirements. In the future, another method such as biometric authentication, including fingerprint or iris scanning, may eliminate this type of issue, although new risks of exposing privacy lurk, as outlined in Sect. 8.4.4.2.3.

Other barriers to registration reported in a study from Goel [9] include lack of information, lack of motivation, negative attitudes toward portals, and computer problems. These issues are more effectively addressed through patient education at the point of service or through outreach programs. Use of mobile technology may partially address the issue with computer problems and provide access to a wider audience, but raises its own set of concerns (e.g. around security and accessibility).

PHRs are a repository of patient-supplied information and there is no interaction between that repository and the medical provider's system. All information that is collected in the PHR is inputted by the patient, either manually or through import of data sent from a provider's system. Patient portals, on the other hand, do interact with a medical provider's system and can offer functionality that a PHR cannot. A survey of popular patient portals shows a wide variety of available features, with a subset being available on most portals. The most common features are:

- Secure messaging with providers
- Refilling prescriptions
- Viewing lab results
- Viewing visit history
- Scheduling appointments
- Reviewing the patient account

Segall and coworkers [21] found that patients encountered significant problems when attempting to use a patient portal for a large university health system. Most problematic was the navigation system, which participants found confusing. When doing other tasks, such as finding a particular lab test, entering data, requesting an appointment, or interpreting a test result, patients were frustrated or made mistakes. These issues point to problems with usability, which we will discuss later in the chapter.

Some functionality might be in limited use at present, but will be more widely available in both PHRs and patient portals in the future. Capabilities that might be more widespread in the future include tracking family tree and family health history, setting and tracking individual health goals, interacting with visualizations of patient data, downloading and transmitting the medical record, and storing omics data. Omics data includes genomics, proteomics, metabolomics, and other biological data. These data can be used to personalize medical care.

14.3 PHRs and Patient Portals in Context

It is important to understand the parts of a patient portal, but it is just as important to understand the context in which it is situated. This section will discuss aspects of the environment in which portals operate that concern policy and individual use.

14.3.1 Political Forces and Meaningful Use

Nationwide electronic health records (EHR) became a main goal of US health care reform in recent years to combat rising health care costs and as a way to increase quality of care. In 2009, US congress passed the Health Information Technology for Economic and Clinical Health Act (HITECH), part of the American Recovery and Reinvestment Act, to promote nationwide adoption of health information technology over the next century. To support this initiative, congress created incentives, in the form of Medicare and Medicaid payments, to providers who made meaningful use of EHRs and penalties for providers who do not adopt EHRs by 2016. To achieve meaningful use providers are required to comply with technical standards set by the Office of the National Coordinator for Health Information Technology (ONC), certification by the Department of Health and Human Services (HHS) ensures that EHR's are compliant, functional, and secure.

PHRs and patient portals are a cornerstone of Meaningful Use (MU). MU is defined as using certified EHR technology as a means by which doctors, patients, and family members can store and retrieve medical information to gain access to their medical records and to more completely engage in their care, to improve quality, safety, efficiency, and for care coordination (www.cdc.gov/ ehrmeaningfulusc/introduction.html). MU consists of three stages, each stage has a set of core functions that providers and hospitals need to comply with in order to receive incentive payments. Stage one primarily requires the sharing and collection of data (e.g., providing patients with electronic copies of their medical records, e-prescribing, and recording of patients aged 13 or older that smoke); stage two, which builds upon stage one, focuses on advanced clinical processes (i.e., to increase secure online health information exchanges between providers and patients, such as secure messaging, imaging results, and electronic notes); and stage three, again building on the previous two stages, aims to improve outcomes (e.g., through prevention care, interventions, and the ability to track and monitor actionable data), final recommendations for stage three are forthcoming ([19]; www.healthit.gov/ providers-professionals/meaningful-use-definition-objectives).

For example, the Institute of Medicine (IOM) formed a committee to identify social and behavioral determinants of health for inclusion in forthcoming recommendations of MU guidelines [18]. However, lower than expected stage one and two compliance rates and achievement deadline challenges resulted in extended deadlines and modifications. A lack of available literature on how to meet these standards and further how to deal with challenges regarding vulnerable populations still need to be addressed [16]. Some health care systems have been making progress towards MU initiatives, such as Group Health:

The Patient Portal at Group Health – Vignette

> *Gwen O'Keefe, MD*
> *October 27, 2014*
>
> "Group Health is an integrated health care system linking care delivery and insurance coverage in order to achieve one goal – affordable, quality health care for all. As a nonprofit organization, Group Health helps nearly 600,000 patients throughout Washington state achieve better health through a focus on preventive care, combined with medical education, a charitable foundation and a nationally recognized research institute.
>
> One of the leading principles at Group Health is that the medical record belongs to the patient. This was a guiding factor in the decision to activate the patient portal BEFORE implementing physician charting tools when Group Health began implementing the EHR in 2002. GHC is likely the only institution to start with secure messaging between patients and doctors prior to physicians using other EHR tools. As part of the initial implementation, the patient record was also populated with lab results, prescription data and diagnoses. Over the years this has expanded to include immediate release of new lab results to patients and all radiology results and pathology results, after a short delay for abnormal results to allow for provider review and communication of potentially serious results. All release is now automatic, and this is felt to also add to patient safety, as patient review of their data adds another level of safety to assure that abnormal results are appropriately followed up. Viewing medical test results, messaging with providers and ordering medication refills are the most popular portal features, followed by viewing after visit summaries.
>
> Seventy percent of adult practice patients access the portal. Messaging and immediate communication of key information regarding their health has become a hallmark of how clinicians practice and partner with patients at Group Health. The ability to have seamless communication is often listed as the biggest reason patients stay with Group Health. Parents of children can also access the records for their children up to age 13. One of the most popular features here is the ability to download immunization records, a frequent need for the parents of school-age children.
>
> Group Health continues to evolve its use of the patient portal to continue to fit the goals of transparency and patient empowerment in their care."

While MU standards, stage requirements, and hospital and provider compliance rates continue to be evaluated and evolve, other considerations such as patients access to the internet, computer self-efficacy , health literacy concerns , acceptance of technology for health purposes , and usability of patient-portals/PHR interfaces, especially those with disabilities, needs to continue to be researched to prevent a possible digital health divide [12, 19]. Also of concern is the validity of measures used to verify compliance. For example, MU law counts a patient's single use of a portal as evidence of adoption whether they use the system again or not.

14.3.2 Access

Patient access to PHRs and portals is an important concern because older adults, those that are ill or disabled, and those at higher risk for illness stand to gain the most from use of a PHR or portal, but often have less access to those resources. Furthermore, studies are showing some disparities in use of patient portals. Goel et al. [8] found that patients at an urban academic medical center exhibited racial and ethnic disparities in portal enrollment. Those differences do not persist among enrollees, however, in the enrolled population, usage differs by age and gender, with those 18–34 showing lowest utilization among any age group, and males showing less utilization than females. Ancker and coworkers ([1]pmid 21647748) studied adoption among a predominantly low-income patient population and found that those with chronic illness were more likely to adopt use of the portal, but groups that showed lower adoption included non-English speakers, non-white patients, and those without insurance. They also showed that these factors were more pronounced than racial disparities. Although some racial disparities were evident, the differences were lower than reported in earlier studies.

However, Zarcadoolas and coworkers [24] show that vulnerable populations (e.g., consumers who are racial minorities, or have low education levels) are enthusiastic about patient portals and found portals as useful and beneficial. The authors also found that to make patient portals successful with these populations and others, designers must ensure that portals are "easy to read, visually engaging, and have user-friendly navigation." Mobile interfaces to patient portals may also increase accessibility to vulnerable populations as mobile internet use becomes more widespread in all communities. Currently, 91 % of Americans own cellular phones and 60 % of those use their phones to access the internet [6].

14.3.3 Use and Usability

Patients are more aware of their health due in part to the growth in access and use of the Internet coupled with the availability of digital medical information [3]. Along with this trend, use of PHRs and patient portals will grow, but functionality must keep up with patient expectations and the tsunami of patient-generated data. These systems must also make it easy for patients to access and use their information. Usability is a measurement of how easy it is for someone to use a technology. A high or low level of usability directly impacts how much benefit a person will gain from using a patient portal. Several studies have investigated the usability of PHRs and their features. Many have found that just the perception of poor usability is a barrier to use [24].

As mentioned earlier, registration and authentication is problematic for many patients. Haggstrom's and Goel's groups [9, 14] both found multiple usability barriers to successful registration and authentication including problems understanding password guidelines, lack of help information, and computer difficulties. Their findings suggest alternative authentication techniques and mobile technology as possibilities for more usable systems.

Segall and coworkers [21] conducted a usability study of a university health system's patient portal, finding several usability issues including problems with navigation, locating a lab test, and interpreting a lab test. A human factors engineer (a professional familiar with human-centered technology design) made suggestions for site improvements, which included new navigation hierarchies and labels, as well as a redesign of how lab results are displayed. Other common complaints include the heavy use of text and jargon, suggesting that improved use of charts and data visualizations as well as precise yet understandable language can further improve usability. These are small improvements, but they can have a large impact on how well a person is able to make use of the system.

Furthermore, researchers have extensively studied provider workflows, but done little examination of patient workflows. PHRs and patient portals do not currently take into account the many facets of patient workflow, including the patient's level of ability, literacy, culture, the many providers and family members involved, finances, outside activities, and transportation needs. Designers must consider all these factors and more when designing for patient workflow. As it stands, PHRs and portals are new technology that are not fitted to the tasks and are therefore disruptive. Future work must focus on how to incorporate the needs and tasks of the patient into the design of the system.

The consumer market explosion of mobile health applications (apps), wearable devices (e.g., fitbit® and Jawbone®), and remote monitoring devices (e.g., monitoring vital signs such as blood pressure) is growing as more consumers gain access to technology and the US health care system advances to a digitally-based health information infrastructure [4, 22]. These various health applications and devices provide patients with immense quantities of data on many types of health behaviors and conditions, such as daily physical activity, blood glucose and blood pressure measurements. Quantified Self is slowly becoming a universal term for a technology use movement that combines self-monitoring and self-tracking technologies for acquisition of data to track behavior, such as physical, mental, or social [22]. For example, the quantified self movement has sparked advances in new wearable and sensor technologies referred to as smart wearable body sensors (SWBS). SWBS include a wide range of wearable sensors, such as sensors to monitor mobility for rehabilitation, physical activity, and seizure activity ([2]). Individuals are increasingly motivated to seek health information, access health information via the Internet, and use health applications, yet how access to health information informs or influences their medical decision-making is still

14.3 PHRs and Patient Portals in Context

being researched [12]. Moreover, health care organizations now offer patients the ability to exchange secure messages with providers through their patient portals and secure text messaging options will be forthcoming for such purposes as health promotion, reminders (e.g., medication), advice from providers, and exchange of vital information (e.g., Florence or Flo in the United Kingdom, www.getflorence.co.uk/).

Therefore, to leverage data from newer modes of tracking and collecting health status information and to monitor changes in health behavior, PHR and patient-portals will need to consider how best to incorporate patient-provided data into their systems and how best to make it useful and actionable (i.e., for effective quality of care, treatment, and behavior change) for patients and health care provider, such as uploading, manually inputting data, or synchronization of accurate information from various types of devices or systems, if multiple systems or devices are used. The implementation of Health Information Exchange (HIE) (www.healthit.gov/HIE) in the United States will accomplish a measure of this synchronization. Visualization tools (e.g., display of an individual's blood pressure data history or public health alerts) and self-tracking/self-monitoring of patient-provided data will need to be easy to understand and interpret, which includes considering comprehension of health information and health literacy of the user. Many additional challenges include usability of PHRs, patient portals, and medical devices, interpretable information, customizable personal health information, incorporating completely consumer-driven information into medical health records, personalized medicine through use of genomics, and confidentiality of information [11]. While these challenges persist, the potential benefits of patient-provided data include aggregation of health behavior trend data that can be used to change or modify health behavior for just-in-time adaptive interventions, inform medical decisions, track health status changes, and provides an opportunity for health care providers and patients to discuss health behaviors to promote prevention and self-management of diseases. Chapters 4 and 5 and the applications in Part II describe various augmented services.

14.3.4 Liability, Reliability, and Accuracy

The PHR and patient portal provide access to immensely sensitive information. Privacy and ownership of that information is of great concern to patients and their families, as well as providers. However, legal ownership of the data is not clear cut. When records were kept on paper, the patient owned the record while the provider had custody. With records kept digitally, providers appear to exercise both custody and ownership of data accessed through a portal, although the patient still has the expectation of ownership. It is unclear if a provider must grant a patient complete deletion of his medical record from an EHR, if requested. On the other hand, for data that is stored in a PHR, the patient has ownership of the data and the host site has custody.

Patients also expect to be able to limit others' access to their data. For example, a patient and provider must have an explicit release form in place in order for the provider to exchange information with another provider. However, there is no provision in the patient portal for the patient to indicate what information they would like to be shared with which other providers. This is not a pressing issue as long as data is tethered to a provider, but will become much more of an issue when Health Information Exchange (HIE) allows collection of all providers' records in one repository. In one case, a patient might desire for her primary care provider to have access to all records, but might not wish for her ophthalmologist to have the ability to access mental health notes.

System designers must also make provisions for ensuring data quality. Patients and providers must be able to view data and request corrections. Revisions should be marked with date and requestor, while leaving the prior version viewable as well. Suspect data or data not yet vetted (as might occur with patient-provided data) should be flagged to avoid confusion and to promote further inspection.

14.4 Conclusion

This chapter explained the differences between PHRs and patient portals as well as the components and functionality of each. We also examined the context of these systems, including the political, accessibility, usability, and legal issues. PHRs and patient portals are going to remain an important part of the health care system moving forward, but we will encounter many opportunities and obstacles along the way. Policymakers must address legal and political roadblocks, and designers must resolve use and usability issues. If developed well, PHR and patient portal technologies have the potential to transform the spectrum of patient work across the lifespan from managing health information to maintaining health to managing chronic illness and end-of-life care.

Acknowledgements This work was supported in part by the National Institutes of Health, National Library of Medicine (NLM) Biomedical and Health Informatics Training Program at the University of Washington (Grant Nr. T15LM007442). The content is solely the responsibility of the authors and does not necessarily represent the official views of the National Institutes of Health.

References

1. Ancker JS, Barron Y, Rockoff ML, Hauser D, Pichardo M, Szerencsy A, Calman N. Use of an electronic patient portal among disadvantaged populations. J Gen Intern Med. 2011;26(10):1117–23. doi: 10.1007/s11606-011-1749-y.

2. Appelboom G, Camacho E, Abraham ME, Bruce SS, Dumont EL, Zacharia BE, D'Amico R, Slomian J, Reginster JY, Bruyère O, Connolly Jr ES. Smart wearable body sensors for patient self-assessment and monitoring. Arch Public Health. 2014;72(1):28. doi: 10.1186/2049-3258-72-28.
3. Archer N, Fevrier-Thomas U, Lokker C, McKibbon MA, Strauss SE. Personal health records: a scoping review. JAMIA. 2011;18(4):512–22. doi: 10.1136/amiajnl-2011-000105.
4. Bonato P. Advances in wearable technology and its medical applications. In: Engineering in medicine and biology society (EMBC), 2010 annual international conference of the IEEE. IEEE; 2010. pp. 2021–24
5. Cimino JJ, Li J, Mendonça EA, Sengupta S, Patel VL, Kushniruk AW. An evaluation of patient access to their electronic medical records via the world wide web. In: Proceedings of the AMIA symposium. American Medical Informatics Association; 2000. p. 151
6. Duggan M. Cell phone activities 2013. Pew Research Internet Project. 2013. Retrieved from http://www.pewinternet.org/2013/09/19/cell-phone-activities-2013/. Last viewed 27 July 2015.
7. Emont S. Measuring the impact of patient portals. What the literature tells us. California Health Foundation, 2011. Oakland. http://www.chcf.org/~/media/MEDIA%20LIBRARY%20Files/PDF/M/PDF%20MeasuringImpactPatientPortals.pdf. Last viewed 27 July 2015.
8. Goel MS, Brown TL, Williams A, Cooper AJ, Hasnain-Wynia R, Baker DW. Patient reported barriers to enrolling in a patient portal. JAMIA. 2011;18 Suppl 1:i8–12. doi: 10.1136/amiajnl-2011-000473.
9. Goel MS, Brown TL, Williams A, Hasnain-Wynia R, Thompson JA, Baker DW. Disparities in enrollment and use of an electronic patient portal. J Gen Intern Med. 2011;26(10):1112–6. doi: 10.1007/s11606-011-1728-3.
10. Goldzweig CL, Orshansky G, Paige NM, Towfigh AA, Haggstrom DA, Miake-Lye I, Beroes JM, Shekelle PG. Electronic patient portals: evidence on health outcomes, satisfaction, efficiency, and attitudes: a systematic review. Ann Intern Med. 2013;159(10):677–87. doi: 10.7326/0003-4819-159-10-201311190-00006.
11. Gibbons MC, Wilson RF, Samal L, Lehmann CU, Dickersin K, Lehmann HP, Aboumatar H, Finkelstein J, Shelton E, Sharma R, Bass EB. Consumer health informatics: results of a systematic evidence review and evidence based recommendations. Transl Behav Med. 2011;1(1):72–82. doi: 10.1007/s13142-011-0016-4.
12. Hall AK, Bernhardt JM, Dodd V. Older adults use of online and offline sources of health information and constructs of reliance and self-efficacy for medical decision making. J Health Commun. 2015;20(7):751–8. doi: 10.1080/10810730.2015.1018603.
13. Halamka JD, Mandl KD, Tang PC. Early experiences with personal health records. JAMIA. 2008;15(1):1–7.
14. Haggstrom DA, Saleem JJ, Russ AL, Jones J, Russell SA, Chubler NR. Lessons learned from usability testing of the VA's personal health record. JAMIA. 2011;18 Suppl 1:i13–7. doi: 10.1136/amiajnl-2010-000082.
15. Goldberg L, Lide B, Lowry S, Massett HA, O'Connell T, Preece J, Quesenberry M, Shneiderman B. Usability and accessibility in consumer health informatics current trends and future challenges. Am J Prev Med. 2011;40(5) Suppl 2:187–97. doi: 10.1016/j.amepre.2011.01.009.
16. Luque AE, van Keken A, Winters P, Keefer MC, Sanders M, Fiscella K. Barriers and facilitators of online patient portals to personal health records among persons living with HIV: formative research. JMIR Res Protoc. 2013;2(1):e8. doi: 10.2196/resprot.2302.
17. Nazi KM, Hogan TP, Wagner TH, McInnes DK, Smith BM, Haggstrom D, Chumbler NR, Gifford AL, Charters KG, Saleem JJ, Weingardt KR, Fischetti LF, Weaver FM. Embracing a health services research perspective on personal health records: lessons learned from the VA My HealtheVet system. J Gen Intern Med. 2010;25 Suppl 1:67–7. doi: 10.1007/s11606-009-1114-6.

18. Committee on the Recommended Social, Behavioral Domains, and Institute of Medicine Measures for Electronic Health Records. Capturing social and behavioral domains in electronic health records: Phase 1. books.nap.edu/openbook.php?record_id=18709 (2014). last visited 27 July 2015.
19. Ralston JD, Coleman K, Reid RJ, Handley MR, Larson EB. Patient experience should be part of meaningful-use criteria. Health Aff. 2010;29(4):607–13. doi: 10.1377/hlthaff.2010.0113.
20. Szolovits P, Doyle J, Long WJ, Kohane I, Pauker SG. Guardian Angel: patient-centered health information systems. groups.csail.mit.edu/medg/projects/ga/manifesto/GAtr.html, 1994.
21. Segall N, Saville JG, L'Engle P, Carlson B, Wright MC, Schulman K, Tcheng JE. Usability evaluation of a personal health record. In: Proceedings AMIA 2011 annual symposium. American Medical Informatics; 2011. pp. 1233–42.
22. Swan M. Emerging patient-driven health care models: an examination of health social networks, consumer personalized medicine and quantified self-tracking. Int J Environ Res Public Health. 2009;6(2):492–525. doi: 10.3390/ijerph6020492.
23. Tang PC, Lansky D. The missing link: bridging the patient-provider health information gap. Health Aff. 2005;24(5):1290–5.
24. Zarcadoolas C, Vaughon WL, Czaja SJ, Jevy L, Rockoff ML. Consumers' perceptions of patient-accessible electronic medical records. JMIR. 2013;15(8):e168. doi: 10.2196/jmir.2507.

Chapter 15
Scrutinized Proof of Effectiveness or Cost Effectiveness Regarding Patient Reported Outcomes

15.1 Introduction

When Consumer Health Informatics services are regarded as medical treatments it is legitimate to ask whether they are superior to known treatments or are equally effective at a lower "impact" or "price". To determine superiority outcome measures have to be defined. These can be hard medical indicators such as HbA1c in diabetes, number of re-admissions in follow-up care of surgeries, or number of infections after a vaccination campaign. Outcome measures can also be behavioral such as compliance to diet recommendations, to medication dosage and intervals, or avoidance of risk taking sexual behavior. Since Consumer Health Informatics is about the client's active role and buy in his perceived quality of life is an equally legitimate outcome target. It may be tested as reduced anxiety in the follow-up care of breast cancer surgery, as feeling safer in an ambient assisted living setting, or feeling in better control of chronic pain. If the client of a Consumer Health Informatics service has experienced improved quality of life and has associated it with his active role as a subscriber of the Consumer Health Informatics service he experiences his self-efficacy improving and, correspondingly, is likely to sustain his compliance with the advice provided through the Consumer Health Informatics service. We encounter positive feedback loops and self reinforcement of healthy behaviors as has been observed for decades and summarized in [3].

For the sake of argument we compare the effectiveness test of a Consumer Health Informatics service to the effectiveness test of a new pharmaceutical agent. This comparison is a necessary baseline because drugs *are* a genuine part of medical care while Consumer Health Informatics is aiming at *becoming* a genuine part of medical care. Consumer Health Informatics services should, therefore, strive to demonstrate their effectiveness in a similar arena as drugs have to. We will have to address a number of shortcomings of this comparison and how they can be dealt with. It should be noted that the following sections do not deal with testing a software for functionality or usability. We rather investigate methods to demonstrate the effectiveness of a Consumer Health Informatics service under the premise that this service has been thoroughly conceived, professionally implemented (including but not limited to the software used), and field tested for practicality.

> **Take Home**
> For Consumer Health Informatics services to become a genuine part of medical care and to become recognized as offers that health plan will pay for, they must prove their appropriateness at the same level of scrutiny as e.g. new pharmaceuticals. Therefore, elements of a clinical trials methodology for Consumer Health Informatics services will be outlined.

15.2 Awareness and Precautions Prior to Beginning a Trial

15.2.1 Nature of the "Active Agent"

When writing about a trial in general or an RCT in peculiar we have so far made the implicit assumption of a phase 3 trial as typically conducted as last step and prerequisite to register a new drug with the FDA or corresponding authorities. As the name suggests there are earlier phases in drug development. They include aspects of the behavior of the drug in the human body including how it is modified and removed from the body (pharmacokinetics) and how it affects body functions in terms of both expected effect and unwanted, potentially toxic adverse effects (pharmacodynamics). None of these notions transfer literally to the preparations of the trial for a Consumer Health Informatics service. Some of the notions in drug development do not even make sense in Consumer Health Informatics service development, such as pharmacokinetics. The common bottom line of preparing a drug and preparing a Consumer Health Informatics service for the phase 3 trial is that everything must be ready for the experiment in a setting like the one where routine application on a broad scale is anticipated and that scrutinized data collection about utilization and effects is in place. For a Consumer Health Informatics service this includes but is not limited to medically correct contents, error free function, error free rollout to clients' environments of use such as diverse platforms, browsers etc. where a web application is to be used, good usability of the GUI, tracking of utilization behavior, measurement of the development of target variables, etc. Once the trial is launched – and this is in agreement with drug development – nothing can be repaired anymore for the duration of the trial.

15.2.2 Change Within and Around

In Sect. 15.2.1 "nothing can be repaired" was purposefully used where one might as well expect "nothing can be changed". The apparently subtle difference is of crucial importance for Consumer Health Informatics. While repair means that something has to be fixed that didn't work properly before, change means the absence of stereotypy. In the approval process of a new drug you can request both: that the treatment does not need a fix and that it can be applied equally for a reasonable amount of time. Consumer Health Informatics services under trial should not need fixes either. However, consider a web portal as a major constituent of the tested service: if it remains the same months over months it will lose all its attraction because one of the reasons to visit a web portal is curiosity, the basic human instinct to spot for something new. Therefore, applying the request to keep the active agent constant – as a prerequisite for the scientific proof of its effectiveness – literally to a "web portal" the service it conveys is doomed to fail because frequencies of clients stopping by will continually decrease. To the contrary, a Consumer Health Informatics service may achieve effectiveness because of a keen sense of its developers for trends in consumers' expectations, resulting in web portal updates that "keep the customer satisfied" (song title by Simon [37]) and hence actively visiting the web portal. Such sensing and reflecting trends in consumer expectations can be done totally opportunistically. In that case it will be hard to argue what is the active agent and why a Consumer Health Informatics service succeeds. Consider, however, that the service delivers a certain medical, behavioral or psychiatric treatment concept such as CBT (against depression or addiction), confrontation (against phobias) etc. through the means of a web portal and updates are within the keeping of that therapeutic model. Then we can argue that "delivering the therapeutic model through the Internet" is being investigated. It goes without saying that the same applies for other technologies such as SMS or apps.

The relative effectiveness of an underlying therapeutic model, the methods to impact behavior, and how this is packaged and delivered to clients has been reviewed by Webb and coworkers [43]. For depression Stuhlmiller and Tolchard have delivered a detailed look at different provisions of CBT and their effectiveness and limitations [39]. Similarly, it has been shown outside the realm of Consumer Health Informatics how a theory of goal setting, motivation, and self efficacy guides the design of therapies [19]. Concretely, task difficulty is systematically increased in their experiments. All such models underlying treatment concepts inform the desirable and permissible range of variations within Consumer Health Informatics services.

Besides purposeful changes that developers implement proactively within a service to preserve its attractiveness, in good apprehension of client expectations, adaptations required to remain operational in changing environments must also fit under the umbrella of a trial. New browser versions, new requests to protect privacy, new pricing policies for text messaging on cellular phones etc. affect the character of a Consumer Health Informatics service from outside. Failing to comply and to adapt accordingly may entail failure; therefore, such reactive adaptations must also fit under the methods of trials for Consumer Health Informatics services.

> **Take Home**
>
> While undergoing a clinical trial a Consumer Health Informatics service has to find a delicate balance between permanence and adaptiveness.
>
> - As a treatment under trial it must deliver a therapeutic "substance", "agent", "strategy" unmistakeably from beginning to end. Whatever it presents to or collects from clients must have a definite and traceable role in the therapeutic concept. In other words: the tested service is tested as an implementation of the therapeutic concept.
> - As an Internet based or mobile service it must show as up to date, entertaining, enticing, encouraging to visit again. To not lose curiosity driven clients it must change its appearance at reasonable speed.
>
> To bridge these two competing requirements a clear therapeutic concept and an architecture that implements it must guide the launch and continuation of a service.

15.2.3 Clients' Behavioral Patterns

Arguments have so far emphasized the quality and the nature of the service. More challenges arise from the fact that the service does not come upon a set of passive objects whose property changes can be objectively observed. The entities of study rather are human beings with all their predispositions, comprehensions and expectations. Their active contribution in terms of transforming Consumer Health Informatics service elements into personal behaviors are not confounders to be removed from the statistics but parts of the desired effects. As we will see they can still not just be taken as is. Certain behaviors have been well investigated to systematically bias patient reported baseline, intermediate, or endpoint data. Such biases will subsequently be outlined. Among these, the biases introduced through the requirement of voluntary participation in trials is analyzed first. Biases in voluntary participation by the way do not only affect trials of Consumer Health Informatics services but are a little known challenge of drug approval trials as well.

15.2.3.1 Volunteering

In [31] it has been pointed out that it is nearly impossible to make sure that those who volunteer for a psychological experiment are a representative sample of the population from which they are taken. Just asking the whole population and

15.2 Awareness and Precautions Prior to Beginning a Trial 299

including who raises their hands may have overrepresented those who are better educated, have higher social status, higher need for approval, higher intelligence and lower authoritarianism. In medical research, volunteers tend to be more maladjusted than the average [31, p. 111]. Offering financial incentives may attract subgroups that are in more severe need of cash although experiments also show that the need of cash is brought up retrospectively as a justification for an apparently insane behavior. Generally, for whatsoever attempt to draw an unbiased sample voluntarily there are experiments that demonstrate that some bias remains. The turnout can be increased by assigning value to an investigation through financial incentives, education, linking it to the career of the researcher [31, pp. 62–63]. IRB emphasis on absolutely voluntary participation in trials and perfect absence of coercion in the process of enrolling for a trial is, of course, indisputable for the sake of protecting the individual's self-determination. The downside is that strictly speaking the results of the trial can only be generalized to that subgroup of the population for which the voluntary sample is indeed representative.

15.2.3.2 Clients' Situation

Once enrolled in a trial the client does not turn into a passive recipient to whom procedures are applied. Rather does he exhibit all the behaviors and has reflections that make up his human nature. These will now be analyzed in several dimensions and their effects upon the presumed results of trials will be analyzed. The first set of effects relates to the client's medical problem and his knowledge about the problem that have to some extent been observed in the services presented in this volume. Then we turn to his reflections about the situation that he is in, referring to a textbook in experimental psychology [32].

What is labeled as learning effect in Table 15.1 can nicely be studied in one of the trials presented below (Sects. 15.3 and 15.6): While a Consumer Health Informatics effect was concluded clients had presumably just learnt to better tell harmless from alarming signs as time passed. This is typically the case when a condition remains equally severe over time and the capacity to manage is continually challenged.

For conditions that heal, like wounds after discharge from surgery, knowledge and attention are high in the beginning and decrease when intervals between events increase. So if a subject in an experimental arm of a trial does not know how to manage a crisis half a year after discharge this is not necessarily a failure of a Consumer Health Informatics patient training but a normal course of affairs.

15.2.3.3 Clients' Reflections and Expectations

In contrast to these object level mechanisms that take influence on collected data and outcomes there are more subtle ones residing in perceptions and expectations that individuals have or develop while being part of an experiment. Some of these mechanisms have occurred and have been described in the literature of

Table 15.1 Human expectations and behaviors and their effects on trial outcome measurement

Common name	Description	Reference/source	Comment
Recruiting			
Volunteering	Readiness to be an experimental subject differs between individuals. Results only valid for the sub-population that would volunteer	[31], Sects. 12.2.1.2[(1)], and 5.2.2[(2)]	(1) Validity of a depression scale, (2) Effectiveness of depression coaching
Selection bias	Due to applied inclusion/exclusion criteria subjects are not representative for the target population	Sects. 8.4.3.2.6[(3)], and 5.2.4[(4)]	(3) Validity of a literacy test, (4) Superior medication compliance
Patient knowledge			
"Learning effect"	Patients apprehend their condition and their need for service decreases	Sect. 15.3[(5)]	(5) Effectiveness of post discharge management
Investigator's and subjects' reflections and reactivity			
Hawthorne effect	Subjects change behavior and may modify outcome solely due to the knowledge that they are being studied	[18, p. 121][(6)], [10][(7)], Sect. 15.6[(8)]	(6) Phenomenon as such, (7) (Negative) medical example, (8) "Therapy" effect in untreated group
Subject expectancy effect	"subject expectancy of direction of change and its effect on the obtained direction of behavior change"; also called "Demand characteristics"	[22, p. 145], Sect. 5.2.2.2[(9)]	(9) Subject reported abstinence from smoking
Social desirability bias	Subject's "concern (to) win positive evaluation from the experimenter or at least (to) provide no ground for a negative one"; also called "Evaluation apprehension"	[28, p. 281], Sect. 9.4.2.4[(a)]	(a) Subject reported step counts
Observer bias	Investigator is preoccupied to expect or want a certain result and treats differently, selects cases differently or observes and records in favor of his expected outcome	[29, p. 182], Sect. 15.3[(b)]	(b) Provider decision about re-hospitalization
Observer expectancy effect	"effect of the experimenter's expectation on the responses he obtains from his subjects"	[29, p. 196], [30], Sect. 15.4.1.2[(c)]	(c) Subject reported physical exercise
Pygmalion effect	Unwarranted "experimentally created teacher expectations resulted in changed performance of the students"	[30, 34]	

clinical procedures and research. A comprehensive outline from the perspective of psychology with a variety of finer grained distinctions has been provided as early as in [32], which still is the foundation of respective research, as evident from the verbatim reprint of the 1969 book in a 2009 series [33]. In the following we adapt [32]'s line of argumentation because the respective names, concepts and mechanisms can be found there together with all the details about experimental evidence. Where existing we also provide the names of mechanisms as used in clinical research.

Since the line of argumentation is borrowed from psychology and sociology we use the term subject here for an individual whose behavior is manipulated and/or studied. Normally in Consumer Health Informatics the client is in the subject role. While in a "clean" experimental situation an object is manipulated and properties or changes are assessed through objective measurements we here find humans in the roles of being investigated, being the investigators and the latter often in the duplicate role of observers. For good reasons is the human object of experimentation called subject. For it cannot be taken for granted that either subject or investigator or observer function objectively according to their assigned roles. Rather, while performing the roles they inevitably reflect their roles, others' roles and the experiment. While it is a characteristic of a clean experiment to deliver objective properties of the object, it is a characteristic of an experiment involving humans that the outcome is a complex composition of the effects under investigation and the reflections of the involved persons. In the following we look at the roles involved in an experiment and major effects that modify outcomes.

15.2.3.3.1 Hawthorne Type Impact of the Measuring Situation

Pretest sensitization [18] means that the sole announcement of an experiment or placement of a measuring device affects those being measured. In situations where human behaviors or self reported judgments of any kind are used to assess effects of interventions, two fallacies can happen. In the case that baseline values of target variables are known upfront changes after the onset of the experiment may be owed to the investigated intervention or through the experimental situation itself. In the second case, without known baseline, the attempt to establish one can inadvertently affect target variables. If they change in the same direction as under a subsequent intervention the effect size of the intervention is underestimated. It is overestimated if the experimental setup works in the opposite direction. In either case results must be interpreted under the assumption that the baseline is gone before the intervention begins. This effect is also called Hawthorne effect owing to the history of respective observations [26]. Since the term Hawthorne effect is better known we use it throughout this volume. Compared to the next two effects it should be noted that the Hawthorne effect can hit without any synchronous interaction between individuals. It can fully reside in the setting.

15.2.3.3.2 Other Subject Reflection Effects

Demand characteristics [22] operate in the subject. His perceptions or beliefs whether he is in the control or experimental arm of an investigation may lead him to report observations that fit this belief. In most experiments we inevitably have volunteer participants and will most likely encounter an attitude to contribute positively. This leads to "good" subject behaviors: behaviors inclined to "give the right responses"; in a medical context "to give the normal response, that is characteristic of healthy subjects" [22, p. 145]. In contrast to interpersonal expectations that will be discussed below demand characteristics operate without an experimenter being visible at all. They are nothing but inferences of what the subject hypothesizes as the purpose of the experiment, its expected effect and how he can contribute for this effect to materialize.

In the medical context this has also been called subject expectancy effect, denoting the subject expectancy of direction of change and how he changes behavior accordingly.

Evaluation apprehension [28] is another mechanism that modifies subjects' behaviors out of their own reflection, i.e. without an observer or experimenter taking influence. In contrast to demand characteristics, however, the subject now tries to be "good" in his own right, displaying attitudes or behaviors that make him look good, irrespective of what aims the investigation may have. This is informally also called the social desirability bias ([8], cited according to [28, p. 281]) which is a form of subject expectancy. It entails that socially accepted behaviors (such as losing weight) are over-reported and socially unacceptable behaviors (such as alcohol abuse) or the breaking of taboos are under-reported. Like the Hawthorne effect this can also effect baseline estimates: If subjects try to shine good upfront they may have no improvements to report during an intervention. The effect has more recently been confirmed and Risko and coworkers – though adding another level of differentiation – also have hope for us: the social desirability bias seems to be less pronounced in home Internet portal settings; maybe another facet of the perceived anonymity of Internet communication [25] that endows us with cleaner data than can be expected from face-to-face settings.

15.2.3.3.3 Observer Biases

By observer bias we denote a set of behaviors of the experimenter – unconscious and not meant malicious – to arrive at the data set that confirms his purpose of the experiment. This includes differences in treating subjects, selecting cases, observation of data etc. ([22], p. 147). While most of these mechanisms that bear the risk of manipulating expected result are nowadays avoided in the designs of serious clinical trials, it may still be the case that an investigator who also is a therapist treats differently and interprets observations differently on subjects in different arms. In distinction from the following interpersonal expectations this can be regarded as unidirectional: the experimenter applies different behaviors toward different subgroups whose members are regarded as passive targets of what the experimenter does.

15.2.3.3.4 Observer Induced Subject Expectations

Interpersonal expectations describe a yet more complicated set of effects that may bias or blur the interpretation of trial results. We now consider what it means that the experimenter or observer has expectations that do not go unnoticed by the subject who acts according to his perceptions of the experimenter's expectations. This has also been called observer expectancy effect, which emphasizes that the experimenter cannot conceal his goals or expectations and unconsciously transfers them to the subjects. While in behavioral research this interaction is target of investigation and source of knowledge in its own right [29] we regard it here as a source of uncertainty asking the question where and when we should be aware that observer expectancy rather than treatment caused an observed effect.

One of the most intricate versions of an interpersonal expectation is the so-called *Pygmalion effect*. Preoccupations in the observers or experimenters – which may by no means be warranted – make them have and transfer high expectations to presumably good performers and low expectations to presumably bad performers. Statistically such expectations have materialized although before the onset of the experiment the groups could not be distinguished as to their prognosis.

Take Home

Even more than in clinical trials clients are not passive matter exposed to an impact named treatment. They rather are human beings with all their reflections about the Consumer Health Informatics service and their role. Their individual ways to react and cooperate are not confounders that we should try to eliminate but part of the process that we need to understand. A selection of important drivers of client behavior and client-service interaction that are most pertinent to Consumer Health Informatics trials are the following:

Volunteering Volunteers differ from non-volunteers; observed effects may not transfer
Hawthorne effect Announcing an experiments creates expectations that change behaviors even if no experiment takes place
Demand characteristics Unconscious inclination to cooperate with the experimenter together with speculations about the expected effect leads to reporting data that support that effect
Observer induced expectations Such latter effects can be initiated or increased through unconscious transfer of expectations from the experimenter to the client
Social desirability Human beings tend to over-report well appreciated and to under-report tabooed or embarrassing behaviors or conditions

15.2.4 Control of the Test Setting

The natural setting of a drug trial is an inpatient or outpatient medical service with certain demographics, primary diagnosis and co-morbidities of its patients. In an in-person encounter with the patient a physician checks inclusion and exclusion criteria, eventually suggests participation, and enrolls those who give informed consent. A patient then is assigned to his treatment arm, an accumulation of baseline data is taken, he receives instructions and the substance, and applies it according to the scheme he is given. Some drugs may even be administered in an inpatient or outpatient controlled setting. Blood tests of the level of the active agent, alongside with other labs and tests that safeguard the patient against adverse effects, allow monitoring of the patient's adherence. The personal relationship between care provider and patient normally entails good compliance and few dropouts. Occasionally patients have to be withdrawn from the trial for clear medical reasons which are then clearly and meticulously documented. To summarize: the typical trial for a new drug is tightly embedded in the traditional provision of medical care and even more tightly monitored than in routine clinical care.

Embedding drug trials into the tightly controlled classical medical care makes sense because the intended scenario of usage after release is a nearly as tightly controlled in-person initiated medical setting with a physician who establishes a diagnosis and a precisely defined set of procedures and regulations that govern prescription, refill, monitoring etc. This makes several of the problems discussed below rare and unlikely.

In contrast, a tight medical setting mostly does not make sense for trials of Consumer Health Informatics services, because their intended future use and purpose requests that they are effective "out in the wild": clients mostly on their own, with at most a lose attachment to classical medical care (cf. Sect. 2.4.5) and no naturally imbedded way to establish inclusion criteria, consequently client personality and devotion varying from labile stopper by to fully committed chronically ill. The necessary absence of a tight medical setting for a trial of a Consumer Health Informatics service has several new challenges and risks for some of which there are methods to control or at least curb.

We have seen mechanisms and reflections that may affect and bias measurement of baselines and outcomes (Sect. 15.2.3.3). These mechanisms are, however, not confined to the measuring situation but a genuine part of human behavior.

At any time during the trial may clients guess and later change their mind whether they are control or experimental arm. As opposed to the control we have over labs that we can calibrate and medical exams that we can standardize and quality check we have no chance to control clients' guesses in which arm they are. Clients may even meet in forums and exchange data that inform guesses. Trying to establish control by intervening with forum use would jeopardize trust in the service under trial, so we have to accommodate to the variation that subject expectancy brings.

Similar concerns relate to social desirability. Patient may not care upfront but at some point in time do, or vice versa, beyond our control anyway. It may even be part of a treatment concept that patients bond with their human or virtual therapists, with increasing vigor to satisfy observer/therapist induced expectations (cf. [1] on therapeutic alliance and its importance in in-person and Internet settings).

The effort to control all this concurrently is prohibitive. So control of the setting is confined to excluding certain personality abnormalities or psycho-pathologies when enrolling a subject, by methods outlined in Sect. 12.3. A sense of proportion has to be applied, though, because, as will be outlined in Sect. 15.8, imposing an overwhelming battery of checks imposed on persons who just want an advice or desperately long for a cure may equally jeopardize acceptance of a service.

Besides uncontrollable features residing in the patient himself we cannot control the environment where he accesses the service either. Alone in the home office versus in the midst of family or friends in the living room, at a large screen or using a small mobile device, at rest or between appointments. Truthfulness, diligence, completeness, comprehension of conveyed information and other quality indicators of a communication can all be affected through such factors. We actually cannot want to exclude such variation. A prospective routine use would profit from allowing people to interact with the service at the best convenience. The same confounders will then be present and therefore we should be prepared to take them into account in the trial. If a trial indeed shows superior effectiveness or cost-effectiveness under such unfavorable circumstances we can the more be sure that it will also be superior "out in the wild".

> **Take Home**
> Clients of Consumer Health Informatics services utilize and enjoy the liberty to connect any time any place under all kinds of environmental conditions. In order to claim at the end of a trial that a service has the desired effect the setting of the trial must concede the subjects exactly that liberty. An effectiveness proof achieved under lab conditions does not have any predictive power for effectiveness "in the wild"!.

15.3 Historical Comparisons

Like in the early age of testing drugs early Consumer Health Informatics service attempts were rolled out and outcomes were compared to the state before the Consumer Health Informatics service in so-called intervention studies or pre-post comparisons. The following example has been published as early as 1998 [35]. For patients having been treated for congestive heart failure a tight monitoring scheme had been set up to support them after discharge from inpatient care. It consisted of equipment ("a digital sphygmomanometer, digital weight scale, and alphanumeric pager"), education ("instructed on use of these devices by a registered nurse."), other disease related, behavioral and diet information in eight packages surface mailed weekly in the first 8 weeks [35, p. 374] and a treatment scheme of automatic pager reminders, weekly telephone calls and escalation management involving physicians when signs such as body weight appeared to get out of control.

The target outcome in the effectiveness study reported was number and duration of re-hospitalizations. 27 patients were included based on their congestive heart failure diagnosis. Some patients with severe heart related conditions and some with known bad compliance with medication were excluded. Hospitalization days had been recorded before the intervention. They provided medically valid baseline data – matter of fact need of a clinical intervention – where Hawthorne, social desirability, or subject expectancy effects (cf. Sect. 15.2.3.3.3) were very unlikely. Hospitalization days before were compared to hospitalization days in the 1 year period after the intervention in a paired design: individual patients' before and after hospitalization values were compared. Both, number of hospitalizations and accumulated days of hospitalization decrease to a variable extent in the intervention period. The strongest effects can be seen with patients of higher severity and with patients who had been re-hospitalized in the three months prior to the intervention. Most differences are reported as significant ($p < 0.05$) including admissions for causes other than cardiovascular. Some differences are impressive, e.g. hospital days in the highest severity diagnosis group being brought down from 15.1 to 1.0 per person year – presumably as an effect of the intervention.

Presumably, because the following other factors may also have caused or contributed to the reduction, i.e. the intervention may not have been causal for the effect. One is the observer bias (Sect. 15.2.3.3.3). Nurses and physicians who served as telephone contacts and made the triage decision for or against re-admission may have applied more care and sophistication to manage cases at home rather than fast summoning to the hospital. Patients themselves may have added subject expectancy behaviors – now knowing that they are part of an experiment and wishing to be good patients. And last but not least anything may have changed concurrently with the trial, not really related and unnoticed, but influential to the outcome. The reader may think of seasonal effects (seasons are not reported in [35]), changes in the environment such as more privately practicing cardiologists, new rules for financial coverage of re-admissions through health plans etc. Last but not least may the patients have learned to tell true symptoms apart from harmless other signs and request a visit less frequently. For the sake of argument we call this a "Learning effect", cf. Table 15.1.

> **Take Home**
> When employing designs other than RCT as proof of superior effectiveness additional attention is required to identify hidden confounders such as patients better understanding their condition and henceforth seeking professional care less frequently.

15.4 Randomized Controlled Trials

The randomized controlled trial (RCT) is a quasi experimental approach which tries to establish a causal relation between different interventions applied and a medical effect observed. It does so by (randomly) drawing a sample of subjects presumed to represent the group that has the medical condition under investigation. This sample is randomly split into intervention arms. One arm may be a "control", where either no intervention or the state of the art intervention for the medical condition is applied. The interventions are uniformly and uniquely applied to all subjects within an arm and an outcome is equally measured in all arms. If the accumulated outcome values differ significantly between the arms the conclusion is that the difference can only be explained and therefore causally attributed to the difference in interventions. "Significantly" has a precise meaning substantiated through statistical test theory. For more details on both the mechanics of statistical testing and on many other necessary assumptions, precautions and requirements for establishing a result as a scientific insight the reader is referred to [12]. This and other articles in the Trisha Greenhalgh's "How to read a paper" series in the British Medical Journal 1997 create the necessary awareness of the temptations and pitfalls of creating impressive results although there is no treatment effect. The whole argumentation most of which can be followed without deep knowledge of the mathematics underlying biostatistics is also available as [13].[1]

While [13] emphasizes *what to avoid* [9] is a practitioner oriented brief guide to *what to do* in seriously planning and running trials. For RCTs for non pharmaceutical treatments [6] should also be considered.

It goes without saying that other practices approved in trials for new treatments should also be paid attention to here. They include disclosure of conflicting interests if there be any, detailed charting of subject demographics and morbidity, tracing of dropouts to the utmost possible extent to get cues whether characteristics of the dropouts are indicative of a bias etc. These precautions equally play a role in all subsequent designs of trials.

In designing trials one should also find a good balance between internal and external validity. Internal validity means that we have a clean experiment with treatments clearly distinguished and crisp, with the target population precisely described, individuals assigned to treatments randomly; with the consequence that the experiment can be replicated and if it showed some effect the first time it is likely to show an equally sized effect the second time. External validity means that when a treatment that is effective in an experiment is taken into the real world it

---

[1] Greenhalgh [13] has chapters on complex interventions which relates to our arguments about Nature of the active agent, Subject expectations and (lack of) Control; on economic analysis, like our section on Cost-effectiveness; on qualitative research and questionnaires which plays a role here whenever subjects self-report qualitative observations; and on getting evidence into practice, like our After the trial.

is effective there as well and to the same extent. In the following we look into the design, conduct and outcome of various example trials.

15.4.1 Effectiveness Trials

Effectiveness trials asks the question whether a treatment modifies a medically meaningful target. Often they do it in comparison: whether some treatment modifies a medically meaningful target more than another treatment. They do not address cost of the intervention or financial consequences of target achievement.

15.4.1.1 Mental Health

Blankers and coworkers [5] present an RCT that strives for high internal validity. For problematic alcoholics they offer three treatment arms and randomize the subjects. Control is a waiting list condition (WL) and there are two treatment arms. The less intensive one is called self help alcohol online (SAO) and operates with automatic media alone. The more intensive one is called therapy alcohol online (TAO) and includes seven text chat sessions of 40 min each with a human therapist who is specifically trained in CBT (cognitive-behavioral therapy). The trial aims at proving that the primary outcome: "number of standard drinks[2] per week" can be reduced after three-month and six-month follow-up.

Visitors of a much visited Dutch information platform for alcoholics who seemed to meet inclusion criteria were invited to participate in the trial. Some inclusion criteria are primarily logistic requirements (between ages 18 and 65, resident of the Netherlands, being health insured, having internet access at home). Persons with a history of drug addiction or former therapy attempts for some mental health conditions were excluded. The procedure to assign 205 individuals randomly to one of these arms is described in detail. The same holds for details of the three therapies.

Seventy percent of participants at three months and 60 % at six months respond to the follow-up assessment, most through Internet, some through telephone. Not every detail can be reported here but expectations are to a certain extent met. Most essentially, the number of standard drinks per week, as reported by the subjects, is reduced significantly when comparing TAO with WL and when comparing SAO with WL. To mention this just briefly: Bonferroni correction for multiple testing is applied. At six month follow-up TAO is also significantly superior to SAO. The most intensive therapy offering, therefore, has the best lasting effect. So why not call this the perfect RCT?

---

[2]Blankers et al. [5] use the European convention for standard drinks – 10 g of ethanol – as opposed to the North American one of 13.6 g.

15.4 Randomized Controlled Trials

Because it has limitations in the design and the interpretation of results themselves which will be discussed here and limitations which are relevant for the attempt to turn it in a routine program which will be discussed in Sect. 15.8.1. The obvious attempts to achieve high internal validity are at a high price. Of the 650,000 visitors of the webpage where the recruiting took place only about 800 qualified upfront and 205 were finally enrolled, i.e. we have a selection ratio of about 1/3200. Nothing can be said about the other appr. 649,800 visitors of the web page, let alone the 30 %, then 40 % dropouts. Therefore, the concern has to be raised whether those finally reporting their behavior actually represent "the problematic drinker" or only a yet to be characterized subgroup.

The following observation puts the validity of measuring the primary outcome variable under question. While the number of standard drinks per week decreases from 46.6 to 22.4 in TAO and from 43.6 down to 27.0 SAO, as can be expected, it also decreases in the virtually untreated arm WL (= waiting list) from 47.2 down to 35.4. How can that happen?

A strong Hawthorne effect (Sect. 15.2.3.3.1) is a possible explanation. It is not proven but it is not excluded either by [5]. It reads: when a visitor to the web site stops by and considers to participate he does not behave like a participant in an experiment yet and reports truthfully. In other words: the baseline is not affected, it is taken before the situation "feels" like an experiment. Once enrolled participants do feel as experimental subjects and Hawthorne hits. In the WL group other explanations such as demand characteristics or observer induced subject expectations can be excluded because that arm receives no treatment, is intelligent enough to notice that and has therefore no reason to come up with "good" or "fitting" self-reports.

If this is true i.e. a Hawthorne effect is present it presumably is equally present in the two treatment arms TAO and SAO. If the Hawthorne effect can be quantified to be 47.2. minus 35.4 equals 11.8 which is the average change reported in WL, this has to be subtracted from the effect sizes of TAO and SAO reducing them from 24.2 to 12.4 (TAO) and from 16.6 to 4.8 (SAO).

The conclusion can then still be: yes, there is a small effect when subjects just get some attention, and there is a larger effect when subjects are truly treated. But for the two treatment arms it cannot be excluded that demand characteristics or subject expectancies (cf. Sect. 15.2.3.3.2) are in effect, too: subjects who have received "good" treatment show "good behaviors" in unconscious appreciation and under-report their drinking behavior after the treatment. Their unconscious reflection is that the treatment they received should have had an effect. And therefore the size of effect they expect to be in reasonable relation to the intensity of the treatment received is the size of effect they report. Taking this argument further we might even have a dose response effect here for the size of the subject expectancy effect rather than the desired dose response effect for the two intensities of the treatment.

To make this clear once again: all this need not necessarily be the case. But it is the obligation of the investigators to address such potential biases. Which they do to some extent only. And it should be the competence of the readers of such papers to reveal such possible points of criticism.

15.4.1.2 Physical Health

Rheumatoid arthritis (RA) is a diagnosis that suggests itself for fostering enhanced physical activity through Internet interventions. A randomized controlled trial conducted in the Netherlands (van den Berg and coworkers [42]) in the years 2002 through 2004 seems to provide evidence that a tailored intervention is superior to static material available on the web.

Guidelines suggest that patients with rheumatoid arthritis should exercise moderately for at least 30 min per day on 5 days of the week and/or 20 min vigorously on 3 days of the week. This criterion is valid unless some cardiopulmonary condition precludes physical exercise. To establish the diagnosis of RA approved criteria by the American College of Rheumatology were applied.

160 patients matching the above profile were enrolled by selection from the electronic health records of three outpatient rheumatology units. Other inclusion criteria were not doing regular physical exercise now, being able to use a bicycle ergometer and having regular Internet access at home. Patients were also physically examined before being enrolled. Patients were randomized either to a treatment consisting of a website with educational material about the value of physical exercise to reduce the complaints of RA (arm: general training; GT) or to a tailored program provided from the same website (arm: individualized training; IT). Individualized training consisted of the suggested program for the exercises of the forthcoming week, e-mailed reporting back about the exercises performed, individually tailored e-mails from therapists, quarterly group meetings face-to-face with therapists, and the possibility to communicate with others in the GT group through a forum within the website.

The trial lasted 12 months, with most outcome measures being taken at baseline, three; six; nine; and 12 months. The major outcome measure was proportion of weeks where patients self-reported moderate 30 min exercise on at least five or vigorous 20 min exercise on at least 3 days of the week. According to this primary outcome the GT arm was clearly inferior to the IT arm: 22 % in GT vs. 38 % in IT exercise above the 5 times 30 min criterion at six months, and correspondingly for all reported checkpoints and criteria. All differences were significant. Another perfect trial, as it appears.

What seems to be a valid proof of superior effectiveness of tailored guidance as a means to modify behaviors has, however, a number of shortcomings. For the first, nobody should wonder that a website that does not change for a whole year loses interest. As a consequence the time spent there is likely to be less than the time spent on the evolving IT website and as a consequence, again, the emerging – not necessarily the planned – "dosis" of the treatment GT is smaller than the "dosis" of the treatment IT. The authors actually substantiate this suspected difference in utilization: percentage of at least once a week users declined from 86 % to 55 % in the IT and from 16 % to 7 % in the GT arm in the nine months following the three month checkpoint.

Therefore, what the authors interpret as an effect of the superior *quality* of IT can as well be an effect of the higher *quantity* of IT consumed.

15.4 Randomized Controlled Trials

For the second, secondary outcomes put the primary outcome under severe doubt. One secondary outcome is the amount of physical activity recorded through an acceleration device attached to the patient's ankle. In contrast to what the patients self-reported the objectively measured exercise that did take place was not superior in IT over GT. Diverse other outcome measures that pertain to rheumatism showed a mixed picture: disease activity, limitations in daily activities, rheuma related quality of life and other varied somewhat between IT and GT, in both directions. The authors have marked up a few differences as significant, doing exactly what [12] warns not to do. The question is: how can the contradiction between self-reported superiority of IT over GT and lack of measured evidence for such superiority be explained?

Likely answers are similar to Sect. 15.4.1.1. It should be noted that in addition to these biases discussed below a Hawthorne effect Sect. 15.2.3.3.1 may be in operation, although we would not find it reflected in the data. Since the acceleration device that records physical activity is only applied three times for 5 days in a whole year these 5-day intervals each create a Hawthorne type experimental situation which may in its own right stimulate more – and less likely less – physical activity. If a Hawthorne effect is present it modifies the baseline equally – at least there is no reason to believe that it does so selectively – for all recorded times and both treatment arms. Therefore, the acceleration device readings, which already fall short of the self-reported activities, may even be boosted above average actual activities in weeks without acceleration device. The over-reporting of activity may be even larger than the difference: "self-report" minus "acceleration device reading" suggests.

Reasons for participants in the IT arm to over-report can be identified easily, and there are many. Concerning self-reported frequencies of activities subject expectancy Sect. 15.2.3.3.2 and observer expectancy Sect. 15.2.3.3.4 may both play a role. Subjects may speculate about desired outcomes. Those visiting the website more often may speculate more intensely or more often and are therefore more likely to report activity levels that comply with their expectations about the outcome of the study. Since this trial also has web mediated human coaching and face to face sessions, rarely though, instructors in these sessions may transfer their expected outcome to the subjects who will react accordingly and in the same direction as implied by their own reflections. Therefore, higher reported activity levels in the experimental condition IT may be an effect of the treatment or as well of subjects' reflections what to report.

All such happens – if it does happen – unconsciously and is not meant malicious. On a micro-level it may happen over again that exercise intervals of borderline length are re-envisioned and reported as above criterion if there is momentum to and as below criterion if there is no momentum. Subconscious momentum, which is not reason, comes from intensity of exposure to either IT or GT. The accumulation of such micro-level imprecisions adds to significant statistics although there is no effect. Some deficiencies in external validity will be discussed in Sect. 15.8.1

> **Take Home**
>
> RCT design and procedures for Consumer Health Informatics services basically do not differ from RCTs in general. Notable specific points of attention have been pointed out in take home messages 15.2.2, 15.2.3.3.4 and 15.2.4. Concretely, the following must be expected
>
> - Hawthorne effects in control groups
> - Subject expectancy and social desirability effects when asking for estimated alcohol consumption
> - Discrepancies between measured and self reported behavior when the behavior is socially appreciated (such as physical exercise)
> - Decreasing visits to a web site that does not change for a year, and hence decreasing "doses" of the Consumer Health Informatics intervention

15.4.2 Cost-Effectiveness Trials

Cost-effectiveness trials need a broad approach and face various challenges of fully accounting for the cost and the benefit dimensions. Tate and coworkers (cf. [40]) provide some good insights into the methodology and into trials published between 1997 and 2008. Here we go into some depth of a more recent investigation described in Sect. 5.2.2.1. Bergström and coworkers [2] compared a standard group Cognitive Behavior Therapy (CBT) setting of treating anxiety disorders with an Internet administered CBT. Their design targeted at first making sure that the Internet arm of the trial was efficient and did not cause harm and second establishing reduced cost for the Internet treatment compared to the group therapy standard.

Mostly logistic exclusion criteria cut the primary sample of 396 down to 54 randomized to the control and 50 to the experimental arm. Both arms received the same amount of information in the form of 10 modules and homework assignments for making their personal use of the information. Each module was intended to be finished within 1 week. The control condition consisted of weekly 2 hour therapy sessions in groups of five to six patients led by two clinical psychologists who were not specifically trained for this investigation. In the group therapy sessions paper printouts of the same material were used as the Internet arm received as files.

The intervention itself and the basic design of an RCT are described in Sect. 5.2.2.1. The bottom line – based on responses from more than 80 % at six month follow up in both arms – is that the percentage cured according to standardized instruments (mainly 40 % improvement at Panic Disorder Severity Scale – PDSS and correspondingly at Clinical Global Impression Scale – CGI subscales pertinent to anxiety) and according to blinded clinical judgment is at the same level in the control and Internet arms and hence the Internet therapy apparently is not inferior to the group therapy. Apart from the fact that the authors do not actually apply the methodology of Noninferiority trials as outlined in Sect. 15.5 we follow their conclusion and subsequently concentrate on aspects of cost and effort saved in a broad sense in the Internet arm.

The major cost factor investigated in [2] was therapist time and respective cost charged to the insurance system. Other cost mentioned are room and travel in the group therapy and Internet development, maintenance, and equipment cost in the experimental. However, when concentrating on the therapists the results clearly favored the Internet arm. Its cost per patient was €68 versus €325 for group treatment; if counting only those patients where PDSS had improved by 40 % or more it was €143 versus €516 at the end of the treatment and €121 versus €500 at six month follow-up. Correspondingly average time spent with a patient in the group was 6 hours compared to 35 min for a patient in the Internet treatment. We will take a more differentiated look at therapist workload below.

Apart from the fact that a Hawthorne effect cannot be excluded – which the authors briefly mention – this is a compelling investigation in a number of aspects. Beyond sufficient effectiveness and superior cost-effectiveness it offers some other results and insights to promote Consumer Health Informatics.

Looking first at patient behaviors and adherence figures we find that Internet patients finished 6.7 (SD = 2.5) modules (out of 10), group therapy patients on the contrary attended 8.1 (SD = 2.1) sessions. Nevertheless, the Internet arm performed better at six month follow-up. This can be seen – optimistically – as empowered behaviors in the Internet setting versus dependent, paternalistic patterns of behavior in the group therapy setting. Those patients randomized to the small group setting know that two therapists are waiting for their (on the average) 5.4 patients and may feel compelled to go. Their motivation is partially extrinsic. This is related to, but different from demand characteristics because here actual behavior must be modified to satisfy assumed expectations of the therapists. Demand characteristics in its basic form means that reported results rather than actual behaviors are modified to satisfy assumed expectations. On the contrary subjects in the Internet arm are mostly on their own, with much less situational bonding with the therapist and therefore feel less compelled to "attend". They are equipped with the necessary means and to a large part grab the opportunity to take control of their process i.e. ideally develop their personally best patterns to work with the material. Having developed such habits more easily extends beyond the 10 week duration of the trial than memories of past group therapy sessions. A possible reason why the Internet arm outperforms the group therapy arm at six month follow-up is that clients have become empowered. Anxiety and panic disorder are a appropriate medical domain where empowerment can develop: compared to depression, metabolic syndrome, high blood pressure, the burden of disease is such that in cases of insufficient response or relapse one can return to the therapeutic material as long as it is there and can try to revive good habits developed during a 10 week intensive therapeutic period.

Next looking at therapist and service provider effort we find tailoring here as well. For the first therapists can allocate their time according to individual needs. They invest more time in patients who need more time and vice versa. Second, they invest the time when the patient communicates needs, be it through assignments with alarming results or through e-mails. Third, patient status is checked and intervention is provided within 24 hours when need be, while, in contrast, in the group therapy setting access to the therapist is available once per week. Looking at this more broadly it may also serve as an example to demonstrate that a service level which is in accordance with the patient's needs can be offered while still reducing overall therapist time. Rather than allocating stereotypical 45 min or 60 min sessions for everybody while some only need 15 min others as much as 75 min this allows for 75 min for those in need because therapist time can be saved at those with lesser needs. Knowing that lack of trained therapists is one of the major problems the reduction in time per patient, taken on average, is an important improvement.

The cost effectiveness of this kind of resource assignment in response to acute need increases with larger units: Load balancing is less exposed to coinciding client emergencies when 200 therapists serve 5000 clients than when two therapists serve 50 clients.

Only one important downside remains: the necessity that the client studies demanding material in the form of web pages requires a certain level of intelligence and education. Therefore, this is one of the many situations where Consumer Health Informatics widens rather than reduces the digital divide. This may be inevitable here because CBT has the C for cognitive in its name, implying that certain cognitive demands cannot be avoided. Therefore, this is not really a limitation of external validity of the trial because prospective clients with insufficient cognitive capabilities would not qualify for the in-person or group CBT either.

> **Take Home**
> Ideally the pre-assigned primary outcome of a cost-effectiveness RCT is cost per achieved benefit. A weaker and often applied – though not scientifically sound – approach is to use the fact that a control could not be shown to be superior in medical outcome to an experimental (Consumer Health Informatics) treatment and from this to conclude that the experimental treatment is equally good. Subsequently control and experimental arm costs are compared.

15.5 Noninferiority Trials

In various places (e.g. Sects. 5.2.2.1, 5.2.2.3, and 10.2.5) we follow authors' arguments that their Consumer Health Informatics services achieve similar medical or behavioral outcomes with lower cost, effort, etc. and should, therefore, be accepted as substitutes for classical in-person delivered care. Arguing "similar outcome at lower cost" where cost is meant in a very wide sense has become common for therapy or delivery of care trials in general when existing approved therapies turned out too costly, resource intensive, adverse effect prone etc. This

15.5 Noninferiority Trials

gave rise to a new sub discipline within statistic test theory: noninferiority trials, often named in conjunction with equivalence trials. In the following we briefly outline how to systematically test noninferiority and precautions and procedures mandated in [23].

Amazingly, the minor difference in wording between superiority and noninferiority testing entails new considerations for nearly every step of the design and conduction of an experiment. The only commonality is that both are pairwise (or multiple) comparisons between therapies targeting the same medical problem. Distinctions include:

Control, waiting list, i.e. doing nothing can ethically be the comparative arm of a superiority trial as long as no effective treatment is known. In contrast, noninferiority trials only warrant the effort and exposure of volunteers to the experiment if there is already an effective treatment and a new treatment tries to come close in effect and has some other advantage to offer, in terms of cost, effort, exposure to risks. Nobody can wish human subjects research to prove that we are as good as doing nothing at an effort or exposure that is more than nothing.

Now we assume that effectiveness has been proven for one treatment and a new treatment strives for noninferiority. Then the noninferiority trial should compete on the same outcome variables. If the to be matched treatment performs well against diastolic blood pressure the "noninferior" candidate should not target systolic pressure or heart rate.

So we use an outcome variable that served the superiority proof of the present standard treatment and turn to the mathematics of testing that this outcome variable by and large has the same value under the new therapy. For the sake of completeness we mention that "by and large" has the following meaning in equivalence testing: we want to confirm that the new treatment achieves an outcome value that deviates less than a to be selected threshold of Δ in either direction from the outcome value in the standard treatment. For most therapy trials such a bidirectional objective is less instrumental than a unidirectional one: to confirm that the new outcome is not more inferior to the standard treatment than a to be chosen Δ.

The reader may have noticed that this reverses the "burden of proof". For superiority testing we must ascertain that the test statistic is large enough to support the conjecture that there is a difference, with a type I error – often called significance level – that a difference be claimed which is not there and a type II error that no difference is claimed although it exists. For noninferiority testing we must ascertain that a test statistic is small enough to support the conjecture that there is no more than a Δ inferiority, with a type I error to claim noninferiority although the new treatment is inferior and a type II error to claim that the new treatment is "good enough" although it is inferior.

"Good enough" or "by and large" must of course be specified. They do not emerge from mathematical but from societal or moral arguments: How much less efficiency of a new treatment do we accept in return for less cost, effort, risk?

Given a Δ that a society has agreed upon we would now have to dive deeper into the mathematics. This goes by far beyond the scope of this volume. So we just mention that it mostly builds on confidence intervals and refer the reader to textbooks such as [27]. However, some ramifications are worth mentioning in support of responsible conduct of noninferiority trials. Generally, by responsible conduct we mean that data that would refute our conjecture must by any means be captured and reported diligently. Superiority trials claim a difference, therefore data that blur or mask the difference require paramount diligence. The reverse is the case for noninferiority trials: they claim a non-difference and therefore data that emphasize the difference require paramount diligence. For example, in superiority trials intention-to-treat analysis is recommended because it includes patients who terminated prematurely and hence delivered scattered, preferably diminished effectiveness data. If a difference is tested as significant it has the safety margin of presumably having been "even more significant" had the drop outs finished. How to handle drop outs in noninferiority trials depends on characteristics of the population – whether dropping out points to premature cure, non-response, interfering other conditions etc.

To summarize: Presently trials for Consumer Health Informatics services claim to prove their (nearly) equal effectiveness in a "we did not see a difference so it must equal" attitude. In the future they are likely to face requests for the scrutiny of true noninferiority methodology.

> **Take Home**
> To proof noninferiority rather than superiority a sound biometrical theory with respective tests exist which puts the usual test theory upside down. Starting with a known effective treatment called control a margin Δ is set up by which the experimental treatment may maximally be lower in effect for noninferiority to be concluded. Now the null hypothesis is that the experimental treatment performs below control by more than a threshold value dependent on Δ and the distribution of the outcome value. The null hypothesis is refuted and the experimental treatment comes out as noninferior when it deviates by less than the threshold.

15.6 Definite Evidence from Non-randomized Trials

The most typical situation for an RCT is that you want to compare a new experimental treatment to an established one and want to be sure that differences in outcomes can be attributed to the different treatments rather than to population characteristics, to other developments during the time of the trial or any type of confounders. Therefore, RCTs are not necessary if we know the effect of the standard treatment precisely enough, if the effect of the standard treatment does not play a role, or if we know securely enough that other factors do not play a role. This is rarely the case. But the following investigation about implantable cardioverters defibrillators (ICD) equipped with a remote monitoring are a good example.

15.6 Definite Evidence from Non-randomized Trials   317

In an investigation in Finland [24] 41 patients with moderate risk of new or repeated cardiac fibrillation, which may lead to sudden cardiac death, who were already using ICD's were provided with additional data collection and transmission equipment. While normally due for clinical visits every three months they were put on data transmission only at three and six months and clinical visits in the beginning and at 9 months. There were scheduled transmissions to test before regular use, at three and six months and the patients could any time initiate nonscheduled transmissions. Support infrastructure was present to assist both in technical problems with scheduled as well as unscheduled transmissions and in need for medical follow-up.

The primary outcome related question was whether the data transmission treatment was safe. This is not a comparative question. It rather means reaching a threshold. If the experimental treatment performs above that threshold it "passes". The intricacy of such an approach does not reside in the comparative experimental design and its implied statistical tests from which one would conclude "better". It rather resides in the ethics of accepting the threshold for "good enough". In the data transmission-based ICD monitoring trial less than 7.5 % of patients suffering unanticipated serious adverse device effects was judged as good enough. Furthermore, a confidence of 90 % was judged as certain enough; therefore, it could be calculated that 7.5 % be in the 90 % confidence interval of 100 % adverse event free operation. The statistical model predicted that this would be achieved with zero encountered adverse effects in a population of 30. To compensate for potential dropouts a sample size for the trial of 40 or more subjects was therefore targeted. It turned out that 41 enrolled subjects all finished the trial and no adverse effects occurred. I.e. the established goal was overachieved.

Secondary outcomes related to user perceptions on ease-of-use and satisfaction. Furthermore, differences in cost between the experimental treatment and the standard – clinical visits at three-month intervals – were evaluated.

User perceptions of ease-of-use and satisfaction can, but need not necessarily be conducted in comparison to the standard treatment. One can argue here as well that if perceived ease of use and satisfaction with the new treatment is high enough we need not care how high it is for the standard treatment. This was the case here for both patients and physicians. Patients were supposed to judge five aspects at set up test, three and six months time and came out with mostly about 90 % very positive or positive on a four valued Likert scale. Knowing that the patients were between 41 and 76, with an average of 62, this is an amazing degree of acceptance. Physician judgments on three aspects relevant to their work were equally positive and even better (100 % very positive on navigation of the website presenting the data). Standard and experimental treatment were compared as to time and monetary effectiveness. For the purpose of comparing time effectiveness on the physician's and nurse's side data were collected how much time they spent on the data transmitted at three and six months compared to data taken in a face to face setting at baseline and at nine months. Data for unscheduled transmission were also compared to data from scheduled visits. Variation was large at all test points but mean values decreased to less than half in the experimental data transmission treatment. It seems that a – from the perspective of the cardiac center – patient free purely data based streamlined process enables fast performance whereas the physical presence of the patient holds things up. On the patient's part the need to travel to the hospital adds to the treatment time in the standard treatment. Since patients lived between 3 and 350 km from the hospital variation was orders of magnitude larger here. But still mean values of time required in the standard treatment was about 50 times higher than in the experimental data transmission treatment.

While time data from the nine-month visit and unscheduled visits could be collected and compared to time data from three and six-month transmissions and unscheduled transmissions, the monetary effectiveness was not established through collected data alone but through modeling expected expenses in the standard treatment and calculating the occurred expenses for the experimental treatment. Expected expenses consist of fees charged to the social health insurance system for visits, travel expenses redeemed to the patients and sickness allowance for those having to stay away from work, all this including for accompanying persons if the patient cannot travel alone. Since definite amounts per unit hold all across Finland the only other factors are the number of events for which payments are due and the likelihood for events to occur. Since most of the follow-up care for ICD carriers is organized in terms of scheduled visits at regular intervals, with few intervening unscheduled visits or transmissions, these numbers are very definite as well. The bottom line of the comparison turns out to be a cost-reduction of €523.60 per patient per year.

Despite a very positive and encouraging result in general a few comments have to be made that restrict the generalizability of the investigation. Some concern the internal validity i.e. mainly the appropriateness of conclusions and comparisons within the investigation. Some concern the external validity that is the degree of trust that what turned out here will happen similarly elsewhere.

The most essential point to consider is the arbitrary threshold of "7.5 % unanticipated serious adverse device effects" that the authors consider "safe enough". In a medical setting, where "doing no harm" is among the highest ranking doctrines (cf. Sect. 17.11.5), tolerating a problem caused through the used technology in 1/12 or 13 patients seems to be a high risk. The threshold does, however, make sense when contrasted to the practice of care in the standard treatment situation. In the latter, events occur in the patient's home or living environment without any immediate access to medical advice or intervention. In the experimental treatment situation medical advice or intervention can be called for any time any place – assuming the necessary equipment is being carried. This allows to argue that the standard treatment situation bears the considerable though not quantified risk of no access to care when needed. So in a discourse outside statistical analysis and experimental design a presumably intolerable risk appears tolerable. In utilitarian or libertarian theories of distributive justice (cf. Sect. 17.11.7) it can be established as a societal norm or granted as an individual right to choose the surveillance and cardioverter service after informing about the risks.

15.6 Definite Evidence from Non-randomized Trials

Time comparisons of physicians' time assume that times spent on one of the four points in time (baseline, three, six, nine months) do not differ systematically. It is argued that times spent on the baseline and nine-month scheduled visits are essentially the same as would have been spent on the three or six month visits hadn't they been replaced by data transmission only events. Regarded in isolation this appears reasonable. However, this may be false in either direction. If the patient does not see the physician for nine rather than three months the agendas of the baseline and the nine month visits may indeed be more packed than they were for more routine like regular three-month visit. In this case the measured times at baseline and nine month overestimate the time that is truly required for a routine visit. On the other hand we can have learning effects (cf. Sect. 15.2.3.2): between the baseline and the nine month face-to-face check the client may have learnt to live with the ICD itself and the monitoring procedures and developed a certain imperturbation. With time passing he becomes more confident in interpreting signs that appeared alarming when they showed for the first time and is hence less worried and less driven to ask and follow up when seeing his doctor. In this case the nine month measured time underestimates the time truly required at three and six months when he still cares.

Since time on the nine-month visit exceeds time for the three and six months consultations based on transmitted data by a factor of as much as 2 there seems to be sufficient margin to uphold the claim that clinicians save work hours in the experimental treatment.

This, of course, raises the question whether the reduced amount of time implies reduced level and quality of care. Observations in the article report two situations where patients would have received better advice if having been seen personally. On the other hand timely unscheduled data transmissions initiated better antiarrhythmic medication in six cases.

Therefore, transmission of ICD data which are then analyzed by specialists and required variations in treatment are summarized is a safe new Consumer Health Informatics service that saves both patient and physician time and reduces costs in a setting such as the cardiological center in Finland. The question still remains whether the results transfer to settings outside Finland and achieved advantages still materialize without the special situation of the trial. The situation in Finland is – for the purpose of this investigation – characterized through long distances and predictable cost for health services and transportation. In countries with shorter distances some of the advantages will decrease if not vanish. Of course the reverse is true in countries with even longer distances. Cost effects are as diverse as payment systems for medical services and benefits for patients having to leave work and travel for seeking medical care are. Such analysis would have to be done country by country.

One of the clear strongholds of the investigation was that no real technical failure occurred and in few situations reported where patients felt insecure about handling the technology technical advice was there within the shortest of time. This has to be seen in light of the fact that two of the authors were employees of the company who produce the data transmission equipment. So there was high interest and momentum to keep the technology side straight, coming close to a conflict of interest. This attitude may have transferred to clinicians (a variation of the Hawthorne effect, cf. Sect. 15.2.3.3.1) such that the favorable results are partially owed to an appropriate technology but partially owed as well to a service-level set up for the purpose and duration of the trial and that both may be fading once it is routine.

Finally, it should be noted that saved physician and nurse time may be a strong factor to allow this treatment to survive beyond the end of the trial. Reduced workload on health professionals is a major emotional factor to promote a service. But it is also among the important drivers from a national economics perspective: it is a means to address the forthcoming shortage of health care workforce.

> **Take Home**
> In some cases when a control to compare with does not exist or is not meaningful performance of a treatment can be assessed other than in an RCT. In an exploratory investigation of an ICD (implantable cardioverter defibrillator) used in distant places together with data transmission and consultation equipment, the number of technical problems was targeted to be below a threshold and number of actual events were counted. In such cases where the comparison is "no equipment" and hence a number of technical problems of control cannot be known such threshold cannot be the results of experimental research but must be consensus of a society.

15.7 Cochrane: Supreme Evidence Fading

Asthma is a wide spread chronic disease where monitoring of therapy compliance is key to good management. Asthma has, therefore, been among the first diseases where a Cochrane review investigated the effectiveness of "telehealthcare" [20]. Published in 2011 it draws on clinical trials published between 1999 and 2009 which necessarily used technologies readily available before the beginning of the trial. The results are underwhelming. Only two studies had significantly reduced inpatient hospital treatments in the experimental arms. All others studies showed marginal if any improvements in self assessed asthma related quality of life and in emergency room visits. Does that mean that Consumer Health Informatics does not work for asthma?

A closer look at the 21 trials reveals that "telehealthcare" means telephone (9) or videoconferencing (2) for more than a half. It is Internet or "other networked system" for 8, and some other including text messaging. Smart phones were for geeks until the first iPhone came in 2007. I.e. for most of the therapy concepts investigated in [20] the convenience of easy multitouch interface, the choice of place and time for access to the treatment, material and intensity or frequency of interactions tailored to actual needs and easy integration of measured or recorded values were not broadly available. The technical environment and user habits and expectations have changed too much for results from the mid of the first decade to be still valid as is. This shows a general problem of Cochrane reviews for treatments that change faster than a review can be achieved.

> **Take Home**
> In a field where technology that was cutting edge 5 years ago is no longer used today systematic reviews with their backlog of publications referenced of several years are not timely to inform present decisions.

15.8 After the Trial: Does It Still Work?

Industry and the finance market know pretty well that not every successful research achievement makes it to the market. The whole field of venture capital investment bets on the fact that among many failures there are few products or services that perform so well that losses from the failures are easily outweighed.

It is the science – or art? – of venture capital investment to aggregate portfolios where the percentage of high performers is large and to develop indicators to identify such.

Consumer Health Informatics has not yet achieved an economic size and penetration that industry specific indicators are available, let alone empirically evaluated. Some investigations have started into that direction [4, 38]. Some risks to regular deployment of successfully tested Consumer Health Informatics services can be demonstrated with reference to examples in this volume and will be provided in the next sections.

15.8.1 Non-representative Study Samples

For the sake of internal validity and logistic ease many researchers delimit their trial populations in a way that dramatically limits the generalizability of results. In some cases this explicitly or implicitly excludes under-served populations thus violating the moral principle of distributive justice (cf. Sect. 17.11.7). This latter drawback applies to trials in Sects. 5.2.2.4 [41] and 9.5.2 [21] where better than average educated, in the case of [41] also much younger, subjects are the exclusive target group. In an investigation where Jacobs and coworkers show for a Dutch sample that cardiovascular prevention is cost-effective [15] they explicitly request that their subjects be highly educated. Regarding the high prevalence of cardiovascular problems in under-served populations this appears somewhat absurd. In Sect. 15.4.1.2

inclusion criteria include having Internet at home (which is becoming more and more normal) and knowing to use a bicycling ergometer (not so normal at all, especially in under-served populations) (cf. [42]).

The selection effect is even much more pronounced in numbers and less precise in the criteria applied in [5] introduced in Sect. 15.4.1.1. Only 800 of 650,000 visitors to a website against problematic alcohol consumption were finally admitted as subjects in the trial of the service.

In either case, replication of the success and offering the service to a general cohort of clients with the respective condition is by no means warranted.

15.8.2 Prohibitive Effort to Maintain Service Level

Some trials operate at an extraordinary level of availability of human resource that will hardly transfer to the routine situation. The success in the trial in Sect. 15.6 [24] depends on two employees of the company developing the used equipment in stand-by for not more that 41 subjects. This certainly does not scale up. In Sect. 10.4.2 we see concerns about the high human workload to clarify situations that start as IVR calls, are supposed to end as IVR, but fall back to in-person telephone calls or fully fail. Therefore, even if such trials prove superior effects of the experimental Consumer Health Informatics service, they are unlikely to establish themselves as routine services.

15.8.3 Arguable Cost-Effect Relation

Several investigation have started to present cost to achievement relations where achievement can be cure, therapy adherence, utilization of needed services, satisfaction, etc. The trial by Jacobs and coworkers [15] mentioned in Sect. 15.8.1 reports cost of €26,910 for its target group of highly educated citizens to achieve 1 QALY. Spontaneously some readers may find that much and other find it not much. The true value of such trials, however, is the sound basis they deliver from which a society can start a transparent discourse along the lines of Sect. 17.11.

15.8.4 Carving Active Agents

Regarding the doubts that some of these observations cast on the sustainability even of very successful trials a different angle of view taken by Schueller and coworkers [36] may help. It suggests and successfully tries methods to differentiate active agents working in different target groups (depressed, high smoker). This suggest a new direction in studying differential effectiveness: parsimonious selection and tailoring of service elements to subgroups of the target population.

15.8.5 Stakeholder Influence

Ball and coworkers [7] provide one example of investigating the visibility and effect of stakeholder funding. During trials research funding agencies often cover expenses, but other funding is required after the trial.

The amount of third party conflict of interest prone funding which remains opaque turns out alarming. The authors do not report any detrimental effect on client trust and loyalty. But the risk of a backlash in case of uncovered misconduct of a donor is there and leads the authors to conclude that self-regulation according to a code of ethics and maybe oversight is recommended. In any case, in the interest of trust providers are certainly well advised to disclose their financial resources from the beginning.

15.9 Further Reading

Many articles meanwhile address evaluation of Consumer Health Informatics services, with JMIR collecting a variety of in-depth trials. The following articles rather address certain aspects in the breadth that this volume also tries to offer.

Glasgow [11] explicitly goes beyond statistically significant improvements of clinical outcomes in handpicked samples. He demands that

- typically under-served populations are included and also benefit (see Sect. 17.11.7)
- cost and quality of life implications are also considered,
- and consequently, that both policy makers and clients value the outcome
- results must be achieved in realistic settings
- behavioral outcomes count, and that
- adverse effects must be attended

There recommendations include that the classical RCT is not necessarily the best design for Consumer Health Informatics services and point to the RE-AIM framework for studies with heterogeneous outcomes.

Gibbons and coworkers [14] on behalf of the AHRQ differ from our services centered approach by asking how "electronic tools, technology, or electronic applications ... interact directly with consumers ... help the patient better manage health or health care." [14, p. 1] Therefore, their subject of studies is technologies, placed in contexts that this volume classifies as Level 1 and Level 2. One definite value of the investigations is the clear distinction of evaluation methodologies for different key questions, such as clinical outcomes, barriers to adoption, cost-effectiveness, etc.

Jones and coworkers [16] go into depth of one aspect of vital importance for realistic evaluation and monitoring of Consumer Health Informatics service performance: They investigate, how Internet conveyed instruments such as questionnaires can be used to correctly collect patient reported outcomes. Finally, Kaplan and Litewka [17] have provided a very broad and inspired perspective of environmental influences and effects of implementing Consumer Health Informatics informatics services.

References

1. Andersson G, Paxling B, Wiwe M, Vernmark K, Felix CB, Lundborg L, Furmark T, Cuijpers P, Carlbring P. Therapeutic alliance in guided internet-delivered cognitive behavioural treatment of depression, generalized anxiety disorder and social anxiety disorder. Behav Res Ther. 2012;50:544–50. doi: 10.1016/j.brat.2012.05.003.
2. Bergström J, Andersson G, Ljótsson B, Rück C, Andréewitch S, Karlsson A, Carlbring P, Andersson E, Lindefors N. Internet-versus group-administered cognitive behaviour therapy for panic disorder in a psychiatric setting: a randomised trial. BMC Psychiatry. 2010;10(54):1471–244X. doi: 10.1186/1471-244X-10-54.
3. Bandura A. Health promotion by social cognitive means. Health Educ Behav. 2004;31(2):143–64. doi: 10.1177/1090198104263660.
4. Buccoliero L, Calciolari S, Marsilio M. A methodological and operative framework for the evaluation of an e-health project. Int J Health Plann Manag. 2008;23:3–20. doi: 10.1002/hpm.881.
5. Blankers M, Koeter MWJ, Schippers GM. Internet therapy versus internet self-help versus no treatment for problematic alcohol use: a randomized controlled trial. J Consult Clin Psychol. 2011;79(3):330–41. doi: 10.1037/a0023498.
6. Boutron I, Moher D, Altman DG, Schulz KF, Ravaud P. Extending the CONSORT statement to randomized trials of nonpharmacologic treatment: explanation and elaboration. Ann Intern Med. 2008;148(4):295–309. doi: 10.7326/0003-4819-148-4-200802190-00008.
7. Ball DE, Tisocki K, Herxheimer A. Advertising and disclosure of funding on patient organisation websites: a cross-sectional survey. BMC Public Health. 2006;201(6). doi: 10.1186/1471-2458-6-201.
8. Crowne DP, Marlowe D. The approval motive. New York: Wiley; 1964.
9. Coggon D. Statistics in clinical practice. 2nd ed. London: BMJ; 2003. E-Book.
10. Fox NS, Brennan JS, Chasen ST. Clinical estimation of fetal weight and the Hawthorne effect. Eur J Obstet Gynecol Reprod Biol. 2008;141:111–4. doi: 10.1016/j.ejogrb.2008.07.023.
11. Glasgow RE. eHealth evaluation and dissemination research. Am J Prev Med. 2007;32(5S):S119–26. doi: 10.1016/j.amepre.2007.01.023.
12. Greenhalgh T. How to read a paper. Statistics for the non-statistician. II: "Significant" relations and their pitfalls. BMJ. 1997;315:422–5.
13. Greenhalgh T. How to read a paper: the basics of evidence-based medicine. 4th ed. Chichester: BMJ Wiley-Blackwell; 2010. E-Book.
14. Gibbons MC, Wilson RF, Samal L, Lehmann CU, Dickersin K, Lehmann HP, Aboumatar H, Finkelstein J, Shelton E, Sharma R, Bass EB. Impact of consumer health informatics applications. AHRQ Publication No. 09(10)-E019. Evidence Report/Technology Assessment Number 188, 10 2009. http://www.ahrq.gov/research/findings/evidence-based-reports/chiapp-evidence-report.pdf.

15. Jacobs N, Evers S, Ament A, Claes N. Cost-utility of a cardiovascular prevention program in highly educated adults: intermediate results of a randomized controlled trial. Int J Technol Assess Health Care. 2010;26(1):11–9. doi: 10.1017/S0266462309990845.
16. Jones JB, Snyder CF, Wu AW. Issues in the design of internet-based systems for collecting patient-reported outcomes. Qual Life Res. 2007;16:1407–17. doi: 10.1007/s11136-007-9235-z.
17. Kaplan B, Litewka S. Ethical challenges of telemedicine and telehealth. Camb Q Healthc Ethics. 2008;17:401–16. doi: 10.1017/S0963180108080535.
18. Lana RE. Pretest sensitization, chapter 5. In: Rosenthal R, Rosnow RL, editors. Artifact in behavioral research. New York: Academic; 1969. pp. 119–41.
19. Locke EA, Latham GP. Building a practically useful theory of goal setting and task motivation. Am Psychol. 2002;57(2):705–17. doi: 10.1037//0003-066X.57.9.706.
20. McLean S, Chandler D, Nurmatov U, Liu J, Pagliari C, Car J, Sheikh A. Telehealthcare for asthma: a Cochrane review. CMAJ. 2011;183(11):E733–42. doi: 10.1503/cmaj.101146.
21. McMahon GT, Fonda SJ, Gomes HE, Alexis G, Conlin PR. A randomized comparison of online- and telephone- based care management with internet training alone in adult patients with poorly controlled type 2 diabetes. Diabetes Technol Ther. 2012;14(11):1060–7. doi: 10.1089/dia.2012.0137.
22. Orne MT. Demand characteristics and the concept of quasi-controls, chapter 5. In: Rosenthal R, Rosnow RL, editors. Artifact in behavioral research. New York: Academic; 1969. pp. 143–79.
23. Piaggio G, Elbourne DR, Altman DG, Pocock SJ, Evans SJW, for the CONSORT Group. Reporting of noninferiority and equivalence randomized trials. An extension of the CONSORT Statement. http://www.consort-statement.org/extensions/designs/non-inferiority-and-equivalence-trials/, 2012. Last visited 23 Mar 2014.
24. Raatikainen MJP, Uusimaa P, van Ginneken MME, Janssen JPG, Linnaluoto M. Remote monitoring of implantable cardioverter defibrillator patients: a safe, time-saving, and cost-effective means for follow-up. Europace. 2008;10:1145–51. doi: 10.1093/europace/eun203.
25. Risko EF, Quilty LC, Oakman JM. Socially desirable responding on the web: investigating the candor hypothesis. J Pers Assess. 2006;87(3):269–76.
26. Roethlisberger FJ, Dickinson WJ. Management and the worker. Cambridge: Harvard University Press; 1939. Citation from [18].
27. Rothmann MD, Wiens BL, Chan ISF. Design and analysis of non-inferiority trials. Boca Raton: Chapman & Hall/CRC; 2011.
28. Rosenberg MJ. The conditions and consequences of evaluation apprehension, chapter 7. In: Rosenthal R, Rosnow RL, editors. Artifact in behavioral research. New York: Academic; 1969. pp. 279–349.
29. Rosenthal R. Interpersonal expectations: effects of the experimenter's hypothesis, chapter 6. In: Rosenthal R, Rosnow RL, editors. Artifact in behavioral research. New York: Academic; 1969. pp. 181–277.
30. Rosenthal R. Interpersonal expectancy effects: a 30-year perspective. Curr Dir Psychol Sci. 1994;3(6).176–9.
31. Rosenthal R, Rosnow RL. The volunteer subject, chapter 3. In: Rosenthal R, Rosnow RL, editors. Artifact in behavioral research. New York: Academic; 1969. pp. 59–118.
32. Rosenthal R, Rosnow RL, editors. Artifact in behavioral research. New York: Academic; 1969. Newly published in 2009.
33. Rosenthal R, Rosnow RL. Artifacts in behavioral resarch – Robert Rosenthal's and Ralph L Rosnow's classical books, volume 1. Oxford: Oxford University Press; 2009.
34. Rubovits PC, Maehr ML. Pygmalion analyzed: toward an explanation of the Rosenthal-Jacobson findings. J Pers Soc Psychol. 1971;19(2):197–203. doi: 10.1037/h0031526.
35. Shah NB, Der E, Ruggerio C, Heidenreich PA, Massie BM. Prevention of hospitalizations for heart failure with an interactive home monitoring program. Am Heart J. 1998;135:373–8. doi: 10.1016/S0002-8703(98)70310-2.

36. Schueller SM, Leykin Y, Pérez-Stable ES, Muñoz RF. Selection of intervention components in an internet stop smoking participant preference trial: beyond randomized controlled trials. Psychiatry Res. 2013;1–2(205):159–65. doi: 10.1016/j.psychres.2012.08.030.
37. Simon P. Keep the customer satisfied. New York: Columbia Records 45079; 1970
38. Smit F, Lokkerbol J, Riper H, Majo MC, Boon B, Blankers M. Modeling the cost-effectiveness of health care systems for alcohol use disorders: how implementation of eHealth interventions improves cost-effectiveness. J Med Internet Res. 2011;13(3):e56. doi: 10.2196/jmir.1694.
39. Stuhlmiller C, Tolchard B. Computer-assisted CBT for depression & anxiety. Increasing accessibility to evidence-based mental health treatment. J Psychol Nurs. 2009;47(7):32–9.
40. Tate DF, Finkelstein EA, Khavjou O, Gustafson A. Cost effectiveness of internet interventions: review and recommendations. Ann Behav Med. 2009;38:40–5. doi: 10.1007/s12160-009-9131-6.
41. van Bastelaar K, Cuijpers P, Pouwer F, Riper H, Snoek FJ. Development and reach of a web-based cognitive behavioural therapy programme to reduce symptoms of depression and diabetes-specific distress. Patient Educ Couns. 2011;84:49–55. doi: 10.1016/j.pec.2010.06.013.
42. van den Berg MH, Ronday HK, Peeters AJ, le Cessie S, van der Giesen FJ, Breedveld FC, Vliet Vlieland TPM. Using internet technology to deliver a home-based physical activity intervention for patients with rheumatoid arthritis: a randomized controlled trial. Arthritis Rheum. 2006;55(5):935–45. doi: 10.1002/art.22339.
43. Webb TL, Joseph J, Yardley L, Michie S. Using the internet to promote health behavior change: a systematic review and meta-analysis of the impact of theoretical basis, use of behavior change techniques, and mode of delivery on efficacy. J Med Internet Res. 2010;12(1):e4. doi: 10.2196/jmir.1376.

Chapter 16
Economy 2: Economic Subsistence of Services When Research Funding Ends

16.1 Introduction

This chapter deviates from most others in the resources and methods used to develop the arguments. Since routine operation and funding beyond the phase of trials is typically not covered through scholarly publications we often take a direct look at the market place, its stakeholders, and extrapolate from carefully selected observations. The reader should be aware of tentativeness of the conclusions.

Sustainability in a wide sense includes economic stability, naturally embedded in a hosting society, which acts responsibly towards the environment. The following considerations start out from business models i.e. the economic core. But when it comes to equitable access to under-served populations or when Consumer Health Informatics establishes services that reduce the need for travel, the outer spheres of sustainability are implicitly addressed as well.

We do not address one important topic in this chapter: scalability. Since explorations of utility of a Consumer Health Informatics service, including trials, normally involve small client samples, resources are required at a small scale. To reach whole populations predictions are required by what factor resources have to be added to serve orders or magnitude more clients. This deserves a thorough treatment which goes beyond the scope of this volume. We rather point to some informal considerations in Sect. 5.5 in the context of those services that have the greatest promise to scale up: Level 2 services.

16.2 Client Membership Fees

Purchasing unlimited or designated period of time access to a service appears to be an appealing model as long as fees are low enough for the client and profitable for the provider. This is even more so for apps than for Internet based services because the distribution oligopoly of very few distributors of apps (cf. Sect. 7.2) has established a payment model that allows developers to effectively collect money. By contrast, on the Internet an "information is for free" feeling is still dominant and payments are only easily accepted for material purchases such as pharmaceuticals. Since medical or preventive information should be associated with some value to prospective consumers – this is one of the few places in this volume where the widely accepted term "consumer" for a person who seeks health related information and guidance through means of information and communication technology is adequate – the question is whether the "for free" or the "value information" notion dominates.

16.2.1 Apps

For apps the answer is mixed and more of an impression than a scrutinized scientific investigation. For the sake of argument we turn to one of the largest distributors, Apple's App Store. Searching for "health" and the German equivalent "Gesundheit" more than 3000 apps are listed, with some overlap. The vast majority is free. Some come with gadgets such as Nike's ^{TM} FuelBand (cf. Sect. 16.5). Some come with a renowned textbook, hypnotist healer and are a by-product without extra charge with a tens of dollars purchase from their "brand" giving initiators' portfolios. The remaining priced services where the app is the only generator of revenue are rare.

Among the health apps smoking cessation is among those with the best financial prognosis. It pertains to a large consumer base. By numbers of apps it also plays a prominent role: more than 700, again with some overlap between the language versions. Smoking cessation apps are also noteworthy because the share of those with a fee are above one third, and some charge tangible amounts, above €5. Smoking cessation apps mostly include a panel in their advertising material about money saved by not having smoked a recorded numbers of cigarettes. It appears that the prospective consumers unconsciously weigh money spent for the app against money saved by not smoking, a kind of a bargain hunter impulse rather than a long term health motivation. Among the priced apps a vast majority is either from the early days (2009–2010) and has never been updated or is brand new. Very few display a history that suggests regular business. A German one, Rauchfrei Pro from Etago stands out. It has seen nine revisions and one price increase, from 0.79 € to 0.99 € one time charge, and has been reviewed by nearly 1500 consumers, i.e. purchased by at least as many. One thousand five hundred reviews, mostly enthusiastically positive, means more than twice as many reviews as the sum over 30 other randomly selected others smoking cessation apps.

So is Etago the one who delivers us from the evil of smoking and makes a fortune? The signs are mixed at best. Medically no evidence has been provided that Rauchfrei Pro actually helps. Regarding all the concerns raised in Sect. 15.2.3 about the validity of patient reported outcomes caution is advised. But economically Etago is the winner in a winner takes all – and the losers lose all – situation: Rauchfrei

Pro's positive reviews and purchases feed back positively and if someone can be profitable in Smoking cessation in Germany it is Etago. We can conclude that the developer has collected at least 1500 times 0.79 € equals appr. 1200 €. That would feed a professional and cover expenses for less than a week but looking at Rauchfrei Pro doubtlessly requires more than a week's work. The owner of Etago is a hard to trace individual in Berlin, with no obvious medical affiliation. No secondary source of funding such as ads are visible. So unless the number of consumers surpasses the number of reviewers by a factor of hundreds it cannot be sustainably be funded. No wander, therefore, that Etago stopped updating Rauchfrei Pro after October 2012 but (mostly) positive reviews keep flowing.

Take Home

Client membership fees for apps are extremely unlikely to be a source of sufficient revenue:

- Even in domains with many affected consumers traffic concentrates on few providers.
- Even if the app rightfully announces financial on top of medical benefits do the leading providers not generate sufficient revenue for sustainable operation.
- Health apps cannot be recommended as a sole source of business.

16.2.2 Internet

For the Internet membership fees that provide access to all contents and services behind a pay wall are very hard to investigate because the space is so vast. However, surveys and interventions described in Sect. 16.3.2 suggest that for apps membership fees alone are an unlikely sustained resource of funding. For the Internet this is supported through one investigations from Switzerland [1].

16.3 Client Fees for Service

16.3.1 Apps

Individual fee for individual service is a very uncommon transactional pattern with mobile apps. Apps are rather considered as ubiquitous companions that deliver information spontaneously once they have been acquired – with or without fee – and where the individual provision of information such as GPS, resource locator, news, communication etc. is not charged for. In contrast, charges for purchase of substantial goods or physical services such as transportation are accepted and the convenience of a built in pricing and payment methods is appreciated. As long as the marketplace is so perceived the acceptance for a price tag for advice should not be assumed to be a reliable resource of sustained funding.

16.3.2 Internet

For Internet based services we find very inhomogeneous and partially contradictory evidence. In investigations cited in Sect. 3.3.1.5 the picture of client payments as a source of revenue is dire. In a survey in the USA and an intervention study in Switzerland requests for payments are turned down by strong majorities of the subjects asked or investigated. In the USA 26 % of information seekers hit a pay wall but only 2 % paid. In Switzerland the utilization of a service of a renowned university hospital went down by 69 % when a fee of appr. 12 € per consultation was introduced for a formerly free service. So we are inclined to conclude that client fees for services are not a sustainable model of funding.

At the same time services introduced in Sect. 5.2.5.4 (www.dred.com, www.healthcaremagic.com, everydayhealth.com) have existed for at least 5 years – some under other than the present names – although they are charging fees the same order of magnitude as the ones turned down in Switzerland. So what distinguishes them? We do not have access to their balance but several explanations come to mind, especially when looking at www.healthcaremagic.com. Their portal is full of ads from industry giants which add a second resource of revenue. Most of their physicians have Indian names and a respective physiognomy. This is not bad in its own right. It rather points to a method of saving labor costs by exporting labor to regions with low incomes. Regarding tightly enforced state licensure in countries such as the USA such services almost certainly violate applicable law if the character of the service qualifies as practice of medicine, as outlined in Sect. 17.4. Generally www.healthcaremagic.com and the likes provides clear evidence that Consumer Health Informatics must be regarded and hence regulated and quality assured as a global phenomenon.

www.dred.com has another incentive for paying their fee: it offers prescriptions at fees between €9 and 29, i.e. the convenience of one stop shop counseling and delivery without unpleasant questions regarding the indication.

Take Home

Client fees for services

- do not fit common perceptions about mobile apps unless transfer of material goods or physical services is incurred
- are not willingly accepted and do not lead to steady funding alone,
- however, when combined with other cost saving or revenue creating elements may lead to long term successful business

16.4 Heterogeneous Co-branding

For certain conditions alliances with partners outside health care may be an option. A Consumer Health Informatics service for flight anxiety or one for travel medicine might be financially sponsored by an airline. In turn, links within the Consumer Health Informatics service take the client to the airline's home page or booking system, maybe luring with some discount. Other natural alliances are all kinds of conditions for which non prescription drugs are commonly used with mail order pharmacies, skin irritations with cosmetics, childhood vaccinations with toy supermarket chains, metabolic syndrome with sport studios or healthy food chains, diabetes with diet producers, and as bizarre ones as cancer with wig producers.

Other combinations may come to the reader's mind easily. For the goal of this chapter they should have in common that the partner outside health care has a solid financial standing and regards the clients of the service a positively selected target group for his business. Having said this risks and disadvantages become obvious. They emerge from the fact that the co-branded Consumer Health Informatics service may no longer be the one or no longer appear as the one that was successfully tested in a trial (cf. Chap. 15). The economically stronger partner – possibly by orders of magnitude – can take influence on the service itself risking to modify or dilute its approved active agents. Even if the partner leaves the service unaffected and just humbly places his link somewhere, the tested ad free service appeared unbiased and gained respective trust which the presence of the link undermines and puts the whole credibility and consequentially effectiveness at risk.

Ironically, a conflict of interest that would normally be avoided under all circumstances, may be the solution here: Involving the partner already in the trial and give him exactly the same role and visibility in the trial as later in routine.

One thing must not be forgotten: Co-branding partners do not fund for charity or corporate social responsibility. They want ROI and they want to measure it. This poses new challenges for trials. Next to demonstrating health benefits Consumer Health Informatics services must also be instrumental to increased business or profitability for the partner. Successes have not become known as yet, however, through private communication the author knows that such plans have been started, then discontinued in a Consumer Health Informatics service in the field of healthy diet with a healthy food chain. Too many factors overlap, too many confounders cannot be safely excluded such that a proof failed that ads and a link from the Consumer Health Informatics service to the food chain improved their business.

Take Home

Partnering with stakeholders from other industries such as a healthy diet service with a food retail chain creates the expectations of a win-win: steady flow of funds to the Consumer Health Informatics service and increased food sales. Even if such effects materialize they are very hard to measure which bears the risk that the retail partner cancels prematurely.

16.5 Service-Device Bundles

The recent boom of self-tracking devices such as (fitbit®, Fuelband,[1] Jawbone®), and the quantified self movement of presenting their signals draws attention to services, mostly mobile apps, that aggregate and display health related behavioral data (step counts, hours of sleep, etc.) and vital signs (heart rate, ...). Other functions are goal setting and monitoring, social network, GPS, etc. Presently self tracking and its associated mobile applications reside in the domain of infotainment and self enhancement although some flavor of health cannot be neglected. For more centrally medical signs devices have also become available for client use, such as blood pressure, blood glucose and insulin concentration, prothrombin activity under anticoagulation treatment, pulse oximetry and flow meters for PEFR or FEV_1 under asthma or COPD treatment etc., cf. Sect. 14.3.3. All these devices have a 6–7 digit customers market in the USA or the European Union including the 110 million German speaking Germans, Austrians and Swiss, i.e. truly large customer bases with enormous purchasing power. Similar considerations apply to the Spanish, Portuguese, Chinese and other large language communities, although characteristics of local populations should by no means be neglected (cf. [3]).

Customers are paying prices in the 100 $ range – some quite a bit more – for self tracking gadgets. Various apps exist to synchronize with the gadgets, some coming one-on-one with a gadget and many more by third parties. It is too early to say, since most of the apps are not older than one or 2 years. However, the margins from device sales may be sufficient to subsidize Consumer Health Informatics services conveyed through mobile apps where a scientifically approved preventive programs such as the ones in Sect. 9.4.2.1 for the metabolic syndrome is offered and the tracked data required in these programs are effortlessly there, transmitted from the gadget through Bluetooth® or WiFi.

The medical devices above have their sales prices as well and some are recommended for use in conjunction with some pharmaceuticals for the underlying conditions (corticosteroids, antihypertensive drugs, anticoagulation etc.) whose sales generate continuous highly predictive cash flows and incomes. Depending on the condition and treatment health plans are the final payers. Again margins from the substantial sales can be used to subsidize the virtual good – the Consumer Health Informatics services – enriched by knowledge and situational advice for control of the condition. Again the apps can offer the convenience of effortless data management on top of their underlying medical treatment concepts. It appears like a win – win – win situation. The Consumer Health Informatics client has a convenient approved service for free. The Consumer Health Informatics service provider has a sustainable resource of funding. The sponsor can openly showcase its device or pharmaceutical core business and enhance its customer relationship because everybody knows upfront that it is a sponsored service.

---

[1] At the editorial deadline Nike's trademark was challenged in a lawsuit.

A provider that comes close to that model is Roche™. They sell devices for blood glucose management (AKKU-CHEK®, cf. http://www.accu-chek.com/us/) and coagulation status (CoaguChek, cf. http://www.site.coagucheklink.com). For blood glucose management an app Accu-Chek 360 from Google play® supports the use, data charting, statistics, and more on insulin therapy. For anti-coagulation a web based service www.site.coagucheklink.com/ supports the client in a similar way. A mobile app game for iPad (it works for iPhone but the print is too small for comfortable use) CoaguGame from App Store teaches the use of the instrumentation required to reliably take INR measurements. Roche with its two device classes and respective suite of Consumer Health Informatics services is a special form of the service-device bundle: the Consumer Health Informatics service provider is in-house rather than third party. Roche does not take, however, the last step: automatic transmission of measured data to the mobile device or computer. No such services with a device producer and a Consumer Health Informatics service provider offering a technically and financially integrated solution have reached the scholarly literature as yet. Concerns about medical device regulation and security [2] may be reasons.

> **Take Home**
> Companies that sell lifestyle gadgets or medical devices made for client use profit from the fact that purchase prices for material goods are regarded as normal while "for free" is regarded as normal for electronically conveyed services. They can fund themselves through adding margins to the device sales prices from which the Consumer Health Informatics services can be subsidized. This is a true win-win because neither service nor device would work without the other.

16.6 Providers' Customer Relationship Services

In Sect. 4.5.1 we see two examples of apps from major hospitals (Mayo Clinic from Google play and App Store and JoHo Dortmund Innere Medizin I from Google play and App Store) with similar portfolios of services both mainly meant for patients they are treating in regular face-to-face services and whom they offer information and convenience implicitly subtly building and maintaining customer relationships. Both Consumer Health Informatics services have been offered and continually updated and expanded since February 2011 (JoHo) resp. May 2012 (Mayo). This alone is not an overwhelming life span but Mayo has a long running Internet based predecessor. However, once such services have started they create expectations. A health care provider that discontinues without very good comprehensible reasons risks loss of credibility. Therefore, there is some immanent urge for extended operation. Furthermore a look at hospital budgets nourishes hope for sustained operation. The yearly transaction volumes of such hospitals are between a half and several billion US$, with between 4 % and 7 % spent on electronic data processing. If Consumer Health Informatics services receive just 1 % of that amount their yearly financial supply is 200k US$, larger by a factor of more than 100 than in the membership fee example in Sect. 16.2.1. In the provider-client situation more benefits may materialize on both ends: Clients may get through to the right specialist faster if they can place their request based on a shared medical history. Hospitals may gain in efficiency due to fewer missed appointments, cf. Sect. 10.2.2.1. A present disadvantage and challenge for future development results from the fact that hospital maintained and centered Consumer Health Informatics services may lead to clients' fragmented medical histories: Their internal medicine record is with provider A, their gynecological one with B etc., without presently existing standards to integrate or bridge.

> **Take Home**
> Technically advanced providers share their medical data, appointments, knowledge resources, etc. with their patients. This can be achieved with a small share of the yearly budget. The offered transparency suggests advantages for the client who is better informed and can proceed more targeted while the provider can hope for fewer missed appointments. A present challenge is the integration of data from different providers' patient portals.

16.7 Online Pharmacies

Online pharmacies are discussed in Sect. 5.2.4, including their similarity to online shopping. They generate revenue through material sales and shipment. Their efforts for provision of the Consumer Health Informatics part of their service can be drawn from their normal operations: the margins of their material sales. Since centralized warehousing and delivery allow economies of scale compared to decentralized retail pharmacies, Online Pharmacy is a self supporting business model as long as sufficient volumes can be processed legally which presently means as a Level 1 service. Required regulations for Level 2 are addressed in Sect. 17.5.

> **Take Home**
> Online pharmacies create large incomes through material sales which easily support respective Consumer Health Informatics portals to their services.

16.8 Employer Sponsorship

Employer sponsorship happens in the private and public sector. Two examples from Sect. 9.4 with notable medical and behavioral effects will now be analyzed economically. They are H.E.A.L.T.H. at a military base and DASH for Health at EMC. Both employers regard it as part of their employee benefits programs and both Consumer Health Informatics services are integrated with other existing programs: H.E.A.L.T.H. with an intranet at the base and DASH for Health with $EMC^{2®}$'s health plan infrastructure. Therefore, their marginal costs are small while their actual benefits are noteworthy and the emotional identification of employees with their caring employers adds intangible benefits. Neither is a guarantee for prolonged operation. But DASH for Health has already been in operation since 2003. H.E.A.L.T.H. is being pushed out army wide through Department of Defense funding, presently until 2016.

Employees who enroll with health related services provided or mediated by their employers either are not aware of or are not concerned about sensitive health data residing in a space that their employer may have or get access to. Risks for future operation of employer sponsored Consumer Health Informatics services may originate from growing privacy awareness on the part of the employee rather than from financial shortage on the part of the employer. The whole Chap. 13 deals with reasonable client interests for privacy and through what kind of methods and at what price privacy and other required qualities of data integrity can be achieved. This scholarly treatment overlays with alarming news popping up in mass media how foundations of the privacy and integrity enabling methods can be breached. If public opinion mounts that no data are safe anymore clients may turn away from Consumer Health Informatics services and employer sponsored ones may be hit first.

> **Take Home**
> Consumer Health Informatics services can be part of benefits that employers offer to attract skilled work force. Services can than be seamlessly integrated with other health benefits, as can the collected and used data. This has been gladly accepted or tolerated in the past but may face client concerns and withdrawals because the awareness for data abuse is growing.

16.9 Third Party Entrepreneurship

In Sect. 16.8 we discuss DASH for Health as it is used at an employer ($EMC^{2®}$). This is just one facet of DASH's broader approach. DASH for Health is provided through a small LLC near Boston University (cf. http://cvs.dashforhealth.com/

pages/clients/cvs/info.php). The LLC guarantees the quality of the Consumer Health Informatics service through specialists in the fields of cardiology and nutrition and offers the software and hosting of the medical contents, client records etc. It has several resources of revenue, including business partners such as EMC^{2}® who lease access for their employees, and some individual clients who pay subscription fees. The DASH LLC also tried but did not succeed to co-brand with food retail, cf. Sect. 16.4 because the co-branding partners' models were based on ROI rather than on corporate social responsibility or charity.

16.10 Charity

Charity and philanthropic donors have been drivers of providing health related information to the public longer than the Internet has existed. In Sect. 6.1 the 60 year old Reach to Recovery is addressed. Komen®'s (http://ww5.komen.org) campaign for breast cancer patients started in 1982, http://www.oncolink.org of Livestrong for cancer survivors (cf. Sect. 5.2.3.3) in 1994. The first roots of Planned Parenthood® (http://www.plannedparenthood.org, cf. Sect. 10.2.3) were planted as early as 1912 and the foundation has since survived mainly through donations although starting 1970 US federal funding has become a second resource.

Of course we mainly see those that are alive and may miss those that defaulted, were forgotten and patient records they kept lost. But still the evidence is impressive that for conditions that have wide attention through the public such as cancer and family planning, charity and donorship are a lasting resource of funding.

> **Take Home**
> Charities have maintained Consumer Health Informatics services on a large scale for quite a while. They tend to flock around conditions that have a large patient base and a positive public perception. When the latter changes they may face hard times to maintain services and assets (knowledge, patient longitudinal data) may be lost.

16.11 Government Organisations

Federal as well as state governments play a role in funding broad coverage basic services. Locators of certified providers are discussed in Chap. 5 (cf. Sect. 5.2.5.2 for physicians or Sect. 5.3.2 for online pharmacies). The US Office of Disease Prevention and Health Promotion provides educational material on healthy behavior at http://health.gov. The NIH offers http://www.ncbi.nlm.nih.gov/pubmedhealth/ and http://www.MedlinePlus.gov whose properties have been described in Sect. 3.5.1.

Of course the client may also go the hard way of reading original scholarly articles referenced in http://www.ncbi.nlm.nih.gov/pubmed/. Rather than further elaborating the character of the Consumer Health Informatics services we emphasize here that the US and likewise the German governments have been committed to fund the provision of information for a broad public for a long time. PubMed's paper based predecessors date back to 1879 when the Index Medicus started and the first electronic form MEDLARS was initiated in 1971. It should, however, be noted that according to the open market resp. Bismarck orientations of the US and German health care systems, authorities do not assume the roles of service providers but only broker information (cf. Sect. 5.2.5.1 or support logistics (cf. Sect. 5.2.5.2).

In contrast the NHS in Beveridge oriented UK initiated similar services but transferred them into private ownership of e.g. http://www.patient.co.uk/, cf. Sect. 5.2.5.1, which depends on other resources of income as the large number of personalized ads on their home pages demonstrates. Only the future can show whether the privately funded UK model in a state funded health care system will sustain in parallel to the publicly funded US and German ones.

16.12 Health Insurance Coverage

Inasmuch as Consumer Health Informatics services can be proven safe and effective as screening, diagnostic, therapeutic, or monitoring services, it should naturally imply that they are covered through health insurance. Few services, though, have so far achieved that state. Two examples from Germany will be used to demonstrate the direction.

The Techniker Krankenkasse social health insurance offers various so called coaches at http://ecoach.tk.de/coaches/. Each is "advertised" by an infotainment teaser which invites to register when the client feels affected. Some coaches are behavioral and well being related such as fitness, nutrition, walking. Two, however, address ICD-10 diagnoses, burnout and diabetes mellitus 2. In any case, to enroll the client has to provide a membership number and to access the service which is free of charge. The burnout service assists the client in identification of stressors and coping strategies. The diabetes mellitus 2 service includes general information about the disease and healthy behaviors plus a sophisticated diabetes diary with convenience functions, graphical displays etc. It is not meant to replace physician visits but suggests to "help the diabetic to gain more autonomy" and to "enhance the retrospective assessment of the treatment plan" (translated from http://ecoach.tk.de/diabetescoach/). These and the other Techniker Krankenkasse coaches add convenience to the patient encounter and some may have preventive effects in the metabolic syndrome arena. As wide and unspecific the clients, the circumstances, the target criteria and an endpoint in time are, sound proofs of effectiveness, cost-effectiveness, or non-inferiority (cf. respective sections in Chap. 15) will be hard to achieve. Therefore, Techniker Krankenkasse offers the Consumer Health

Informatics services as what they are: additional services to strengthen their customer relationships.

The DAK deprexis Consumer Health Informatics service is different in this respect. It offers a German version of the http://deprexis.com/ treatment by Gaia AG (plc) in Hamburg. DAK has started in 2012 to invite members for large clinical trials. The character of the treatment is not fully clear. Deprexis has a patient and a therapist portal. From the therapist portal therapists can monitor their patients' progress. However, whether deprexis is Level 1 or Level 2 design is not fully clear.

An advanced US example is Kaiser Permanente®'s My Health Manager at http://healthy.kaiserpermanente.org/health/care/consumer/my-health-manager which, however, does not go quite as far: Its symptom checker has pre-screening functionality.

> **Take Home**
> Depending on the character of the health care system the government or health plans are the ultimately responsible stakeholders in charge to fund approved Consumer Health Informatics services. Advances in this direction are very slow and to some extent paradoxical: UK's service has been privatized while health plans in open market US are less advanced than in socialized Germany.

References

1. Brockes MC, Neuhaus Bühler RP, Schulz E, Neumann CL, Schmidt-Weitmann S. Medizinische Online-Beratung im Universitätsspital Zürich vor und nach Einführung einer Bearbeitungsgebühr (in German). Dtsch Med Wochenschr. 2010;135:231–5. doi: 10.1055/s-0029-1244838.
2. He D, Naveed M, Gunter CA, Nahrstedt K. Security concerns in Android mHealth apps. In: Proceedings AMIA 2014 annual symposium; 2014. http://www.amia.org/amia2014. Download proceedings...Papers; Accessed 07 Dec 2014.
3. Hartzler A, Wetter T. Engaging patients through mobile phones: demonstrator services, success factors, and opportunities in low and middle-income countries. Yearb Med Inform. 2014;182–94. doi: 10.15265/IY-2014-0022.

Chapter 17
Towards Future Consumer Health Informatics Adapted Health Care Legislation

17.1 Introduction

Among the many facets of Consumer Health Informatics we have sometimes addressed legal issues. We have looked into legal notices – inasmuch as they existed – of service providers (e.g. in Sect. 7.4). We have analyzed challenges and methods to protect privacy, authenticity etc. in Chap. 13. In this chapter we assume that such aspects as legal nature of providers and privacy are sufficiently addressed and turn to the core questions of legality and legitimacy of Consumer Health Informatics as such.

To the most part we regard Consumer Health Informatics as a new way of delivering health care and therefore analyze how Consumer Health Informatics fares under the ethics underlying the codes regulating medicine. This primary process sets the stage and transfers legal assessment for other individuals and professions. In Sect. 17.9 we briefly address how the perspective of health informatics professionals, one large and pivotal other profession, and their code of ethics modifies judgments.

17.2 Frames of Reference

In Chap. 2 we show that the future holds a significant shortage of adequate health services. If we ignore this development we will face triage and denial of medical services decisions on a broadening range in not more than a decade. Society can decide to direct a greater share of resources towards the health care industry at the cost of diverting funds from other economically important activities. Or we can seek alternative ways within health care to allocate the available funds. One way of mitigating this imminent shortage is that, while the shortage draws near, new technologies and services develop at sufficient speed, affordable price and sufficient

© Springer International Publishing Switzerland 2016
T. Wetter, *Consumer Health Informatics*, Health Informatics,
DOI 10.1007/978-3-319-19590-2_17

quality to fully compensate for the emerging shortage. Consumer Health Informatics is advocated here as a discipline of new services wrapped around new technologies that may take a respective role.

But no technologies have ever come without risks. Through Chap. 8 and others we have an idea about risks of Consumer Health Informatics services that presently we are not sufficiently able to understand let alone control. As long as we do not know how safe they are it is legitimate to not release them for routine use. But we will also show that even some services that are safe enough are illegal under present law because legislation and professional codes do not yet follow up on the opportunities of Consumer Health Informatics. Likewise, some promising IRB, Ethikkommission[1] or alike supervised research projects, as successful as they may turn out, cannot make it into routine services under present law, because certain risks still remain.

Depending on the field of legislation laws reflect a balance between benefits and risks accepted or tolerated in a society. For instance in the field of traffic laws speed regulations balance the benefit of covering distances with the risk of accidents. Thirty-five miles per hour or 50 km/h are the present defaults in town in the USA respectively Germany. Those limits enable people to reach goals but tolerate a small minority being hurt and even killed in accidents. Only 0 speed would fully exclude risks, but nobody would reach any goal any more. Would the limits be changed to 40 mph or 65 km/h with the same cars and streets and drivers the majority would reach their goals earlier, while a larger minority than before would become victims of accidents. Since there is no definite and undisputed value of covering distances as there is no definite and undisputed value of human lives and physical integrity, societies can assign utilities to either and from these utilities can come to the conclusion that a certain speed limit optimizes the portfolio of its values. Later (cf. Sect. 17.11.8) we will analyze whether such a utilitarian or other evaluation is morally acceptable.

Here we consider first what it means when society invests into novel or better ways to convey required services. Assuming resources were not limited and waste of natural resources were tolerated more streets, straighter and wider streets could be built throughout. More efficient means of street use could be developed and made available to achieve more transportation without increased risk.

This is as unlikely for the necessary additional amount of transportation as it is unlikely for the necessary additional volume of medical services as derived in Chap. 2 and summarized in Table 2.2. For the field of Consumer Health Informatics we will, therefore, argue that we should advance in two directions. One is to investigate methods designed to enhance the safety of current Consumer Health Informatics services such that they may meet the current legal safety bar under an unchanged balance of benefits and risks. The second is to investigate appropriate acceptable risk/benefit ratios informed by public opinion, government, and professional associations. Professional organizations play a key role to move the legal acceptability of services. If they follow a rationalist utilitarian attitude, the

---

[1] Institutions in German medical research that corresponds to IRBs in the USA.

basics of which are outlined in Sect. 17.11.8.1 they can encourage certain services to be justly provided society wide at the price of some compromise in the balance of achievable benefits and incurred risks. For this to be seen as progress a public debate about the weight of the different ethical principles of medicine should be moderated by trusted professional organizations such as the American College of Physicians, the American Medical Association and its House of Delegates, the German counterpart "Deutscher Ärztetag" or alike.

For some major Consumer Health Informatics medical domains such as psychiatric and counseling services the argument can even be simpler. In some health care systems such as the US one such services are presently only available after a long wait and at cost or with insurance premiums that are prohibitive for large population groups. For them it is no service at all vs. a somewhat approved Consumer Health Informatics service. Quite some sophistication and scrutiny is already applied for ever better approval, cf. Chap. 15 and Sects. 4.4.2 and 5.2.2. Distributive justice i.e. equal access for all of equal need can be achieved through scalable – mainly Level 2 – Consumer Health Informatics services.

> **Take Home**
> The following assumptions and considerations underly the outline of this chapter:
> - The demographic development leads to scarcity of the medical workforce fast.
> - Medical legislation reflects societal consent about balancing benefits achieved through forms of service such as cure with incurred risks such as adverse effects.
> - Consumer Health Informatics services suggest themselves as a complement, even a substitute, for some service presently conveyed through humans.
> - Both, technical and demographic development call for a new ethical assessment.

17.3 Legislation, Ethics and Research

Ethical principles inform how ideally legislation should regulate societal processes. Though partially or temporarily overlaid through political party and pressure group tactics they should and will in the following be respected as basic principles.

Following the widely respected approach of Beauchamp and Childress (cf. [2]) four principles guide medical ethics: respect for autonomy, nonmaleficence, beneficence and distributive justice. Since in a complex field as medicine there is hardly ever a procedure (diagnostic, therapeutic, preventive, etc.) that only increases benefit, reduces harm, increases justice and autonomy, ethical considerations have to address whether we are willing to trade increased risk of harm for better or more justly distributed outcome or whether we want lower risk at the price of reduced service coverage. In asking such questions we implicitly take a utilitarian stance whose moral acceptability will be analyzed and compared to other moral judgments of benefits and risks in Sect. 17.11.8.

In recent history (cf. Fox and Swazey [6, Chap. 11]) this rational approach is competing with a conservative principlism backed up through non-compromising theological positions which are more outspoken in the USA than in other countries explicitly covered in this volume. Such principlism – although often widely publicly controversial as Fox and Swazey point out – is easier to apply to individual cases in clinical ethics. In the utilitarian approach, by contrast, a clinical and a public health perspective mutually fertilize each other. Some of the arguments later in this chapter actually are more public health than medical.

To inform specifications of the four principles research is required before something becomes law. Inasmuch as medical and health care delivery research involves patients or patient data and hence holds the risk of patients being harmed or patient data becoming exposed Institutional Review Boards (IRBs) or respective institutions in other countries assess the expected benefits and impending risks, as further outlined in Sect. 17.10.

> **Take Home**
> For medical legislation to be in accordance with the state of medical knowledge and common morality ethics plays a mediating role. Publicly favored moral theories co-determine the direction that health care takes.

17.4 Present Regulations

Consumer Health Informatics services are offered in a vast variety of settings through individuals and organizations of an equally vast variety of types and qualifications, located in different countries and regions. Therefore, it does not come as a surprise that regulations that pertain to Consumer Health Informatics have different origins and legal cultures. As a consequence it may not always be crystal clear what does and what does not apply and we may encounter contradictory permissions or obligations. Therefore, the following section can by no means be exhaustive. It rather uses two countries, the USA as an open market inspired and Germany as a socialized medicine Bismarck[2] type model, to illustrate how Consumer Health Informatics services can principally be assessed from a legal

---

[2]According to Otto von Bismarck, 1815–1898, First Imperial Chancellor of Prussia, who 1883 drafted the still prevailing German health insurance system with premium parts being paid by employers and employees and where all inhabitants of Germany are covered, be it as family of employed citizens or through other subsidies.

perspective. In few places the UK Beveridge[3] model is also addressed. This includes judgments of the author that some of the services described in this volume presently are unlawful.

17.4.1 Structures and Resources in the USA

The structures that provide, enforce and further develop the laws and codes of physician professional conduct in the USA are somewhat fragmented. A framework for payment, privacy, quality assurance etc. comes from Washington, DC. Then we have the state medical boards as the sites of certification, applicable law, and enforcement. Principally, this allows quite some variation which can only marginally be covered here. We will use some examples from the pioneering California Rules of Professional Conduct. For Consumer Health Informatics's neighbor discipline telemedicine there is a central resource at www.medlicense.com/telemedicine_license.html where the state practices can be found, while regulations for Consumer Health Informatics are still absent.

As a side note on Consumer Health Informatics relevant regulations for other major health professions we observe that pharmacies and drug dispensing are regulated nationwide by the Federal Food, Drug and Cosmetics (FD&C) Act and that nurses have the Interstate Nurse Licensure Compact for practicing across states (cf. [14]).

In the sequel we look beyond the horizon of present fragmented legislation and at the American Medical Association (AMA) as an umbrella organization where all physicians can be members and depending on federal state of practice are compulsory members. Also, medical specialty associations are formally affiliated with AMA. AMA represents and lobbies for the mind set of the "good physician". Its surveys and comments are very broad in range on developments that concern the practice of medicine and the role of physicians in society. Part of its work is day to day lobbying reaction to national politics. But in its ethics opinions, its health policies and its directives it conveys a clear stance about what physicians' services should and should not be. All these documents reflect the majority vote of elected representatives in the House of Delegates or of committees that those install. Therefore, AMA positions provide a clear image of what physicians certified in the United States think and plan.

It should be noted that Consumer Health Informatics services inevitably make use of information and communication technology and may make use of medical devices. It is FDA's role to supervise safety of medical devices including medical software. We appreciate an important role of assuring safety of used software and devices. However, we do not go into the depths of this part of regulation because here as throughout this volume we want to emphasize the client perspective. We

---

[3] According to William Henry Beveridge, 1879–1963, British social reformer who drafted the UK welfare state model with public authorities in charge of organizing and financing health care.

are not so much interested in whether a technology can *principally* be used safely – which FDA checks. We are rather interested whether a technology in the hands of real lay Consumer Health Informatics service clients with their limitations and inherent risks as they are addressed in Chap. 8 improves, maintains, or deteriorates outcomes. This relates to the distinction between functionality and fitness for use. We regard it as the responsibility of a provider of a Consumer Health Informatics service to scrutinize the quality and safety of technology that he employs in view of client side risks.

17.4.1.1 Level 0

Publishing on the Internet is essentially governed by the same rules as publishing in print or public speech. The First Amendment to the U.S. Constitution gives authors virtually unlimited rights, including advocacy of unpopular ideas. In the medical domain well researched and perfectly described effective therapies may find themselves competing with scientifically unfounded medical advice and ideologically or irrationally incubated fairy tale such as anti-vaccination campaigns [19].

This right to free speech holds in its full extent when laypersons publish online. When physicians assume the role of writers the AMA has some recommendations though not directives for good professional conduct. Through Health Policy H-455.998 the AMA[4] principally encourages to speak out as "responsible physicians" and H-478.999 supports the development of an international code of ethics for medical Internet sites. In Ethics Opinion 9.124 Professionalism in social media – in good appreciation of their opportunities – is spelled out as "maintain(ing) appropriate boundaries of the patient-physician relationship ... just as ... in other context" and bringing apparently "unprofessional content ... to the attention of the individual". The most concrete guidance comes from Ethics Opinion 5.027 which request to "ensure that the information is accurate, timely, reliable, and scientifically sound, and includes appropriate scientific references". In summary: physicians are requested to behave as diligently as they are in-person. Concerning the recipient end the AMA "support(s) efforts to address the economic, literacy, and cultural barriers to patients utilizing information technology" in H-478.996.

17.4.1.2 Level 1

Legally the most important feature of Level 1 services is that they are initiated through an in-person provider-patient contact. When such services are provider driven they are also called telemedicine. In this case everything is legal as long

---

[4]All up to date versions of subsequently referred to AMA policies can be searched at AMA's freely accessible Policy finder at http://www.ama-assn.org/ama/pub/about-ama/our-people/house-delegates/policy-finder-online.page?

as it is done diligently and in appreciation of the special opportunities and more so risks of telecommunication.

Concretely, H-160.937 on "Quality Telemedicine" requests that "(t)he physician is responsible for, and retains the authority for, the safety and quality of services provided to patients by nonphysician providers through telemedicine." Elements of how to implement such responsibility (supervision, inspection, reporting ...) are then spelled out. They all explicitly or implicitly assume that qualified, though not medical, staff is involved at the patient end of a telemedicine setting.

That is not always the case in Consumer Health Informatics services. It is obviously not the case when patients e-mail their physicians and vice versa. For such situations H-478.997 first mandates that "(n)ew communication technologies *must never replace the crucial interpersonal contacts*[5] that are the very basis of the patient-physician relationship. Rather, electronic mail and other forms of Internet communication should be *used to enhance such contacts*." It then mainly offers detailed guidance about establishing rules of communication (turnaround times, privacy, archiving, ...). While explicitly referring to e-mail alone the following sentence suggest that other transactional forms of electronic communication such as a patient writing and a physician commenting on a diary would be judged similarly: "Patient-physician electronic mail is defined as computer-based communication between physicians and patients *within a professional relationship*, in which the *physician has taken on an explicit measure of responsibility* for the patient's care."

17.4.1.3 Level 2

Health policy H-478.997 rules how to use e-mail and Internet have already been presented in the section above about Level 1. When analyzing Level 2 the preamble of this policy sets a concluding negative signal for the practice of medicine: "New communication technologies *must never replace the crucial interpersonal contacts ... Treatment through the internet alone is illegal*."

Prescribing through the Internet is one way of treating patients, and it is a common phenomenon with many involved stakeholders. In a Health Policy H-120.956 on Internet Prescribing the AMA publishes an updated action plan meant to foster safe prescribing through the Internet while also enforcing "action against physicians who fail to meet the local standards of medical care when issuing prescriptions through Internet web sites". Partners addressed are state medical societies and the Federation of State Medical Boards, the National Association of Boards of Pharmacy and federal and state regulatory bodies. Regarding that this Policy underwent its most recent revision in June 2005 the final sentence to "keep pace with changes in technology by continually updating standards ... " demonstrates the gap between perceived regulatory need and the capacity of institutions to respond to a changing technological landscape.

---

[5] All emphasis in this and the next sections by the author of this volume.

While this is a recommendation only, authoritative though, an example of how one of the addressed authorities turn such recommendations into legislation is the California Business and Professions Code which at law.onecle.com/california/business/2242.html declares in an uncompromising formulation: "Prescribing, dispensing, or furnishing dangerous drugs as defined in Section 4022 without an appropriate prior examination and a medical indication, constitutes unprofessional conduct." According to Code 4022 dangerous drugs essentially are prescription drugs. Code 2242 lists various process exemptions which, however, all recur to another health care professional with whom the patient is mandated to have a provider-patient relationship. Internet prescribing is only the tip of the iceberg of virtual therapy but a very large tip. This does not change as of today that the whole iceberg is illegal unless a health care professional is involved in-person at some point.

In its Ethics Code Opinion 5.027 (last endorsed June 2003) AMA hesitantly and indecisively looks ahead, requesting that "services through interactive online sites ... with not ... a pre-existing relationship or ... decision-support programs that generate personalized information ... to users, should be consistent with general and specialty-specific standards. ... include ... disclosures such as limitations inherent in the technology."

Medical specialty associations are not clearer or more specific either. Gynecologists and obstetricians, whose domain is very strongly represented in Consumer Health Informatics through all kinds of breast cancer related services (cf. Sects. 12.2.2.3 and 6.1) and online prescription of contraception and menopause hormone replacement therapy, do not have "Internet" as a searchable term on the American Gynecological Obstetrical Society (AGOS, at http://www.agosonline.org/) and American Congress of Obstetricians and Gynecologists (ACOG, at www.acog.org) home pages. The American College of Physicians (ACP) has a comprehensive policy statement at http://www.acponline.org/advocacy/acp_policy_compendium_2012.pdf. It addresses fair payment of services conveyed through electronic media, certification of online pharmacies, direct-to-consumer drug advertising but unmistakably commands that "direct physician patient relationship remain(s) inviolate and ... Internet for prescribing should facilitate, not circumvent that relationship" (last endorsed by the BoR in 2010). Andrologists with their blockbuster representation of Viagra and erectile dysfunction at online pharmacies and pre-screening services (cf. Sects. 5.2.4 and 5.2.5.3) and the American Society of Andrology, http://andrologysociety.org/ do not mention Internet either. Similarly, pediatricians (American Academy of Pediatrics, (AAP) at http://www.aap.org) just address some privacy, media impact on child and adolescent health, and use of e-mail issues but do not cover the role of online communication for diagnosis and therapy. In a 2009 letter to the editor of Journal of Rheumatology Lacson and coauthors urge the scientific and professional public to define its place and rules of conduct for what they call "facebook medicine" [9].

Psychiatrists should be most attentive to the development because for many diseases there is no logistics necessity for psychiatrist and patient to meet since physical examination, lab and imaging often play a subordinate role.

17.4 Present Regulations

Despite all precautions and sanctions and the slow motion in response to present practice the AMA has also endorsed and renewed in June 2007 the visionary policy H-160.975. It encourages to invest in "individual lifestyles that promote good health", to introduce "innovative and cost-effective health care services", with "government at all levels" encouraged to take an "integral role" and "not unduly restrict" and "ensure ... continuum of supportive health care services for special populations". The central encouragement to advance legislation that will be used as an argument in the later Sect. 17.12 comes from (3) in H-160.975: "Decisions concerning the use of health care services, including the selection of a health care provider or *delivery mechanism*, should be made by the individual." Furthermore (4) addresses the ethical principle of justice by requesting "incentives ... (to) give care to those who otherwise would not have access to such care. In addition, existing short-comings in the current public system for providing access need to be addressed." H-373-997 tries to balance between market forces and the patient advocate role the physician should assume, ending with a plea to "preserve patient's freedom of choice". This is where the US open market conception of the medical industry finds its clearest expressions.

The regulation in the DF&C (Drug, Food & Cosmetics) Act on drug dispensing is as crystal clear as AMA policy H-478.997 against treatment through the Internet alone. The core sentence of a long law is in section 353 and mainly says that "a drug ... shall be dispensed *only upon* written *prescription of a (licensed practitioner)*,... an oral prescription ... which is reduced promptly to writing, or ... refilling ... if refilling is ... authorized". This is upheld in the process towards regulation of Internet pharmacies as visible through testimonial originating from the FDA (e.g. Hubbard 2004, http://www.fda.gov/NewsEvents/Testimony/ucm114792.htm]): no drug dispensing without prescription, be it written or through a auditable process of ex post charting of an orally conveyed order. Since it may be important in situations where physician and pharmacy identities cannot be checked easily organizations such as the American Board of Medical Specialties (ABMS) holds respective lists about board certified physicians, e.g. http://www.certificationmatters.org/. To find about license search can be done by state such as at http://www.mbc.ca.gov/lookup.html for California. On the other hand pharmacies certified for safe drug dispensing initiated through the Internet can be found at the US (NABP) at http://www.nabp.net/boards-of-pharmacy under programs, VIPPS. Thirty-two US based pharmacies are listed here. NABP also links to the respective organizations in Canada, Australia, and New Zealand.

17.4.1.4 Level 3

A patient lay member of a general or medical forum, social network etc. is allowed to post everything within his country's free speech range. He risks exposure of information meant private but he does not risk prosecution or interrogation concerning his conduct.

In Sect. 4.3 we touch upon recommended health professional behavior with their patients in social networks, mostly addressing privacy and trust and advocating reluctant and cautious use because of too many uncontrolled risks of exposure. Regarding the fast growth of social network membership and use it nevertheless happens and has been investigated by Munson and coworkers [11] and a group including the authors of Chap. 6 [8]. Munson and coworkers mostly apply a computer supported cooperative work perspective and assess flow of information and the extent to which communicational goals are achieved. In one paragraph they touch upon HIPAA and other reasons that let provider-client communication in social networks appear as a "legal grey area" [11, p. 5]. Huh and coworkers categorize roles and contents that holders of different roles convey using subspaces of WebMD as an example. Their results includes that "90 % of all health professional moderator responses contained clinical expertise" [8, p. 631]. Certainly there is a temptation for a health professional such as a physician to not withhold advice that comes to his mind in response to a poster's problem. But the border not to be transgressed to practice of medicine is near. A physician who acts as a moderator must also pay good attention to not abuse the moderating role to choke patient wisdom that is unknown to or seems strange from the perspective of scientific medicine, cf. Sect. 6.3.3.

Legally this is a dark grey area, equally in the USA as in Germany. To shed some more light we must first clarify the distinction between the practice of medicine and the provision of information, cf. Sect. 17.5. We will, therefore, come back to the problem and summarize constellations in Table 17.1 in Sect. 17.6.2.3.

17.4.2 Structures and Resources in Germany

Historically, German lawmakers, (the Bundestag – Federal Parliament and Bundesrat – Federal Assembly) have delegated the majority of legislation for professional conduct of physicians to elected representatives of all physicians, the Ärztetag (German Medical Assembly). The Ärztetag continually updates by majority vote of the representatives the Musterberufsordnung,[6] a ~30 pages document that regulates many aspects of physicians' professional behavior. Compliance with the Musterberufsordnung is overseen by the licensing organizations (Ärztekammern, Medical Associations) which also have the authority of sanctions up to including lifetime withdrawal of the privilege to work as a physician. When physicians act on

---

[6]http://www.bundesaerztekammer.de/downloads/MBOen2012.pdf for an up to date English version; (Model) Professional Code (subsequently just "Professional Code") for Physicians in Germany. It is called (Model) because of the federal structure of Germany: the nationwide model is the blue print from which the federal states Medical Assemblies derive their regional Professional Codes. The state Professional Codes do not differ in essentials of physician conduct. All subsequent quotes including those referring to a report relate to the 2010 Ärztetag.

17.4 Present Regulations

the borderline between the roles of practicing their profession and being lay citizens general legislation such as the Grundgesetz (Constitution) may also apply.

For the software and devices part of Consumer Health Informatics services BfArM is involved, a federal office which supervises safety of medical products and has the authority to release or withhold. For reasons already outlined in Sect. 17.4.1 we do not address that further here.

Online pharmacies are registered at http://www.dimdi.de/static/en/amg/var/index.htm by Deutsches Institut für Medizinische Dokumentation und Information (DIMDI), a federal office in charge of various medical informatics and HTA resources. Pharmacies authorized for mail order services are listed here and clients can connect to one through DIMDI to gain additional trust that hyperlinks have not been corrupted (cf. Sect. 13.3) and take them to fraudulent providers. Details about delivery across European borders follow in Sect. 17.8. The DIMDI source (German only) also takes the reader directly to the German Arzneimittelgesetz (Pharmaceutical Substances Bill).

17.4.2.1 Level 0

Level 0, which from the client perspective is searching and trying to make sense and draw conclusion, from the perspective of the service provider is free speech. §5 of the German Constitution grants the right to everybody to freely express and publish his opinion in speaking, writing or imagery (Recht der freien Meinungsäußerung). §5 excludes censorship but allows some balancing of free speech against other personal rights or offenses such as libel, sedition etc. These exceptions are wider in Germany than those of the US First Amendment. But the US-German differences do not affect Consumer Health Informatics because in Germany as well as in the USA everybody can post medical opinions as unwarranted or even obviously false they may be. This holds without further restrictions for lay persons.

When physicians assume the role of Level 0 providers the (Model) Professional Code imposes some farther reaching rules of good professional conduct. As soon as they identify themselves or are identifiable in their capacity as Dr. med. (German MD) or with their specialty (surgeon, pediatrician, etc.) the preamble requests that their "conduct in public" is supportive of "maintaining and promoting confidence between physicians and patients". §2(3) requests to act in "compliance with the accepted state of medical knowledge" as an ingredient of "conscientious practice". The word "practice" seems to confine that obligation to the closed situation of a treatment contract. Judging, however, by the spirit of that part of the Berufsordnung it extends to the open situation of addressing a non circumscribed public such as writing in consumer periodicals or giving public speeches. As long as physicians comply with the above regulations they can legally be Level 0 providers of Consumer Health Informatics services. The Internet, by the way, is not mentioned in the Berufsordnung at all.

17.4.2.2 Level 1

§7(4) of the (Model) Professional Code prohibits "individual treatment, in particular medical counselling, exclusively via print and communications media. It must also be ensured that physicians treat patients directly in the case of telemedicine procedures." This is as unclear in the English translation as in the authoritative German original: Does it mean an in-person initiated relationship or a physical presence throughout all treatment steps? A report that was endorsed by the same Ärztetag that also endorsed the present Professional Code (http://www.bundesaerztekammer.de/page.asp?his=0.2.23.8260.8265.8432.8433&all=true) clarifies: Telemonitoring with devices such as heart rate monitors that the physician suggest after in-person contact and that the patient carries in his home and work environment is one major form. Another is tele consultation where a centrally localized specialist assists another physician who investigates the patient in a remote place and where data are transmitted through means of communication technology such as images, video etc. For the latter it requests local presence of physicians while specialist advice comes through the distance.

17.4.2.3 Level 2

Level 2 Consumer Health Informatics services are truly problematic. In §7(4) the Professional Code commands for the practice of medicine that "physicians may not perform individual medical treatment, particular medical counseling, exclusively via print and communications media." This is in accordance with §8 which for a valid consent of the patient to a treatment requests "personal communication". These two regulations mean a blunt definite prohibition of purely virtual services (cf. Sect. 5.2.5.4). Other negative obligations do not address Consumer Health Informatics services explicitly. But behaviors prohibited play a marginal role for classical settings of care, while they are common if not typical ingredients of commercialized Level 2 services. One group of sanctions relates to advertisement. Different paragraphs preclude advertisement that is "praising, misleading or comparative" (§27(4)), advertising that promises success, or which just tries to add credibility to a commercial by harnessing it through names of physicians or the medical profession as such.

Another group of prohibitions regulate concrete economic behavior. Competition through price is not allowed; rather do German wide regulated fees have to be charged. Third-party commercial interests must not interfere with the welfare of the patient. Physicians are not allowed to "supply goods and other items" unless they are genuine part of an ongoing treatment. They are "not permitted to recommend or refer patients to specific physicians, pharmacies," etc. They may also not "aid abuse of their prescriptions".

17.4 Present Regulations

Finally it should be mentioned that in some aspects that are important for Consumer Health Informatics the Professional Code is very liberal. According to §17(1) "ambulatory physician's activities outside hospitals" are permitted under rather unconstraining conditions. German statutes even admit physicians from other member states of the European Union to "temporarily and occasionally perform their medical activity on a *cross-border* basis in the territory covered by this Professional Code ... they must observe the provisions of the Professional Code" (§2(7), cf. Sect. 17.8)

Concerning the delivery of drugs the Arzneimittelgesetz (Medicinal Products Act, English version at http://www.gesetze-im-internet.de/englisch_amg/index.html) in its § 48 unmistakably contends that prescription drugs may only be handed to patients who present the prescription. All kind of detail regulate what is a prescription drug, the delivery to research institutions, pest-control authorities, vessels on international travel etc. in a bill of approximately 100 pages. But none of the exceptions touches the core obligation that no prescription means no drug. Mail order delivery is as clearly regulated in § 43(1).1 and §11a of the Pharmacies Law (Apothekengesetz, German only at www.gesetze-im-internet.de/apog/) and as clearly commands processes to be set up that guarantee timely safe delivery if and only if a valid written prescription is presented securely. Pharmacies from the EU can register for delivery to patients in Germany based on prescriptions issued by physicians in Germany. For them the same non-negotiable obligation exists to securely collect the client's prescription. Therefore, any online convenience described in Sect. 5.2.4 limits itself to non-prescription drugs or is illegal without a written prescription. Means of telecommunication to validly transmit a prescription instead of surface-mailing have to be seen in the light of the risks outlined in Sect. 13.3.

Coming back to physicians, all the above is present applicable law. It implies that physicians licensed in Germany who offer Consumer Health Informatics services as personal treatment (Level 2) and not just as publishers of information (Level 0), violate their professional code. In Sect. 17.5 we analyze how to distinguish Level 0 and Level 2.

17.4.2.4 Level 3

Level 3 regulations in Germany precisely correspond to those in the USA. The governing bodies of law carry different names but agree in spirit. For lay persons the German right to free speech (Recht auf freie Meinungsäußerung) does not set any limits that would affect Consumer Health Informatics. Health professionals, besides being aware of potential breeches of privacy and trust, are requested to behave as to maintain the confidence into medicine and the medical profession which includes to write in accordance with the accepted state of medical knowledge. While this is obvious in principle the lines are much harder to draw whether a physician's contribution is legal provision of information of illegal practice of medicine.

> **Take Home**
>
> Professional associations maintain a conservative attitude towards Consumer Health Informatics.
>
> - For publishing or moderating in the Internet or mobile networks health professionals must apply equal diligence as when publishing in any other medium. "Friending" and conveying personalized advice is strongly discouraged.
> - Extending and enhancing a treatment through means of telecommunication is encouraged as long as high safety and quality standards for procedures applied to the distant patient are fulfilled.
> - Many such "telemedicine" standards do not transfer to Consumer Health Informatics. Other ways of providing sufficient safety for the client have to be found.
> - Medical treatments solely through means of telecommunication are illegal.

17.5 Practice of Medicine, Provision of Information, or Business?

In Sects. 17.4.1 and 17.4.2 we have seen clear designations of legal and illegal physician conduct which draw on the distinction between providing information available for Level 0 type search and entering an accountable Level 1 or 2 type provider-patient relation. Therefore, criteria to distinguish whether a Consumer Health Informatics service is Level 0, 1 or 2 are of paramount importance to tell apart whether it is legal or illegal. The latest scholarly analysis[7] of this distinction dates back to 2008. Derse and Miller [5] discuss the recent developments in professional practice, incorporation into health plans and funding, and recommendations of authoritative institutions such as the Institute of Medicine. They provide a definition of the Practice of Medicine Online and criteria how to distinguish from less binding patterns of providing and exchanging information.

> **Take Home**
>
> The legal assessment of a Consumer Health Informatics offering depends strongly upon whether it practices medicine, conveys information, or sells a non-medical service.

---

[7]An equally inspiring somewhat earlier outline is [10]. Lewis' expression Telemedicine corresponds to our Level 1, her Cybermedicine relates to our Level 0 or Level 2.

17.5.1 Criteria for Practice of Medicine

Referring to traditional medical practice Derse and Miller see a patient-physician relationship established when "there is implied or express consent by the patient and the physician to the relationship, the provision of medical advice, and foreseeable reliance by the patient on advice extended". These three criteria do not require a particular setting. The legal practice of liability suits has, however, used "payment for services ... (as) decisive evidence of the relationship" (both citations [5, p. 455]).

Nevertheless, new patterns of flow of information in new media make the line between practice of medicine and other forms of communication harder to draw. Derse and Miller maintain the points made in Sects. 17.4.1.1 and 17.4.2.1 that publication of medical information alone does not establish a provider-patient relationship but rather falls into legal categories of free speech. Therefore, the following three criteria dig deeper into making the distinction. They are

(1) direct or personal communication between patient and physician,
(2) the provision of professional judgment tailored to the patient's particular medical circumstances, and
(3) closure to the encounter or foreseeable reliance by the patient [5, p. 455].

(1) is further differentiated as: "Information posted ... even if highly specific and targeted to patients with a particular medical condition, is unlikely to generate a doctor-patient relationship in the absence of one-on-one or other personal communication that creates a duty to the particular patient." Implicating patient duties is a major distinction because clients or customers who buy services normally do not have duties. For (2) "the extent to which physicians render the professional judgment tailored to the patient's medical history, social circumstances, personal concerns etc.," are important criteria to establish a pattern of medical practice. For (3) the specificity and degree of detail of the advice and whether it is sufficient for the patient to follow up without requiring further medical advice is taken as a criterion for practice of medicine.

Derse and Miller also address the contrast between an interface of a service that clearly suggests that it practices medicine and that charges a fee versus its sometimes well hidden disclaimers where it denies to provide medical advice or to establish a patient-physician relationship. "These disclaimers will not withstand judicial scrutiny if they fly in the face of the facts of the online encounter between patient and physician." (all citations in this section from [5, pp. 455–7]).

Pharmaceuticals often are the core part of a suggested treatment. Hence the processes of prescription and of delivery of pharmaceuticals require attention. While prescription is explicitly covered in the legal analysis of practicing medicine above delivery is an economically large gray zone where a legal analysis is still due, but should follow along the lines of practicing medicine for two reasons: like medicine pharmacy is a health profession with high ethical standards and like medical treatments application of pharmaceuticals bears high risks alongside with high potential benefits.

Derse and Miller [5] also provides a well considered outline of other crucial aspects of medical advice or practice without in-person encounter such as assessment of quality and effectiveness, conflict of interest etc. Some of these aspects are covered elsewhere in this volume drawing on other and partially newer (e.g. in Sect. 15.4 ff) resources. Therefore, we will mainly use the criteria outlined above to assess the nature and hence legal state of Consumer Health Informatics services introduced in Chap. 5.

> **Take Home**
>
> Practice of medicine is characterized through
>
> - Personal communication
> - Advice tailored to the patient's medical circumstances
> - Closed deal with foreseeable patient compliance
>
> Services of that character cannot escape from being judged as practice of medicine through disclaimers.

17.5.2 Criteria for Business

There is, however, a large segment of Consumer Health Informatics that does not fall under criteria and hence regulations of medicine: the segment of prevention and well-being. Sports studios, super market chains, and many others offer services or goods that presumably lead to better health. Medical professions legitimately are among such service providers. For these, rules of professional conduct still apply concerning state-of-the-art information and promoting confidence in their professions (cf. Sects. 17.4.2.1 and 17.4.1.1). However, when their is no disease there is no pressing need for personalized advice and closure of a transaction to the end of foreseeable reliance. Rather does the client take initiative to achieve added value for himself and chooses the means. This is a typical open market situation where good business conduct in a general sense reigns. This holds, e.g. for the myriads of different diets recommended for weight reduction or behavioral approaches to control stress.

The legal discourse for this kind of Consumer Health Informatics services is reigned by the caveat emptor principle. It is meant for contracts where all partners have the capacity to investigate the consequences of a planned contract and hence can be assumed to make an informed decision and cannot legitimately request a return. The only requirements on the part of the vendor are that "goods must be fit for the particular purpose and of merchantable quality" (Wikipedia: `caveat emptor`).

In borderline domains it depends on the circumstances whether a Consumer Health Informatics service would be regarded as medical or business. These include screening programs and how clients at excess risk for a condition can choose or should be urged to screen regularly (cf. Sect. 12.2.2.3). They include hazardous behaviors such as severe overeating or smoking. Is a person with BMI 35 being treated or does he try to manage himself, and likewise for a smoker of 40 cigarettes per day? There is no firm legal ground as yet. A heuristic that suggests itself is whether there is an ICD-10 code for the condition. We see some examples where this heuristics would help to assign services to either medicine or business (cf. Sects. 5.3.4.1 vs. 17.6.2.3 and 9.2 vs. 16.12).

> **Take Home**
> Services for well-being or prevention can follow rules of business conduct as long as no immanent risk has to be attended.
> A heuristics for distinguishing practice of medicine from business is that a named disease, represented e.g. through an ICD-Code, is treated.

17.6 Present Legislation Meets Present Practice

17.6.1 US: German Commonalities and Differences

Section 17.4 has shown that the free market oriented US and the social welfare oriented German health care systems agree to the most part in the legislation and codes of conduct for physicians when utilizing the Internet or other forms of operating other than face-to-face with the patient.

17.6.1.1 Commonalities

The two systems agree that

- Physicians have to write diligently and responsibly and comply with other rules of professional conduct when they author content on the web
- The author-reader relationship is not a physician-patient relationship to which various farther ranging requirements of professional conduct apply
- Treatment through the distance alone, without in-person encounter, is "illegal", "unprofessional", "not allowed"; the wording varies but the meaning is crystal-clear
- Specialist advice conveyed through the distance, often called telemedicine, requires local presence of a health professional
- Even in in-person initiated treatments that continue into services provided through the distance physicians still have far ranging responsibilities. They are for instance responsible for the quality of monitoring devices attached to or implanted into the patient's body
- Dispensing a prescription drug necessitates a prescription

The two systems also agree that laypersons as writers of medical content are cleared by the right to free speech. Minimally differing restrictions which do not play a role for Consumer Health Informatics content relate to criminal content.

17.6.1.2 Differences

The two systems differ in the role they assign to decision support programs that generate personalized information: The AMA Ethics Opinion Code 5-027 briefly mentions them requesting high general and specialty-specific standards and disclosures of limitations to prospective clients. German regulations do not mention automated decision support programs.

AMA also stands out in encouraging support of individual healthy lifestyles, a continuum of supportive health care, patient selection of delivery mechanism, access for those who otherwise would not have access; without undue restrictions (AMA H-160.975). In all US legal sources online prescription plays a much wider role than in the German ones.

German regulations generally prohibit typical behaviors of business oriented delivery of services such as comparative advertisement, commercial use of credentials, sales oriented behaviors (competition through price, sales trusts) as they are often associated with online offerings.

German regulations allow, however, physicians to practice on a much larger geographic scale. A federal state based license qualifies for nation wide practice and even beyond national borders – inbound and outbound – as long as mutual authorities are informed and mutual regulations are respected.

17.6.2 Legal Assessment of Present Approaches

17.6.2.1 Level 0

Since Chap. 3 focuses on the hazards of searching rather than on behaviors of publishing we do not have a lot of material to take a fresh look at through the lens of law and ethics. There are, however, some noteworthy observations. They are related to communicational behavior and responsible contents.

17.6.2.1.1 Appropriate Communicational Behavior

All following patterns are inappropriate under any circumstance but would not be prosecuted when the authors are lay persons since they are protected through the constitutional right to free speech. We will argue, however, that some patterns violate rules of good professional conducts set for health professionals.

In Sect. 3.3.1.4 we report on findings in the past[8] that Wikipedia information on pharmaceuticals was not written by independent experts but could be traced back to pharmaceutical industry owned IP-addresses. Such behavior camouflages the interests behind a contents published which is certainly not a behavior to promote confidence in the medical profession.

In Sect. 3.3.1.2 we analyze the group dynamics of authors claiming authority for themselves and denying others' authority. The used example could not be traced back to authors who were or were not medical professionals. Medical professionals, however, would certainly put the confidence in their profession at stake through bullying behavior.

The third aspect is more intricate. We see in Sect. 3.4 which subtle communicational means of the service provider build trust in the seeker. These include color photographs of the authors and other graphical elements, ease of use etc. and, somewhat behind, that the resource has references to scientific articles. What can be seen often, too, are long lists of abbreviations alluding to academic or professional qualification that the reader has hard times to verify. None of these alone is bad. However, responsible professional providers have to find a good balance between a trust-building shell, intelligible presentation, and a sound kernel.

17.6.2.1.2 Responsible Contents

In the lights of Chap. 3 where decreasing comprehension of medical contents meets increased inclination to change behavior anyway (Sect. 3.2.2) and where an error rate of 59 % of self-diagnosis based on Internet searches (Sect. 3.3.1.5) is observed, both investigations in large samples, the likelihood to cause bad outcomes, even with good contents, is anything but small. This does not mean that authors of respective contents violate laws. Well researched and well presented knowledge cannot give reason for prosecution. However, the above facts increase the responsibility of medical professionals on the Internet – and in any means of mass communication for that matter – to also have AMA's health policy H-478.996 to "address...literacy and cultural barriers" in mind and to avoid any wording that may be understood as implicating harmful client behaviors.

Take Home

Limited comprehension on the part of the client adds to the challenges of diligent writing in openly accessible media.

- Professionals should avoid any prepossessing rhetoric or display of credentials.
- Rather should they try to anticipate potential misunderstandings and hazardous behaviors in response to information delivered.

---

[8]To the author's knowledge no follow-up investigation has been published whether the conduct at Wikipedia has changed.

17.6.2.2 Level 1

In Chap. 4 on Level 1 Consumer Health Informatics services we distinguish two major streams: the condition independent enhancement of regular face-to-face provider-client relationships through incorporation of electronic media and condition specific dedicated services, such as for chronic pain, asthma, etc.

17.6.2.2.1 E-Mail and Social Networks

Incorporation of e-mail and social networks is explicitly addressed both in this chapter and in Chaps. 4 and 13. The US AMA health policies (cf. Sect. 17.4.1.2) mention and encourage e-mail and request rules of conduct, e.g. turnaround times, in the spirit of a reliable accountable professional. From Chap. 13 we know the requirements and methods to protect privacy, establish authenticity etc. Section 4.3.1 lists other process of care aspects that should be paid attention too. Generally, however, e-mail as enhancement of client-provider relations becomes accepted legally.

All structural and quality requirements apply to the German situation as well. The "Professional Code" for Physicians in Germany does not mention e-mail and Internet. Therefore, there is no safe legal ground but reason to believe that with all technical precautions thoroughly made it is accepted as an enhancement of provider-patient-communication.

Social media are regarded equally reluctantly here as in Chap. 4. Arguing again with a spirit of good professional conduct and the image of the responsible physician in mind risks are listed that should be avoided but cannot safely be avoided, mainly that data become known to persons unintentionally. Therefore, even if there is a trusted in-person initiated patient-provider relationship and the patient wants to communicate about his treatment in a social network the physician should encourage other means instead, as clearly pleaded in a medical ethics journal article [7]. If the patient insists and the provider concedes it is not clear whether the provider can be charged legally.

17.6.2.2.2 Condition Specific Services

In the expedited discharge after carotid endarterectomy (Sect. 4.4.1) project frequent photo and video communication was in place through equipment safeguarded by the providers. Other structurally supportive factors (fast landline network, distance from hospital below a threshold) had been controlled ahead of time. Therefore, although being ambitious in its time frame, the project appears as a consequent enhancement of an in-person treatment and would by US and German standards pass legally. Of course, Italian standards would apply here. This demonstrates one of the challenges of Consumer Health Informatics that are only marginally covered: the potentially international reach of services and the national regulations of health care systems.

17.6 Present Legislation Meets Present Practice   359

In the two Consumer Health Informatics services for management of chronic conditions, pain and hypertension, we find very different approaches to intertwine the virtual and the in person parts.

The *Pain Course* intervention enrolls with minimal in-person clearance upfront: Patients come with a diagnosis of stable chronic pain and their treating general practitioners or specialists receive a surface mail letter about their patients' participation. The intervention consists of study material online only and weekly human phone call of planned 15 min length, shorter or longer upon need. Therefore, intermittent in-person attendance – by telephone, but this has not been legally challenged for conditions where essential aspects can be communicated through spoken language and do not need a visual impression – is guaranteed and the service can legally be regarded as to "enhance...interpersonal contacts" (cf. Sect. 17.4.1.2 (USA)). The German legislation does not cover the situation. Note, however, that *Pain Course* was developed in Australia.

The antihypertensive intervention starts in full accordance with the requirement to root a service in an established in-person patient-provider-relationship. During the Consumer Health Informatics intervention with automated uploading and communication of blood pressure readings in-person transactions are mandated in a detailed scheme for therapy changes. The anchor point of all this is the fitness for use of the blood pressure readings and communication equipment. Safety of devices is a large topic of or adjacent to Consumer Health Informatics, which is not covered in this volume. Therefore, a comprehensive legal judgment about services such as this one cannot be provided.

17.6.2.3 Level 2

The majority of the approaches in Sect. 5.2.1 comply with both US and German regulations because they do not satisfy the prerequisites for practicing medicine in the sense of Sect. 17.5. This includes the health awareness services because they do not solicit client compliance; their advice, though medical in content and tailored as it may be, remains without obligation on the part of client.

The somatic diseases dealt with in Sect. 5.2.3 require a more differentiated analysis. For the urinary continence advice Sect. 5.2.3.1 the same arguments hold as above: it remains unbinding and therefore is not practice of medicine. The cancer survivors service Sect. 5.2.3.3 is not binding either. Another feature also exempts it from being practicing of medicine: the core advice is not medical but organizational and behavioral; it relates to assembling one's patient medical record, attending individual risks and taking preventive measures.

The asthma example Sect. 5.2.3.2 is more problematic. The way it is presented it is Level 1. It is initiated face-to-face. Automatically generated aerosol dosage advice based on patient's symptoms and flow-meter readings is double checked by a physician before transmission to the patient. The service, therefore, complies with telemedicine type regulations. Its core ingredients, however, are a flow-meter device and a rule-based system. For flow measurements a client owned flow-meter could as well be used, or a public respiration checkpoint like public blood pressure checkpoints exist. The client could spontaneously enroll for the rule-based system advice. So the service can be envisioned as a Level 2 one. The client enrollment is an implied consent to the treatment relationship, the advice is medical and tailored and repeated visits to the site reporting the development of symptoms can be interpreted as a signal of compliance. The question now is – as it will also turn out in various of the following services – whether the advice appears as conveyed by a machine or by a human professional. In the latter case that professional violates rules of good conduct because he practices medicine without having seen the patient in person. When the advice appears as conveyed by a machine present regulations don't apply. For Germany we don't find any authoritative source of judgment. For the United States the Ethics Code Opinion 5.027 provides some guidance: "...Decision-support programs...(s)hould be consistent with...standards...include disclosures such as limitations inherent in the technology". This does not really save the case but rather opens a loophole. Providers of such systems are cleared when they do their work properly; they cannot be made accountable personally for inappropriate advice. Therefore, the risk resides with the client. He has to be made aware of the hazards of the technology, which, paradoxically, may raise doubts in the clients and reduce their compliance hence jeopardizing the potential of a service that was proved effective if clients comply.

Most mental health Consumer Health Informatics services as outlined in Sect. 5.2.2 can logistically be established as Level 2. For the anxiety service Sect. 5.2.2.1 we can easily have the assessment of clients' assignments in the CBT treatment program and an automatic staging before and after the therapy fully automated. The presently also offered therapist response to e-mails, which was indeed used once per week on an average of all subjects in that treatment arm, makes a difference under several aspects. If it is done by therapists it breaks the rules because it has all ingredients of practicing medicine without in-person contact. It could be done through automatic analysis of client reports and automatically generated or canned text responses, as has been shown by [4]. In their setting outgoing messages went through the hands of a research assistant. Logistically it could be done fully automated and might fall into the so far not regulated category of automated decision-support programs as long as it can make unmistakably clear to the client that the treatment is conveyed automatically although it appears like conveyed by a human being. We have a similar dilemma as in the asthma situation above where the attempt to create trust through human-like behavior of algorithm and the necessity to clearly reveal the fully automatic nature of the service compete. The controversy is hard to resolve because emotional trust is dealt with in the discourse of psychology while compliance with rules of conduct is dealt with in the discourse of law.

This controversy hits even harder in the addiction service in Sect. 5.2.2.2. The most effective variant of the smoking cessation program which was the most personalized one included a photograph of the therapists team and their signatures. Detailed statistical analysis showed that this was not the strongest factor of personalization but still it was present and obviously a photograph and a signature are among the strongest cultural tokens to indicate a personally conveyed service. This shows that a proof of effectiveness that builds on show casing the personal though not in-person nature brings the provider into trouble when the trial is over. Whenever a service addresses the cure of a diagnosed disease it cannot be launched legally unless an in-person entry point is established which takes the service back into Level 1 and sacrifices some of the cost-effectiveness that Level 2 can have. In the case of smoking this is borderline: ICD-10 WHO-2013 lists "toxic effects ... of tobacco and nicotine" as code T65.2 and F17.x for different forms and severities x of behavioral disorders (psychiatric diagnoses) caused through tobacco.[9] An argument may pass that as long as a toxic effect or a genuine behavioral disorder has not become diagnosed a smoking cessation is prevention and by that token cleared legally as being business rather than medicine (cf. Sect. 17.5).

In Sect. 5.2.2.3 we have already analyzed the treatment of mild depression in elderly as done cost-effectively in [16]. Level 2 appears feasible when further research demonstrates the validity of online versions of depression staging questionnaires. In that case questionnaires could replace the voice-to-voice prescreening before granting access to the service. Apart from this entry check the service avoids the impression of advice being tailored to the client situation and conveyed through a human therapist. It may therefore pass as a true Level 2 service offering that is not practice of medicine.

"Online pharmacy" as a type of Consumer Health Informatics service is too broad and to differentiated for unified judgment. If within one country pharmacies ship substances for which they have been presented a valid prescription by a physician licensed in this country they basically operate legally in both the USA and Germany. Both countries make lists of authorized pharmacies available at http://www.nabp.net/programs/accreditation/vipps respectively https://www.dimdi.de/static/en/amg/var/apotheken/index.htm. Additional challenges when physician, pharmacy, and client reside in different countries are briefly addressed in Sect. 17.8. Online resources become available where licensed physician identities can be looked up which is especially important for transactions across borders.

If pharmacies ship prescription drugs without having received the prescription they violate laws (Sects. 17.4.1.3 and 17.4.2.3). Some nevertheless do. We analyze the legal character of the workarounds for within nation transactions here. International transactions are analyzed in Sect. 17.8. Most online pharmacies work with sophisticated disclaimers. For practicing of medicine and the patient-physician relationship we have seen in Sect. 17.5 that such disclaimers may not withstand judicial scrutiny. It may be hard, though, to transfer this argument to purchasing of pharmaceuticals. Online pharmacies that emphasize that the client declares that he has a prescription or offer to inform the client's physician upon client's request emphasize the underlying medical rather than shopping experience character of the transaction. This may invalidate their disclaimers. The more online pharmacies present themselves through a shopping cart metaphor the more may

---

[9]ICD-9 has code 305.1 for nicotine abuse.

the legal argument sustain that the buyer should know what he wants (the caveat emptor legal maxime) and henceforth their disclaimers may withstand lawsuits. The most sophisticated approach of juggling with responsibilities comes through www.euroclinix.net. They offer that "registered physicians check your medical data and then prescribe". Thereby, they enact a scenario of safe medical conduct for the client while at the same time violating the rules of good professional medical conduct because the doctors who prescribe do so without an in-person encounter with a client. Doctors may still be clear because their service has not been invoked by a patient but by a dealer of pharmaceuticals. Let alone when the client resides abroad, see Sect. 17.8.

The four types of online counseling in Sect. 5.2.5 differ in their legal nature. The *information broker* is obviously no practice of medicine because information is not personalized and no behavioral consequences on the part of the client are implied. Physician authors who contribute to information broker services have the obligations of diligence as in other public writing (cf. Sect. 17.6.1.1), while when lay clients contribute by their experience the free speech regulatory frame applies. Physician "undercover" writing, i.e. without revealing their professional credentials, would probably not be accepted as good professional conduct.

The directory rather than provision of care nature of *logistics support services* (cf. Sect. 5.2.5.2) with their additional options to select by region, sex, health plan that a physician contracts with leads to more considerate utilization of classical health care resources but it is not a health care resource in its own right. Therefore, in the first place the request for good business conduct in general as would be expected by other service directory sites applies here as well. Physician ratings that clients can deliver need to be monitored to distinguish bad ratings because the doctor did not find an existing cure from bad ratings because there was no cure or there was parking place. Patient ratings are presently being investigated in courts of justice in Germany because physicians have sued against bad ratings.

For the German situation the premium membership option with preferred presentation of respective physicians' profiles may be in conflict with the prohibition to advertise (cf. Sect. 17.4.2.3).

Pre-screening services (cf. Sect. 5.2.5.3) certainly cross the border towards practicing of medicine (cf. Sect. 17.5). Their process of first presenting a questionnaire to be filled by the client, then using this information in a telephone conversation, then proceeding to prescription, under the premise that the client has paid – and even more so when the provider builds a dedicated medical record – satisfies all necessary ingredients for a service to represent practice of medicine. Then obviously it violates regulations if an in-person element is lacking. The crucial point, therefore, is whether a telephone conversation is in-person enough to render such a service legal or illegal.

The *virtual services* (cf. Sect. 5.2.5.4) fully abstain from synchronous provider-client communication. Therefore, if they are practicing medicine, they are doing it illegally. For DrEd's service the conditions for practicing medicine seem to be given. Provider and client express their consent through the payment made. The advice is medical and tailored since based on disease-related information that the client delivers and in the case of an extended relationship the patient medical record that the provider builds and maintains. Advice turns into transactions in forms of prescriptions. The provider furthermore enacts a trust building online encounter by referring to physician credentials from the UK health care system and by mentioning potential coverage through the health insurance system. On top of that the provider declares himself liable. This suggests but does not imply that the client complies. In the case of accepting and processing a prescription it is highly likely that he does.

The client has to look very closely to find loopholes. Health care coverage does presently not apply, as disclaimers reveal. Liability regulations refer to the delivering of physical goods rather than the provision of advice, let alone personalized medical advice. I.e. DrEd's terms and conditions hide the absence of any responsibility that DrEd takes so perfectly that the normal health advice seeking individual will not be able to penetrate. It certainly is a case that legal scrutiny might find fault with.

Healthcaremagic's legal assessment shares some properties with DrEd's. It collects disease-related information from clients where the free text description of symptoms suggests that the patient's concern is taken full personal account of. The client chooses whether he wants GP or specialist advice and pays a price that depends on this decision. Healthcaremagic's GP's then delivers "medically correct health information", specialist delivers "specialist opinion". Healthcaremagic does not name its information as treatment related although the client may get this impression through the way he delivers information and makes choices. Healthcaremagic does not deliver prescriptions. Therefore, closure of the encounter or the foreseeable reliance are less obvious here and the practicing medicine is not so obvious. The disclaimer and hint to the client that Healthcaremagic "is not responsible for the results of *your decisions*" may pass as in agreement with what the client perceives.

Finally, justanswer® has a whole bunch of types of advice that you can purchase there: health, computers, law etc. Justanswer® passes the client through i.e. might appear like a logistics support service. However, a payment is due, which is an indicator of actually providing a service oneself. A closer look reveals that it is not justanswer® but a subcontracting person who a client contracts with. This person to person implementation of the advice giving within justanwser® makes the encounter appear personalized while the final rating that the client provides can be interpreted as an indicator that the client will rely on the advice. On the other hand, while contracting the client accepts that he is not expecting personal and advice but should seek the advice from professionals. These terms and conditions are the same for health, computer, law or other advice. Medicine is marginalized as just one other field where advice can be purchased. Whether this marginalization is sufficiently obvious for lay clients to realize the nonbinding character of what they receive is the critical point in the judgment of justanswer®'s legal character.

> **Take Home**
> - Level 1 Consumer Health Informatics services can be grounded in various ways with classical in-person services and client side safety can be addressed specifically.
> - Pure Level 2 services presently are illegal. To make approved ones legal calls for action.
> - Some providers seek and find loopholes to blur the true character or their services and keep selling advice and pharmaceuticals without in-person contact.

17.6.2.4 Level 3

In Chap. 6 we analyze the value and methods to utilize patient delivered contributions to (mostly) medically oriented social networks. The chapter stands under the implicit assumption that only lay persons contribute and do not intentionally use the medium for any criminal purposes. In that case nearly everything goes, as will become evident. However, physicians (and likewise other health profession) may also act as authors of posts. For them, their professional codes of conduct apply to the open Level 3 setting equally as for levels 0 through 2. Analysis for Level 3 , therefore, essentially is replication of the arguments in Sect. 17.4, and is summarized in Table 17.1. Additionally privacy and confidentiality need increased attention in the open social network setting, as outlined in Sect. 4.3.2.

Table 17.1 Legal status of level 3 posting in social media

Qualification	Disclosure of professional role	Service type	Relation to client	Legal state	Comment, keyword
Lay person	(N/a)			Legal	Free speech
Physician[a]	No			Illegal	Confidence[b]
	Yes	Information		Legal	Conduct[c]
		Well-being			
		Prevention		Varies	cf. Sect. 17.5.2
		Practice of medicine	In-person initiated	Legal	Level 1[d]
			Virtual only	Illegal	Explicitly excluded in professional codes

[a]Likely transfers to other core health professions such as nurse, physiotherapist; needs separate research, though
[b]The requested promotion of confidence in the medical professions is in conflict with an opaque role
[c]Professional conduct required, mainly state of medical knowledge. Also needs high attention to preserving privacy and confidentiality
[d]Responsible for safe operation

> **Take Home**
> The legal character of Level 3 posting to social media varies in many respects and is summarized in Table 17.1.

17.7 Side Entries

We have so far provided a legal framework and classifications of Consumer Health Informatics services into classes and by doing so have come to conclusion whether services are or are not legal (Sect. 17.6). We have also seen attempts to purposefully blur or unconsciously violate the distinction between legal provision of information and illegal online only practice of medicine (cf. Sects. 5.2.5.4 vs. 5.2.2.2). We now address two ways to convey personalized advice in Level 2 settings that are legal according to the framework.

17.7.1 Well-Being

It has already been addressed in Sect. 17.5.2 that well-being services underlie other legal principles (the caveat emptor maxim) and can be offered freely through provider organizations as long as general rules of good business conduct are respected. Health professionals still have to comply with their professions' codes of conduct. Well-being as field of application may appear as playground and not serious at first and in a way it is. However, an estimated 20% of the services in this volume fall under that category. They are in the fields of the metabolic syndrome (Chap. 9), smoking cessation, uncontrolled drinking etc. In many cases the border to practice of medicine is near. It is crossed when diabetes mellitus 2 has been diagnosed and its management is part of a metabolic syndrome Consumer Health Informatics service. It is crossed when it is not the behavior of uncontrolled drinking but one of the ICD-10 F10 diagnoses has been established.

The reason to propagate well-being Consumer Health Informatics services is that they can function as door openers. When it becomes publicly known that they safely achieve desired targets the readiness to accept them for medical conditions rises. Wrapped in the ethics vs. law discourse of this chapter this is an appeal to empirical ethics (cf. Sect. 17.11): That which becomes accepted in a society as moral behavior is not deduced from general principles but from observations and experiences made.

17.7.2 C-Referral

While above we have a side entry of a whole discipline from a less regulated into a highly regulated field, we now discuss individual patients' side entries to legally receiving medical Level 2 Consumer Health Informatics services. van Voorhees et al. [18] in Sect. 5.2.2.4 test just that successfully in an RCT. Primary care physicians usher patients whom they treat face-to-face and where they get an impression and preliminary confirmation through PHQ-9, into a virtual only moderated support group.

If taken from IRB supervised research into routine use this would formally satisfy the AMA health policy H-478.997 (cf. Sect. 17.4.1.3) resp. §7(4) German Professional Code request that technology may never replace interpersonal contact. Two questions remain. One is whether this *would* withstand legal scrutiny; it might be unmasked as deliberate confusion of the intention of the professional codes. The other is whether it *should* withstand. In the light of Chap. 8 where we argue that a responsible family physician would notice all kinds covert risks that the best Consumer Health Informatics services have hard times to detect, c-referral adds a critical amount of additional safety and control of risks before Consumer Health Informatics takes over. Therefore, ethical arguments in Sect. 17.11 to allow more Consumer Health Informatics services where risks are well curbed, find additional support in c-referral situations.

Take Home

Two opportunistic approaches to improve public and professional perception of Level 2 Consumer Health Informatics services are

- Starting with well-being services and preparing for later upgrading towards medical treatments.
- Referral to a Consumer Health Informatics service for a co-morbidity while treating a main problem in-person.

17.8 Transactions Across Borders

The medical industry is still highly fragmented nationally and to some extent by state. This relates to licensing, professional codes etc. and can have as a consequence that within one town a physician can treat patients on one but not on the other side of a river. In strong contrast and language problems put aside for a moment, once approved a Consumer Health Informatics service can serve and scale up world wide. This causes numerous problems and friction some of which will be mentioned here but not solved.

In an article about various aspects of telemedicine Singh and Wachter [17] describe an example that provides insight for Consumer Health Informatics, too.

17.8 Transactions Across Borders

At NightHawk Radiology (Florida, according to legal notice) half the radiologist have overseas affiliations and the average radiologist holds 38 state licenses. For teleradiology with compliant health professional presence where the patient is this likely satisfies legal requirements. After all NightHawk Radiology has survived under the same name in the USA since 1999. For Level 2 Consumer Health Informatics services licensing physician in the states where the patients live would be a convincing sign of good will but would not satisfy the AMA H-478.997 claim of interpersonal contact. However, from a different perspective it is a huge waste of effort. From Singh and Wachter 2008 we learn that 35 employees at NightHawk Radiology do nothing but licensing and credentials.

Healthcaremagic's http://www.healthcaremagic.com approach is to list their physicians with Indian licenses and to declare in their terms and conditions, with explicit mention of the United Sates, that "(a)ccess ... may not be legal by certain persons or in certain states or countries (and that) you do so at your own risk and are responsible for compliance with the laws of your jurisdiction." – "(E)xclusive jurisdiction ... resides in the courts of India ... Bangalore ...". Since healthcaremagic offers Level 2 medical service, Derse's verdict outlined in Sect. 17.5.1 certainly applies. But in the case of a problem it will not help the client because he will fail to prosecute before an US American court.

In a bundle of cross-border medical consulting and initiating the delivery of prescription drugs we find a more sophisticated plot to suggest legal operation and at the same time to exploit the ignorance or to satisfy the needs of clients who want to circumvent their country's health care regulations and safeguards (cf. Sect. 5.2.5.4). The bundle consists of providing evidence that the involved physicians are licensed in the UK, not mentioning that this applies to in-person treatment in the UK alone, and to deliver through a German-approved mail-order pharmacy,[10] not mentioning that this kind of transaction is not mail order.

Together the different plots of acting across borders demonstrate a need that the whole field of Consumer Health Informatics brings up: international harmonized legislation and judicial assistance. Initiatives such as the Interstate Nurse Licensure Compact (cf. Sect. 17.4.1) or the German and neighboring European Union countries permission to practice across national borders (cf. Sect. 17.6.1.2) can be recommended for study.

Take Home
The locality principle of licensing for the medical professions adds to the legal challenges to smooth implementation of Consumer Health Informatics.

---

[10] https://www.dimdi.de/static/en/amg/var/apotheken/index.htm is the official German register of approved mail order pharmacies.

17.9 Health Informatics Professionals Ethics

Throughout until this point we have taken the perspective that Consumer Health Informatics services are medical or health related services and naturally the masterminds behind and officers responsible for such services are health care professionals. Obviously, however, hardly any described service can exist without informatics contributions. We therefore briefly take an ethics of health informatics perspective on Consumer Health Informatics.

In health informatics we have the favorable situation that a nearly 50 year old international organization, IMIA, at http://www.imia-medinfo.org, endorsed the IMIA Code of Ethics for HIPs (http://www.imia-medinfo.org/new2/node/39 in 2002 and since then propagated its translation and its adaption in national associations of health informatics and to adapt it to new developments in society and science. It covers both practice and research and is in that respect more versatile than the Declaration of Helsinki [20] http://www.wma.net/en/30publications/10policies/b3/index.html) which provides international ethics guidance mainly for research with human subjects and respective materials and data.

Although not world-wide endorsed the IMIA declaration is widely respected and without explicit counter-designs. Some criticize that it is too abstract for day to day problems but it certainly helps in sketching how HIPs can ethically contribute to Consumer Health Informatics. At its core it subscribes to the basic principles that Beauchamp and Childress advocated for mentioned in Sect. 17.3 and further outlined in Sect. 17.11. To the principles of respect for autonomy, beneficence, nonmaleficence and distributive justice IMIA adds the principles of impossibility and integrity. By upholding the first four principles health informatics lines itself up with the health professions and how they are devoted to patient outcomes. The classification of health and medical informatics as a health profession is in accordance with other leaders of the field, cf. [13].

The principle of impossibility denotes that rights and duties are only binding inasmuch as it is possible to fulfill them. So if e.g. a duty to conceal true identities exists and even with the best means and highest effort it can happen that some identity becomes known this would not be regarded as a breech of duties. This is certainly a relief for health informatics professionals in times of ever new privacy breeches becoming known (cf. Sect. 12.5).

The principle of integrity denotes that whoever has an obligation "has a duty to fill that obligation to the best of his or her ability". This implies that HIPs cannot just deliver as ordered by physicians or other domain experts but take own responsibilities in being best-possible trained for their tasks and to take initiative towards better solutions than come to the minds of their medical project partners or – more generally – to make sure that services are not only medically but also technically in accordance with accurate timely knowledge.

> **Take Home**
>
> Health Information Professionals' (HIP) ethic guidance is provided through the IMIA code of ethics.
>
> - In regarding HIPs as Health Professionals it transfers the four moral principle of health professionals to HIPs.
> - It adds the principles of integrity and impossibility thus demanding paramount professionality and at the same time to clear activities where minimal risks cannot be safely excluded.

17.10 Research Under Ethical Supervision

Except the reference to the Declaration of Helsinki in Sect. 17.9 all legal analysis in this chapter pertains to routine use of Consumer Health Informatics services. On the other hand numerous services in this volume are presented at the stage of a trial. Legally trial and routine are two clearly distinct situations. While routine use is governed by public legislation and professional rules of conduct, research and therefore trials are supervised by IRBs, Ethikkommissionen and the like subsequently called ethical safeguard institution. Such ethical safeguard institutions draw on publicly accepted frameworks for weighing the potential benefits of an investigation against its potential risks to human subjects, be it to their health or to exposure of identifiable data or properties of biomaterials. The Declaration of Helsinki is the most widely accepted framework.

Ethical safeguard institutions are affiliated with medical and other research institutions. Societies delegate decisions whether research is ethical or not to these institutions. Institutions receive applications from researchers and use the best expertise – internal or in case of need external – to weigh risks and benefits and then to approve, disapprove, or request changes to research proposals. Their decisions are binding. Under their supervision treatments or procedures can be tested that may be illegal otherwise, including Consumer Health Informatics services. Reporting the trial results is recommended, if not mandated. An increasing number of trials for Consumer Health Informatics services (about one third of those described in this volume) is meanwhile registered with ISRCTN at http://www.isrctn.com/ (e.g. [12]), with ClinicalTrials at http://clinicaltrials.gov (e.g. [1, 15, 18]) or other trial registries (e.g. [3]).

Beyond becoming publicly known through publication a research result does not have immediate consequences. Risks are mostly still present and denoted through figures for their probability or magnitude. Uncertainty also is an explicit element of the decision making about novel therapies. Uncertainty is lack of knowledge. Research tries to add knowledge, but rarely without a residual risk of erring. The 95 % confidence level is usually accepted as a normative judgment coming from outside science about the tolerable level of risking that an experimental result is false. Even for approved technologies new uncertainties may arise through interaction of the technology or through inappropriate use. Reduction of uncertainty is a central challenge for Consumer Health Informatics.

For superior new pharmaceuticals formal approval processes with authorities such as the US FDA at http://www.fda.gov/ or the German BfArM at http://www.bfarm.de/EN/Home/home_node.html in charge are well defined and eventually lead to release for routine use. For Consumer Health Informatics services such institutions and procedures do not exist yet. Therefore, even in the case of a highly successful trial a Level 2 Consumer Health Informatics service that implements a practice of medicine, cannot legally be offered in routine.

> **Take Home**
> Consumer Health Informatics has an emerging methodology to prove effectiveness and safety of its services but lacks a transition path into routine.

17.11 Ethical Considerations for Future Consumer Health Informatics Legislation

Starting out from AMA's encouraging health policy H-160.975 (cf. Sect. 17.4.1.3) we now seek for arguments in ethics to pave the way for future legal Consumer Health Informatics.

17.11.1 Moral Behavior

Laws and policies are a codification of what societies hold as being moral behaviors. Ethics systematically investigates principles of moral behaviors and dilemmas that may arise between conflicting claims as to how to behave under certain circumstances. Expectations as to what is moral behavior may be different for societies in general and for groups within the society that play special roles. The medical professions, i.e. physicians, nurses, and paramedical professions are prominent subgroups of a society where different, typically higher standards for moral behavior are present. We will subsequently use arguments from a standard textbook of biomedical ethics [2] to outline central principles and considerations how future legislation that assigns an appropriate role to Consumer Health Informatics can be developed. This endeavor is based on the assumption that morality is a genuine part of human nature and that at a very basic level there is social consensus that being part of society includes to normally behave according to their shared moral principles.

We will use arguments from normative and nonnormative ethics. Normative ethics focuses on the formulation of moral rules and theories. Nonnormative ethics includes empirical or descriptive ethics, which attempts for example to explore the variation between individuals concerning moral intuitions. Normative ethics derives what should be called moral behavior and may but need not necessarily draw on prevailing empirically observed ethics and how they are judged in societies. Once a behavior has intellectually been found as being moral it can be left to the discretion of the individual to comply or not to comply. We call such claims nonnormative. Or it can be turned into law; we then speak of normative claims. We will later (cf. Sect. 17.11.8) distinguish different approaches whether and how empirically moral behaviors can be turned into codified norms for professional conduct.

17.11.2 Behavioral Codes

Medical codes of conduct serve two purposes: to delineate what expectations society can legitimately have towards medical professionals and to protect medical professionals in situations where their behavior is truly meant to benefit the patient but has an inherent and unavoidable risk of harming the patient. Medical professionals may also require protection in the wider context of public health and health care delivery where to benefit many – such as in vaccination campaigns – harming few through side effects of the vaccine is an unavoidable harm which may be morally tolerable, depending on frequency and severity of the harm. In analogy we will later ask whether it is also morally tolerable for physicians as contributors to Consumer Health Informatics services to serve many while failing to serve few or even harm few where it goes unnoticed that for them a Consumer Health Informatics service is not appropriate.

17.11.3 Principles Underlying Medical Professional Codes

We first introduce four widely accepted principles of biomedical ethics and extend the meaning of three of them inasmuch as it is required to provide argument how these principles as such can be maintained but professional codes – and where required laws – can be further developed that bring to bear the potential of Consumer Health Informatics while fairly incorporating its risks.

The four principles are

- Respect for autonomy
- Nonmaleficence
- Beneficence
- Distributive justice

Some authors in the field of biomedical ethics comprise nonmaleficence and beneficence into a continuum of actions with smaller or higher risks of harming and larger or smaller potentials of benefiting the patient. However, for such dilemmas as assisted suicide it helps to treat nonmaleficence as an independent concept. Such dilemmas are typically not those of Consumer Health Informatics. That is why nonmaleficence will take the least space in the subsequent analysis.

The four principles are too vague and to general to inform day to day behavior or legislation. Ethics provides guidance in that direction by offering the structure of

substantive rules what ought to be done
authority rules who ought to do
procedural rules how can those who ought to do do systematically what they ought to do

Such specification takes us closer to being able to make provisions for prototypical situations. It is mainly helpful in legislation. Another method that is also often required is balancing between the conflicting conclusions that one arrives at when trying to comply with specified yet conflicting behaviors. Balancing is mainly helpful to inform judgment in individual cases.

Although the principles may be the same specifications may differ in different societies reflecting different priorities and socially accepted moral behaviors. European and US attitudes towards autonomy and justice may for instance differ with consequences on (social) insurance and financial affordability interfering with medical judgment. Therefore, nonnormative ethics can emerge first and after some while set the stage for normative ethics to take different routes in different countries. Such moral diversity and moral disagreement are neither good nor bad but a fact of life. It will be a challenge for Consumer Health Informatics which can operate and does operate across national borders which typically have different laws and professional codes to decide which legislation to apply and at whose discretion it is to decide.

Before we go into the details of the four principles it should be noted that one aspect will not be covered but be taken for granted: the moral character. It means that we assume that the agents to whose professional roles the codes apply are moral individuals endowed with basic attitudes to be beneficent, empathetic, respectful, but not heroes ready to sacrifice their own lives for a small chance to do something good. In short: we assume that our agents are not more and not less than "good physicians".

> **Take Home**
> The medical professions play a special role with special responsibilities which are reflected in specific codes of conduct and moral principles.
> Four moral principles are widely recognized as meaningful for medical professions:
>
> - Respect for autonomy
> - Nonmaleficence
> - Beneficence
> - Distributive justice

17.11.4 Respect for Autonomy

Respect for autonomy is not among the historically oldest principles. However, through Enlightenment and the development of democracies it is now widely accepted that a person should not be the means of another person's decisions but rather an agent interacting at par with other agents around him. Two basic and very general constituents of autonomy are

liberty independence from controlling influences
agency capacity for intentional action

[2, p. 102].[11] Exerting choices always depends on information and a space of options. Neither is ever complete and therefore autonomy cannot be an absolute but has to be a relative notion. Autonomy includes the right to delegate i.e. to identify and authorize individuals to choose in one's place. On the part of the patient autonomy is a right to choose and not a duty to choose.

On the part of the provider it is an obligation to offer options and to provide the conditions for the client to make meaningful decisions and to make decisions meaningfully if he so wishes. It requires various considerations how to fulfill that obligation.

Among those, the notions of capacity (as a property inherent to the client) and competence (an authority assigned to him and hopefully reflecting the capacity appropriately) are central. The capacity can be lacking due to insufficient communication, comprehension of information, and reasoning. The restriction in capacity is widest if the client cannot even communicate a wish. He may be able to communicate but there is empirical evidence from surveys in Consumer Health Informatics that this often happens without drawing on available information. Or the client can recall information but cannot make use of it in rational consideration instrumental to his personal aims (cf. Sect. 3.2.2). Agreement is required whether it

---

[11] Many arguments in this and the next sections follow the outline by Tom L. Beauchamp and James F. Childress [2] whose work is gratefully acknowledged.

be sufficient that the client just communicates or whether it must be assured that he also understands and provides reason [2, p. 114f].

It can be argued but has stirred controversy whether the capacity may be allowed to vary with the importance of the decision, such as the severity or likelihood of unwanted effects: Is a low level of capacity tolerable if the consequences of the decision are not severe? This argument would help providers of Consumer Health Informatics services a lot. Primarily medical Level 2 services with low intensity, impact, and risk, which presently are illegal, can become frontrunners in becoming legal.

It still remains an obligation of the provider to set up procedures that equip the client with the required information and make sure that the client understands. For the scenarios of clinical trials the "reasonable person standard" is now applied in the majority of the US states. Rather than requesting that the provider only performs standardized information procedures it imposes the obligation to actively make sure that the client comprehends the significance of what he is about to decide. Technically, reading level assessment of presented information and reading capacity tests of clients address that challenge in Consumer Health Informatics. Beauchamp and Childress put forward that the sophistication of gathering evidence about clients' capacity to comprehend a planned procedure is in proportion with the risk of the procedure [2, p. 120]. If this request becomes law or professional conduct it sets a standard for Consumer Health Informatics which is not easy to meet, regarding all the risks and loopholes in Chaps. 8 and 12.

The challenge to respect the autonomy of patients whose ability to communicate and comprehend is very low but who will not be regarded as incompetent in the full sense to make their own choices is especially high. It may require personal creativity of the physician to argue through analogies etc. to enable the client to develop his personal comprehension and based on that make his personally best choice. When transferred to Consumer Health Informatics this truly is a dilemma. On the one hand highly individualized personal contact and the respective consumption of resources is adverse to the aims and nature of Consumer Health Informatics (cf. Chap. 2). On the other hand, to comply with the principle of distributive justice outlined in Sect. 17.11.7, persons whose capacities are most limited deserve the highest effort to enable them to participate as clients of Consumer Health Informatics services, cf. [2, p. 132]. Regarding high percentages of illiterate not only in developing countries (cf. Sect. 8.4.3.2) it does not suffice for Consumer Health Informatics providers to do the core medical part well. The customer assessment part cannot be neglected.

Ironically, by implementing procedures of utmost sophistication (cf. Chaps. 8 and 12) to detect prospective clients' capabilities to comprehend and make choices and then to offer or not to offer the Consumer Health Informatics service perverts the intention into its opposite: We sacrifice client autonomy for the sake of client safety.

Most considerations so far have dealt with the personal intellectual capacity of the client to comprehend his options and to communicate his choice – and procedures and responsibilities when those capabilities are borderline, under doubt etc. One totally different threat to autonomy is the potential denial of choices for financial reasons. If the price of the option the client has chosen is prohibitive this voids all prior considerations. One could argue that the client was autonomous earlier in buying insurance that would or would not cover what is now being denied. However, for truly expensive treatments either all health plans will at some time refuse payment or the policies of those who keep paying will themselves be prohibitively expensive. For Consumer Health Informatics the problem may pose itself the other way round: if cost-effectiveness trials for Consumer Health Informatics services are absolutely convincing health plans may decide that they terminate paying the classical services and only cover Consumer Health Informatics services. This would coerce clients into Consumer Health Informatics whose autonomous choice would be classical personal service.

Yet another totally different set of challenges arises with Ambient Assisted Living (AAL). As a matter of fact it violates all kinds of confidentiality aspects of autonomy. It works under the consent that clients agree to privacy intrusions. Empirically, in balancing the asset of confidentiality with the asset of bodily safety, most clients of AAL services in the trials run so far easily agree to the various supervision functions installed in their home environments (cf. Sect. 11.3). A point not so well covered as yet is what happens to their consent when their capacity to consent gradually degrades but the instruments and procedures of intrusion remain in place. Can this be covered through advance directives or would surrogates have to be brought into the game?

> **Take Home**
> Respect for autonomy is a relatively new and apparently non-disputable moral principle. It may, however, get in conflict with other equally non-disputable principles such as beneficence showing in safety concerns that prohibit some patient choices. It may also face challenges of insufficient patient comprehension of the consequences of his choices and of availability and affordability.

17.11.5 Nonmaleficence

"At least, not to do harm" or "noli nocere" is one of the most well-known words of guidance or maxims for the medical profession whose being rooted in Hippocrates' writing is not so clear, though. Nonmaleficence in a somewhat broader sense includes not to do wrong as well but here and mostly for the medical field harm is the more pertinent concept. Nonmaleficence and beneficence can be regarded as populating a continuum of prohibitions and obligations, namely

- Avoiding actions that cause harm
- Performing actions that

- Prevent harm
- Remove harm
- Promote good

Most schools separate the first – nonmaleficence – from the next three – beneficence – for several systematic reasons including that nonmaleficence is a negative obligation while the three stages of beneficence are positive obligations.

Normally everybody owes nonmaleficence to everybody; it is an impartial moral duty. Failing to abide can be punished. Beneficence, in contrast, can be selectively granted depending on societal roles such as normal citizen or a holder of a professional role. Moral citizens would typically be beneficent towards their family, friends etc. It is not an expectation of everybody to be a hero who extends his beneficence to unrelated others, to situations of high own risk etc. Failing to be beneficent will, therefore, normally not be punished.

Physicians in their professional role face other expectations concerning their beneficence that will be further analyzed in Sect. 17.11.6.

There are few exceptions to the gross pattern of legal versus illegal behavior outlined above. As a physician or public health worker in a vaccination campaign a professional may cause the harm of adverse effects of the vaccines to very few while preventing or avoiding harm for a vast majority. When done in due diligence i.e. careful checks of contraindications for the vaccination according to standards of infectious disease professional associations the action is not punishable although it actually causes harm. Conversely, if a normal citizen can prevent or remove severe harm at minimal personal risk or effort – for instance when witnessing an accident and having the opportunity to easily remove helpless victims from the danger zone – it can be punishable to fail to do so, irrespective of whether the victims are family, friends, or totally unrelated strangers.

Of a moral person it is expected that he applies due care such that through his actions no harm is caused. This underlying safeguard of behaviors is called diligence, its absence is negligence. We distinguish advertent negligence or recklessness when risks are intentionally or knowingly imposed from inadvertent negligence where risks are actually imposed but have escaped the attention of the agent. The due amount of care to avoid harm or the risk of causing harm depends on both the amount of harm potentially incurred through one's behavior and on one's qualification, often associated with a professional role. Within the professions standards of due care may have to be complied with. Day to day examples of inadvertent negligence in medical care include disclosure of information where the act of disclosure may harm an emotionally fragile patient. This may actually be a point to consider in Consumer Health Informatics. Much deeper and more controversial debates of nonmaleficence are mostly outside the realm of Consumer Health Informatics; they relate to decisions of offering, withholding, or terminating care in futile situations, in assisting in or not preventing suicide for terminally ill patients or patients with futile prognosis such as with a diagnosed Chorea Huntington etc. This will not be further considered here. We will now move on to the more pertinent subtle distinctions within beneficence.

> **Take Home**
> Nonmaleficence is a legal principle that applies to normal citizens as well. In its interpretation for health professionals it commands for not knowingly taking actions that may harm the patient. This is mostly undisputed but may face controversy in situations such as vaccination campaigns where isolated adverse reactions have to be weighed against population level infection control.

17.11.6 Beneficence

For a productive use of the four moral principles it is important to clearly distinguish definite beneficence (an absolute notion; to provide benefits) from utility, a relative notion that balances benefits and drawbacks to produce the best overall result. Utilities versus other methods to evaluate client needs, claims, and outcomes in a continuum of options are compared in Sect. 17.11.8.

Beneficence in the major forms listed in Sect. 17.11.5 is undisputed as a moral principle to guide physicians or other health care providers. Still technical problems, dilemmas and intricacies exist. Some that also play a role for Consumer Health Informatics will now be brought up.[12]

First, benefit itself is not an absolute notion. Different actions may achieve different types or levels of benefit. When undisputed discrete good outcomes are achieved, e.g. a surgery that fully restitutes former physical capacities, we apply cost-effectiveness analysis. Often, however, benefits are multidimensional. For informed choices values have to be assigned to benefits. If societal decisions on approval or coverage of a treatment are due then we apply cost-benefit analysis.

17.11.6.1 Cost-Effectiveness and the Role of Risks

Cost-effectiveness allows three possible constellations: more effective and more costly, less effective and less costly, and, ideally, less costly and at least as effective. Consumer Health Informatics typically is less costly. Typical benefit are diagnoses made early enough to treat, successful treatments etc. Cost-effectiveness analysis is not meant as a mechanism. Like in Sect. 17.10, where a positive trial result does not entail a release of a treatment for routine use, application of cost-effectiveness informs, but does not force societies into implementation. Unwanted or non anticipated effects alongside a service must first be weighed,

---

[12]The general character of the listed challenges uses [2, chapter 6]. The applications to Consumer Health Informatics have been achieved by the author of this volume.

too. A Consumer Health Informatics example is described in Sect. 11.4 ("high tech hermits").

It should be noted that risks have different nature and are therefore approached differently both in the ethics discourse as in medical practice and research. Briefly we distinguish manageable from necessarily inherent risks. Managing and reducing manageable risks increases the benefit in the sense of the list in Sect. 17.11.5 and therefore falls under beneficence. All kinds of risk control methods from Chaps. 8 and 12, but also infectious disease (cf. Sect. 10.5.2) or insulin dosing control (cf. Sect. 9.5.4) which reduce client side risks play a role in Consumer Health Informatics. Presently not manageable risk are part of the weighing process of Sect. 17.11.8. Vaccination campaigns are an example already mentioned in Sect. 17.11.5. This example nicely demonstrates the temporal nature of the distinction between manageable and non manageable risks: Today, with present vaccines we have a certain number of severe adverse effects that we cannot avoid today through the best diligence. Ten years down the road vaccines may be much safer or a disease may be extinct. Applied to Consumer Health Informatics: today we have no safe methods to detect client suicidal ideations. With progress in sensor technology and NLP we may be able to in 10 years. Well, not fully safe certainly. But both, ever safer vaccines and ever more precise detection methods for mental states may turn respective risks into "de minimis risks": risks too small to be taken into account in societal decisions.

17.11.6.2 Moving the Scale Between Benefits and Risks

Historically, two major turnovers in US approval or at least tolerance of emerging procedures allows further insights about the nature of beneficence, also in balance with respect for autonomy. In both the FDA played a major role. Its procedures of approving new treatments and health technologies is generally acclaimed. It can be noted that in some fields its emphasis has "shifted to the possible benefits of clinical trials, while de-emphasizing their risks" [2, p. 250]. The change of mind was accomplished in the 1990s through AIDS advocates who fought for access to new pharmaceuticals before the final evaluation of clinical trials. Presently the Consumer Health Informatics service http://www.breastcancertrials.org/bct_nation offers women with breast cancer an easy fast access to knowledge about recent trials.

A similar approach may also help Consumer Health Informatics as a discipline to achieve wider penetration faster, although often the arguments are somewhat different. AIDS as a life-threatening disease implies a certain urgency to gain access to new therapy concepts. For Consumer Health Informatics services it may rather be the desire to avoid waiting lists or to get access to therapy at all. Some Level 1 services may also fall into the category like AIDS, for instance cardiac pacemaker home monitoring. FDA has also assumed other procedures that suggest to be considered for Consumer Health Informatics services, the "fast-track" for expedited approval and the "parallel track", access to new therapies on the premise of thorough disclosure of the risks.

The movement initiated by AIDS activists to gain access to new treatments before a finished systematic trial poses new challenges to the approved procedure of randomized controlled trials. If subjective reports from volunteer users of the new treatments are overwhelming they may stand in the way of further data collection and statistical testing although biases of the types introduced in Sect. 15.2.3 blur the self-reports. On the other hand, with very large numbers of satisfied clients true effects may be found through non RCT methods described in Sect. 6.3.3.

In another major FDA case that may also be a blueprint for Consumer Health Informatics FDA had been blamed for an overly paternalistic approach which it had meant as a beneficence. Breast augmentation implants, i.e. with no medical history of breast cancer, breast surgery etc. were severely restricted in 1992 after hundred thousands of successful implants the years before. FDA's argument was that in the absence of a medical benefit the small but not certainly known risk of the implants, for instance in circumstances of having to screen for breast cancer was decisive to discontinue silicone breast implants. Among the criticism of this decision is that it unduly restricts the autonomy of those seeking an implant and that, though not curing a disease an implant may improve the quality of life. This latter point implicitly relates to values and expectations in a society that honors good bodily appearance and beauty. Failing to meet these expectations reduces the experience of participating in that society which takes good-looking breasts into the neighborhood of lifestyle signatures. Maybe access to Consumer Health Informatics services can be promoted as a future lifestyle signature and would then follow the routes of breast augmentation implants whose use was released again in 2000 with mandating manufacturers to provide patients with more comprehensive information about risks such as pain, infections, and replacement rates. Informing about risks equally is among the obligations that Consumer Health Informatics service providers have.

17.11.6.3 Cost-Benefits and the Role of QALY's

After having studied risks and uncertainties we now turn to benefits where quality of life plays an important role. QALYs (Quality Adapted Life Years) are a whole family of attempts to quantify the value of a year of life with quality reduced through health issues. Assuming that QALYs can be determined in agreed upon ways they can help with arguments to prefer one health care program or individual intervention over another. They do, however, not solve such problems as moral obligations to save "identified lives" immediately and obviously at stake versus rationally assigning the same amount of resources for preventive or more sustainable programs promising to save "statistical lives". They also do not address the aspect of how care is being provided to achieve a certain amount of QALYs. Regarding Consumer Health Informatics it could be a disadvantage that it achieves its QALYs in an impersonal manner while patients might prefer personal empathetic care. On the other hand patients could feel good by knowing that what they get in terms of cure and QALYs is equally available to all others having the same problem; i.e. it would appeal to a moral sense of justice. One risk associated with the mechanical approach through QALYs is that it adds to a tendency and respective fears to transform a so far traditional moral language of helping the needy into an economic language where consumers calculate how many units of QALY they can buy at what price from which providers.

17.11.6.4 Conflicts Between Beneficence and Respect for Autonomy

The clearest paradigm to illustrate this conflict is suicide prevention. Spontaneous beneficence commands to intervene which violates autonomy. Moral judgment of intervening versus not intervening has to consider the whole spectrum from patients with knowingly futile prognosis to momentarily confused.

With other such conflicts lurking the conflict between beneficence and respect for autonomy is a major theme of the general ethics debate but a minor theme in Consumer Health Informatics because Consumer Health Informatics services typically offer a high degree of autonomy by design. Inasmuch as they also live up to the requirements of Chaps. 8 and 12 they take a good intermediate position on the scale.

> **Take Home**
> Beneficence is without doubt central to medical action. Giving meaning to beneficence poses various questions, including
>
> - how something is good, as a measurable effect or a perceived improvement
> - how good something is, the size of an effect
> - who determines what is good, citizens for themselves or authorities
> - who determines what risks are tolerable to achieve something good

17.11.7 Distributive Justice

In the discourse of biomedical ethics justice primarily means distributive justice i.e. fair, equitable, and appropriate distribution of the scarce resources of health care. When talking about clinical trials it may also mean fair distribution of the burden of risk but the last section has already shown that fair access to new therapeutic options plays a role here, too. A definition attributed to Aristotle: "Equals must be treated equally" seems easy but various questions arise when trying to specify "Equals", "treated", and "equally". "Equals" are sometimes specified as those belonging to a certain class such as the poor or the elderly but that again requires specification. In health care "treated" cannot mean getting everything; attempts to specify use the concept of fulfilling fundamental needs as treating.

Different criteria for "equally" have been brought up in a more general philosophical context, including offering every person an equal share, or serving a person according to his concrete need, his effort or made contribution, his merits in a more general sense, or following rules of free market exchanges. Examples of all can be found in historical and present health care system implementations, including combinations.

17.11.8 Consumer Health Informatics in Utilitarian and Other Theories of Justice

Different starting points can be taken to construct theories of justice.

17.11.8.1 Utilitarian Theories

Utilitarian theories attempt to maximize the overall good at minimal cost and risk of harm achievable for a society and claim that the individual receives distributive justice because he participates in the favorable situation of being member of a society which reaches its optimum.

Utility is here not regarded as the absolute preeminent principle residing above all other moral principles. It rather is a method to balance when actions can cause both, benefit and harm. By assigning utilities a serving role they cannot be abused to argue that generally society's interest overrides individual interests.

The vaccination example already mentioned in Sect. 17.11.5 allows to demonstrate the subordinate nature of utility: depending on the harm that the disease causes, the harm of adverse vaccination events and the likelihood of adverse vaccination events together form a setting where for some disease vaccination campaigns may be moral and should therefore become law while others are immoral. Where the balance is made legitimately varies between societies.

Questions remain as to the care for the sickest and most vulnerable where the ratio of effort and benefit is typically not favorable and as a consequence care might be denied. Also, social utility of subgroups may vary over time and as a consequence patterns of distribution may change over time with some subgroups being innocent victims negatively affected and without a chance to modify to their favor. Therefore, utilitarian theories maintain the advantage of outlining the best use of the resources spent but should be restricted in scope to avoid morally unacceptable withdrawal or malallocation under certain circumstances. As long as objective assessment of the diverse needs and impartial choices how to maximize the overall outcome are installed utilitarian theories can claim to be moral because as a major consequence they promote welfare and by that argument are beneficence-based. Utilitarian theories might help to promote Consumer Health Informatics services because they can often be offered to theoretically unlimited numbers of patients at low cost.

17.11.8.2 Communitarian Theories

Communitarian theories of justice emphasize moral obligations that communities have towards their citizens and that citizens have towards their communities to commonly provide services or procedures that are vital for the functioning of the community. Specification of such theories requires to define what is vital for whom. It may also pose the challenge of financial coverage when the lines of the vitally necessary are drawn too wide. This is part of the problem of some European health care systems. Promises might be easier to hold when Consumer Health Informatics services can take up some of the bulk load of routine yet necessary services provided to all citizens in need.

17.11.8.3 Libertarian Theories

Libertarian theories, in contrast, assign hardly any role to the society except providing the frame where individuals can freely exert their choices. A just society in the libertarian sense is one that protects the rights of property and of using property to purchasing according to one's preferences and the right of liberty for both patients and providers to seek or not to seek or to offer or not to offer services at freely negotiable prices. As a consequence society does not assume the role of a health care provider or organizer. In this theory distributive justice is the lack of regulations and mechanisms that would hinder free offering and free purchasing of health care, and as a side note purchasing or not purchasing health insurance. Consumer Health Informatics services fit here as well, especially because they could reach mass markets and compete through price. Interestingly, the US presumably open market oriented health care system has major impediments through its state based licensing and respective practice restrictions, overly conservative professional policy regulations and an equally overly cautious FDA, which all hinder Consumer Health Informatics to fully exploit its potential, see also Sect. 17.8.

17.11.8.4 Egalitarian Theories

Egalitarian theories emphasize equal shares available to everybody. It does not help to specify equal share as equal amount delivered to everybody. Providing fair opportunity is a more productive approach. It emphasizes that wherever the patient stands in terms of talents, handicaps, diseases, personal support structures such as family, society should grant him that which takes him forward best according to his personal aspirations and reachable assets. This may include that disadvantaged and vulnerable parts of the population receive additional support, at least in as much as unfair disadvantages are compensated for. This poses specific challenges for Consumer Health Informatics services. Making them accessible for persons with all kinds of physical and mental limitations requires such efforts that the cost part of Consumer Health Informatics cost-effectiveness may no longer materialize.

> **Take Home**
>
> For bringing the portfolio of existing services to bear regarding benefits, risks, scarcity and cost, societal mechanisms of distribution and allocation have to be considered.
>
> - Utilitarian theories attempt to maximize the society wide differential of achieved benefits and suffered harms. Utilitarianism is favorable towards many Consumer Health Informatics services since they can offer their benefits to virtually unlimited numbers of clients.
> - Communitarian theories regard their citizens as responsible to give and entitled to take according to their potentials and needs. Consumer Health Informatics can enrich this situation of a deal through an easily achieved supply.
> - Libertarian theories see a society as a place where the citizen can choose without undue limitations and where he consequently is responsible for risks. In such a place Consumer Health Informatics would be one of many providers, with the options to scale up and compete through price.
> - Egalitarian theories want citizens to receive services in fair appreciation of the needs and potential. Since this requires highly individualized delivery especially to low literacy target groups Consumer Health Informatics cannot draw on its potential.

Whatever the theory of distributive justice, it can be argued that morally there is a right to a minimum amount of health care. Not even this is the case in many developing countries and also not in the USA. Special considerations are generally necessary when resources are genuinely scarce, such as donated organs. Since this is not the field where Consumer Health Informatics has its virtues we will not follow-up on that topic.

17.12 Directions for Legislation

Through the contrast between Sects. 17.4 and 17.11 and the non-existence of a transition path from research into routine, as evident from Sect. 17.10 we learn that for Consumer Health Informatics to become a regular branch of the health care industry many stakeholder must contribute. Consumer Health Informatics itself must provide strong evidence of its effectiveness through trials that avoid the confounders and biases discussed in Chap. 15 and in many more places in this volume. Consumer Health Informatics must also demonstrate its safeguards against client inherent risks. Consumer Health Informatics, of course is not meant here as one large monolith but as a discipline that develops services for each of which the above has to be achieved.

Once such has been achieved for a Consumer Health Informatics service it would be a societal waste of effort and in some sense immoral to not take that service forward and eventually into practice. Therefore, it is not an opportunity but an obligation for other stakeholders to assist with that transition.

Medical domain specialist are in charge to clearly identify the achievable benefits and remaining risks. If benefits are marginal or risks large they should intervene, backed up through their professional codes and moral principles of medicine. If, however, benefits are large and risks small they should content themselves with having taken care and then to usher a service further, eventually leading into a situation where the immanent dependency ratio effects of demographic developments described in Chap. 2 are bolstered.

Public health and delivery of care specialists should assess opportunities and limitations to reach populations, whether all in need of a service benefit equally and whether a Consumer Health Informatics service enhances, is neutral to, or limits client autonomy.

Equipped with these assessments societies as a whole or their guild of ethics specialists are in charge to weigh the whole bundle of achieved benefits, potential harms, equal or unequal distribution and client choices or their absence to come with a recommendation that matches their society's perception of and expectations towards health care delivery.

Such recommendations may and will vary between utilitarian, communitarian, libertarian, egalitarian and other theories of justice. While the former emphasize equal distribution with risks safeguarded publicly the latter encourage individuals to seek opportunities and apply their personal evaluation of risks. Affordability and payment overlay this mixture.

All mentioned above are moral theories that are not good or bad by themselves but accepted or not accepted in societies. Consumer Health Informatics as a science that develops services has to face the fact that, although universal and universally effective in its active agents, some service may be welcome in some and not welcome in other countries. This, again, is a waste of effort that a good society should avoid. Therefore, I would like to close this volume with the hope that a decade from now harmonized transition paths from inception to release for routine use have emerged and that Consumer Health Informatics can deliver its successful services world wide without legal or administrative barriers. This volume is meant as a set of methods and perspectives to achieve this aim.

References

1. Bergström J, Andersson G, Ljótsson B, Rück C, Andréewitch S, Karlsson A, Carlbring P, Andersson E, Lindefors N. Internet-versus group-administered cognitive behaviour therapy for panic disorder in a psychiatric setting: a randomised trial. BMC Psychiatry. 2010;10(54):1471–244X. doi: 10.1186/1471-244X-10-54.
2. Beauchamp TL, Childress JF. Principles of biomedical ethics. 7th ed. Oxford/New York: Oxford University Press; 2013.

References

3. Blankers M, Koeter MWJ, Schippers GM. Internet therapy versus internet self-help versus no treatment for problematic alcohol use: a randomized controlled trial. J Consult Clin Psychol. 2011;79(3):330–41. doi: 10.1037/a0023498.
4. Bauer S, Okon E, Meermann R, Kordy H. Technology-enhanced maintenance of treatment gains in eating disorders: efficacy of an intervention delivered via text messaging. J Consult Clin Psychol. 2012;80(4):700–6. doi: 10.1037/a0028030.
5. Derse AR, Miller TE. Net effect: professional and ethical challenges of medicine online. Camb Q Healthc Ethics. 2008;17:453–64. doi: 10.1017/S0963180108080572.
6. Fox RC, Swazey JP. Observing bioethics. Oxford: Oxford University Press; 2008. doi: 10.1093/acprof:oso/9780195365559.001.0001.
7. Guseh JS, Brendel RW, Brendel DH. Medical professionalism in the age of online social networking. J Med Ethics. 2009;35:584–6. doi: 10.1136/jme.2009.029231.
8. Huh J, McDonald DW, Hartzler A, Pratt W. Patient moderator interaction in online health communities. In: AMIA Annual Symposium Proceedings. American Medical Informatics Association; Nov 2013. pp. 627–36.
9. Lacson SM, Bradley C, Arkfeld DG. Facebook medicine. J Rheumatol. 2009;36(1):211. doi: 10.3899/jrheum.080750.
10. Lewis CE. My computer, my doctor: a constitutional call for federal regulation of cybermedicine. Am J Law Med. 2006;32:585–609.
11. Munson SA, Cavusoglu H, Frisch L, Fels S. Sociotechnical challenges and progress in using social media for health. JMIR. 2013;15(10):e226. doi: 10.2196/jmir.2792.
12. McManus RJ, Mant J, Bray EP, Holder R, Jones MJ, Greenfield S, Kaambwa B, Banting M, Bryan S, Little P, Williams B, Hobbs FDR. Telemonitoring and self-management in the control of hypertension (TASMINH2: a randomized controlled trial. Lancet. 2010;376:162–72. doi: 10.1016/S0140-6736(10)60964-6.
13. Shortliffe EH, Cimino JJ. Biomedical informatics: computer applications in health care and biomedicine. 4th ed. London/Heidelberg/New York/Dordrecht: Springer; 2014. doi: 10.1007/978-1-4471-4474-8.
14. Simpson RL. State-based licensure: are we regulating away the promise of telemedicine? Nurs Admin Q. 2008;32(4):346–8.
15. Stockwell MS, Kharbanda EO, Martinez RA, Vargas CY, Vawdrey DK, Camargo S. Effect of a text messaging intervention on influenza vaccination in an urban, low-income pediatric and adolescent population. JAMA. 2012;307(16):1702–8.
16. Spek V, Nykliček I, Smits N, Cuijpers P, Riper H, Keyzer J, Pop V. Internet-based cognitive behavioural therapy for subthreshold depression in people over 50 years old: a randomized controlled clinical trial. Psychol Med. 2007;37:1797–806. doi: 10.1017/S0033291707000542.
17. Singh SN, Wachter RM. Perspectives on medical outsourcing and telemedicine – rough edges in a flat world? N Engl J Med. 2008;358(15):1622–7. doi: 10.1056/NEJMhle0707298.
18. van Voorhees BW, Hsiung RC, Marko-Holguin M, Houston TK, Fogel J, Lee R, Ford DE. Internal versus external motivation in referral of primary care patients with depression to an internet support group: randomized controlled trial. JMIR. 2013;15(3):e42. doi: 10.2196/jmir.2197.
19. Wolfe RM, Sharp LK. Vaccination or immunization? The impact of search terms on the internet. J Health Commun. 2005;10(6):537–51. doi: 10.1080/10810730500228847.
20. World Medical Association. WMA declaration of Helsinki – ethical principles for medical research involving human subjects. http://www.wma.net/en/30publications/10policies/b3/index.html, 2013.

Trademarks

Microsoft, HealthVault and Bing are registered trademarks of Microsoft Corporation
BlackBerry is a registered trademark of Research in Motion Limited
Amazon is a registered trademark of amazon.con, Inc.
Yahoo! is a trademark of Yahoo! Inc.
Epic and MyChart are registered trademarks of Epic Systems Corporation
Kaiser Permanente is a registered trademark of Kaiser Permanente
Group Health is a registered trademark of Group Health Cooperative
Cerner is a registered trademark of Cerner Corporation
fitbit is a registered trademark of Fitbit, Inc.
Jawbone is a registered trademark of Jawbone
Planned Parenthood is a registered trademark of Planned Parenthood of America Inc.
Susan G. Komen is a registered trademark of Susan G. Komen
justanswer is a registered trademark of JustAnswer LLC
everyday HEALTH is a registered trademark of Everyday Health Media, LLC
Google and Android are trademarks of Google Inc.
TSA is a trademark or EMC Corporation
Wikipedia is a registered trademark of Wikimedia Foundation, Inc.
iOS is a trademark of Apple
Drugs.com is a trademark of Drugs.com
WedMD is a registered trademark of WebMD, LLC
SF12 is a registered trademark of Medical Outcomes Trust
EMC^2 is a registered trademark of EMC Corporation
Accu-Chek is a registered trademark of Roche Diagnostics GmbH
Coagu-Chek is a registered trademark of Roche
Accu-Chek 360 is a registered trademark of F Hoffmann-La Roche Ltd
Nintendo is a registered trademark and Wii is a trademark of Nintendo of America Inc.

Nomenclature

AAP	American Academy of Pediatrics
ABMS	American Board of Medical Specialties
ACOG	American Congress of Obstetricians and Gynecologists
ACP	American College of Physicians
ACT	Acceptance and Commitment Theory [15]
ADE	Adverse Drug Event
ADHD	Attention Deficit Hyperactivity Hisorder
advance directive	(also: advance health care directive) written instructions ... that specify what actions should be taken for ... health, if ... no longer able to make decisions ...; source: Wikipedia
agoraphobia	Obsessive, persistent, intense fear of open places, MeSH term
AGOS	American Gynecological Obstetrical Society
AHRQ	Agency for Health care Research and Quality
AMA	American Medical Association
AMIA	American Medical Informatics Association, meanwhile merged to form the WG Consumer and Pervasive Health Informatics
ART	Antiretroviral Therapy
BDI	Beck Depression Index
BfArM	Bundesinstitut für Arzneimittel und Medizinprodukte (Germany) – Federal Institute for Drugs and Medical Devices
BMI	Body Mass Index: $\frac{weight(kg)}{height(m)^2}$
Borg Scale	a rating scale to measure perceived exertion (Wikipedia)
BRCA	Breast cancer genes named BRCA1 and BRCA2

carotid endarterectomy	surgical correction of a stenosis of the carotid artery
caveat emptor	Latin: buyer beware. Legal maxim that holds a vendor free from having to recover damages to a buyer as long as the vendor does not conceal latent defects to the buyer
CBT	Cognitive-behavioral therapy
CDC	Centers for Disease Control and Prevention
CDISC-R	Computer-Based Diagnostic Inventory Schedule for Children – Revised
CES	Curious Experience Scale [2]
CES-D	Center for Epidemiological Studies Depression scale [7]
CMS	Centers for Medicare & Medicaid Services
COPD	Chronic Obstructive Pulmonary Disease
CPOE	Computerized Physician (or Provider) Order Entry
CWD	Coping With Depression
DASH	Dietary Approaches to Stop Hypertension
dependency ratio	in a population: size of age group that needs service devided by size of age group that can provide service
digital divide	TBD
DIMDI	Deutsches Institut für Medizinische Dokumentation und Information
DSM-5	Diagnostic and Statistical Manual of Mental Disorders 5th Edition 2013
DTC	Direct-To-Consumer; offering medical service for purchase without associated counseling
EDS	Edinburgh Depression Scale
eHEALS	eHealth Literacy Scale
ER	Electronic (Health) Record
EU	European Union
FAQ	frequently asked question
FD&C	Federal Food, Drug and Cosmetics Act
FDA	Food and Drug Administration
FEV_1	Forced Expiratory Volume in 1 sec
functional health literacy	the degree to which individuals have the capacity to obtain, process, and understand basic health information and services needed to make appropriate health decisions
GDP	Gross Domestic Product
GP	General Practitioner
GPS	Global Positioning System
HbA1c	glycated hemoglobin; an indicator of average plasma glucose concentration in the weeks prior to measurement
HHS	Department of Health and Human Services

HIE	Health Information Exchange
HIP	Health Information Professional
HITECH	Health Information Technology for Economic and Clinical Health Act
HON	Health On the Net
HTA	Health Technology Assessment
ICT	Information and Communication Technology
IMIA	International Medical Informatics Association
INR	International Normalized Ration, a laboratory test measure of blood coagulation
IOM	Institute of Medicine
IRB	Institutional Review Board
ISRCTN	International Standard Randomised Controlled Trial Number
IVR	Interactive Voice Response
JMIR	Journal of Medical Internet Research
K10	Kessler psychological distress scale
kg	kilogram, a mass unit; 1 kg = 2.205 lbs
lb, lbs	pound, pounds, a mass unit; 1 lb = 0.454 kg
LMIC	Low and Middle Income Countries
MCMI	Millon Clinical Multiaxial Inventory
MEMS	Medical Event Monitoring System
MeSH	Medical Subject Headings, NLM controlled vocabulary thesaurus used for indexing articles for PubMed
MHV	My HealtheVet
MSM	Men having Sex with Men
MU	Meaningful Use
NABP	National Association of Boards of Pharmacy
NCI	National Cancer Institute
NHS	National Health Service
NICE	National Institute for Health and Clinical Excellence
NICU	Neonatal Intensive Care Unit
NLM	National Library of Medicine
NLP	Natural Language Processing
noli nocere	Latin: At least, not to do harm. Maxim of medical ethics above all to avoid harm
NVS	Newest Vital Sign
ONC	Office of the National Coordinator for Health Information Technology
PCHR	Personally Controlled Health Record
PDSS	Panic Disorder Severity Scale
PEFR	Peak Expiratory Flow Rate
PHQ-9	Patient Health Questionnaire 9
PHR	Personal Health Record
PID-5	Personality Inventory for DSM-5

RA	Rheumatoid arthritis
RCT	Randomized Controlled Trial
RE-AIM	Reach Effectiveness Adoption Implementation Maintenance
REALM	Rapid Estimate of Adult Literacy in Medicine
remote consultation	consultation via remote telecommunications, generally for the purpose of diagnosis or treatment of a patient at a site remote from the patient or primary physician (MeSH)
ROI	Return On Investment
RTMM	Real Time Medication Monitoring
SMS	Short Message Service
SNP	Single Nucleotide Polymorphism
SNS	Social Network System
SSN	Social Security Number
STI	Sexually Transmitted Infection
TAN	transaction authentication number
telemedicine	delivery of health services via remote telecommunications, including interactive consultative and diagnostic services (MeSH)
TLS	Transport Layer Security
URAC	Utilization Review Accreditation Commission
VA	US Department of Veterans Affairs
VSA	visual analog scale

General Index

Ä
Ärztekammer, 348
Ärztetag, 348
"East Germany", 42
"West Germany", 42
"friend", 86, 139
"good physician", 343
"patient specialist", 182
"prescription free", 115

A
AAP, 346
ABMS, 347
acceleration detector, 58
ACOG, 346
ACP, 346
ACT, 209
acting on behalf, 183
action plan, 208
adaptivity, 252
ADE, 55, 136
adherence, 198, 203
　　medication, 208, 232
adoption, 289
advance directive, 183, 375
adverse event, 199
advertisement, 350
advice, *see also* recommendation, 123, 126
aerosol, 111
African American, 230, 238, 240
age, 42
　　old, 42, 46, 48, 50, 57, 246, 252
　　working, 42, 46, 48, 50
　　young, 42, 46, 48, 50
age pyramid, 39, 47

AGOS, 346
AHRQ, 77, 107, 323
ALED-I, 194
alert, 285
allergen, 165
allergy, 285
AMA, 45, 69, 84, 343
   directive, 343
   ethics opinion, 343, 344
   health policy, 343, 344
      H-160.975, 347
      H-478.997, 345
   House of Delegates, 343
   nonphysician provider, 345
   rules of communication, 345
Amazon®, 148
ambulatory physician's activity, 351
American Recovery and Reinvestment Act, 287
American Society of Andrology, 346
AMIA
   WG Consumer Health Informatics, 76
Android, 79, 148
Android™, 148
anesthesia, 174
anonymous, 195
Apothekengesetz, 351
app, 79, 290
app developer
   Amazon®, 149
   Apple, 149
   Google™, 149
App Store, 148
App store, 148
Apple, 148
application
   addiction, 104
   ADHD, 71, 102
   agoraphobia, 104
   asthma, 102, 111, 128, 232
      brittle, 256
      childhood, 266
      severe, 256
      steroid-naïve, 256
   BMI, 198
   burnout, 337
   cancer
      breast, 113, 262, 336
      colorectal, 229
      prostate, 113
   cancer screening, 71
   cancer survivor, 135
   cardiac surgery, 233
   carotid endarterectomy, 90
   chronic pain, 92, 164

COPD, 97, 256
coronary artery disease, 198
depression, 104, 106, 108, 211, 236, 257
diabetes, 128, 135, 206, 236
diabetes mellitus 2, 189, 198, 200, 202, 203, 207, 238, 240, 242, 337
    insulin dependent, 200
drinking, 105
eating disorder, 105
emergency logistics, 96
erectile dysfunction, 121
eye screening, 211
falls, 245
family planning, 235
HIV, 219
    ART, 235, 238
    testing, 237
hypertension, 94, 197
hypoglycemia
    incident, 204
influenza, 226
influenza pandemic, 139
injury, 102
iodine deficiency, 219
isolation, 245
lab test, 228
malaria, 219
male circumcision, 219, 232
medication management, 245
melanoma, 129
metabolic syndrome, 189, 198, 337
mobility, 245
obesity, 127
overweight, 127, 194, 195, 197, 202, 207
panic disorder, 104
psychiatry, 341
respiratory disease, 164
retinopathy, 210
sensory impairment, 245
sexual behavior, 219
smoking, 102
smoking cessation, 71, 105, 127, 227
STI, 103, 219
STI testing, 228
substance abuse, 238
sudden infant death, 102
syphilis, 221
television overuse, 102
tropical infection, 124
tuberculosis, 219, 239
urinary incontinence, 110
vaccination, 226
    childhood, 232
appointment scheduling, 286
article, 196, 212

artificial intelligence, 252
Arzneimittelgesetz, 349, 351
assessment
   dimension, 159
      cognition, 161
   method, 159
   resource, 159
   sub dimension, 159
assessment scheme, 159
assessment, client
   dimension
      cognition, 171, 266
      identity, 183, 267
      medical risk, 163, 257, 262
      personality, 167, 264
   method
      Borg scale, 255
      CDISC-R, 257
      CES, 264
      CES-D, 258
      Coopersmith Self-Esteem Inventory, 264
      FEV_1, 256, 257
      gene scan, 261
      genetic counseling, 262
      HEXACO, 264
      informed consent, 170, 266
      K10, 258
      Likert scale, 163
      mammography schedule, 263
      MCMI, 266
      medical ancestry form, 165
      NEO Five-Sector Personality Inventory, 264
      NVS, 177
      online form, 163, 166, 171, 257, 258, 260
      PEFR, 256
      personality inventory, 168, 259, 264
      PID-5, 265
      psychometric instrument, 169
      pulse oximetry, 257
      questionnaire, 168
      rescue medication need, 256
      STOFHLA, 267
      symptom self-report, 256, 257
      TOFHLA, 176
      torso image, 163
      tumor marker scan, 261
      visual analogue scale, 163
   resource
      age, 267
      airflow meter, 164
      biometric authentication, 185, 268
      blood glucose meter, 164
      blood pressure cuff, 164
      client memory, 164

General Index 397

        curricular level, 176
        electronic signature, 184
        ER, 164, 256, 260
        family history, 263
        gene scan, 165
        graphical display, 260
        heart sound recorder, 164
        ID, 183
        image, 163
        knowledge, 184, 276
        legal notice, 183
        micro-array, 165
        mutation, 263
        online activity, 170
        physical token, 268
        possession, 184, 276
        social network trace, 166–169
        URI, 183
        video, 163
        xml, 260
        years of education, 267
    sub dimension
        addiction, 264
        attitude, 169, 266
        behavior, 260
        emotional stability, 168
        familial risk, 259
        family medical history, 260
        functional health literacy, 159, 267
        genetic risk, 165, 259, 262
        Internet addiction, 264
        maladaptivity, 265
        medical history, 164
        medical knowledge, 159
        mental health, 265
        physical exposure, 165
        physical impairment, 170
        religious background, 170
        social exposure, 166
assistance
    cognitive, 249
    sensory, 249
    social interaction, 249
Association of American Medical Colleges, 45
attendance
    visit, 220, 221
attrition, 208
authentication, 290
    SSL-Client, 276
authenticity, 103, 275, 276
automated facial recognition, 185
automatic bedroom light, 246
Aware Home, 246
awareness, 102, 191, 192

B
baby boom, 39
barrier, 208
battery management, 152
Bayes, 97
BDI II, 107
Beck Hopelessness Scale, 257
behavior, 112
    change, 63
    pattern, 208
    recommendation, 194, 202
    unhealthy, 190
behavioral theory, 190
best case scenario, 44
Beveridge
    William Henry, 337, 343
BfArM, 349, 370
Bildung, 175
Bing®, 77
biological family, 165
birds of a feather style, 137
birthrate, 49
Bismarck
    Otto von, 337, 342
blog, 138
blood glucose, 190, 201, 209
blood glucose monitor, 285
blood glucose reading, 129
blood pressure, 190, 196, 201, 208
blood pressure monitor, 285
Bluetooth®, 97
BMI, 194, 196
board certified physician, 347
botnet malware, 277
BRCA, 262, 263
breathing capacity, 255
Bundesagentur für Arbeit, 47
Bundesrat, 348
Bundestag, 348
burden of disease, 190, 205
Bureau of Labor Statistics, 45
business model, 132, 327

C
c-referral, 108
California
    Business and Professions Code, 346
    Rules of Professional Conduct, 343
calory calculation, 194
cancer survivor, 112, 262
car accident, 212
CBT, 92, 104–106, 127, 195, 209, 227
CDC, 48, 151, 260

Censusscope, 45
certification
    ISO27001, 279
charity, 336
Child Depression Inventory, 258
child-safety seat, 172
chip card, 276
cholesterol, 208
claims data, 197
classification
    automatic, 211
client, 6
clinical decision support, 204
closed loop decision support, 204
closure, 353
cloud, 57
Cloze item, 177
CMS, 281
coaching, 201
Cochrane review, 320
commercial institution, 74
community, 140, 195, 208
    virtual, 197
competition through price, 350
complication, 212
confidentiality, 250, 274
confirmation bias, 67
conflict of interest, 350
consent, 353
conservative principlism, 342
Constitution, 349
consumer, 6
contact time, 54
contraception, 170
contract, 122
controlled substance, 117
convenience, 115, 120, 121, 126, 148, 200, 229
    therapist, 132
coping, 210, 212
corporate social responsibility, 336
corroboration, 74
cost
    health care, 197
    reduction, 211
cost-effectiveness, 92, 194, 197, 313
counselor, 209
country
    Australia, 93, 221, 228
    Austria, 122
    Canada, 115, 206, 233, 264
    Denmark, 232
    EU, 32
    Finland, 246, 247
    France, 246, 248

country (*cont.*)
    Germany, 41, 46, 49, 96, 119, 122, 185, 192, 278, 328, 337, 342, 348
    Haiti, 143
    Honduras, 231, 242
    India, 211
    Iran, 219
    Ireland, 246, 247
    Japan, 248
    Kenya, 225, 232, 235
    Korea, 202
    Lithuania, 246, 247
    Mexico, 231
    Netherlands, The, 97, 106, 109, 203, 248, 264
    Norway, 209, 246, 247
    Peru, 103
    South Africa, 237, 241
    Sweden, 246, 248
    Switzerland, 70, 122, 220, 329, 330
    Taiwan, 111, 223
    Tanzania, 222
    Thailand, 239
    Turkey, 200, 227
    Uganda, 218
    UK, 94, 116, 119, 122, 124, 221, 246, 247, 291, 337, 343
    USA, 32, 41, 45, 49, 62, 67, 96, 108, 112, 115, 119, 123, 173, 177, 196, 201, 204, 224, 226, 230, 235, 238, 245–248, 266, 282, 330, 336, 342, 343
CPOE, 54
credibility, 74
cross-border, 351
cryptography, 276
cultural community, 169
culture, 290
customer relationship, 96
CWD, 107, 109

D
DAK, 338
DASH for Health, 182, 196
dashboard, 195, 196
data, 56
    access limitation, 292
    client-provided, *see also* patient-provided, 164
    client-reported, 197, 208
    custody, 291
    historical, 89
    omics, 287
    ownership, 291
    patient-generated, 136, 143
    patient-provided, 88, 89, 128, 212, 285, 291, 292
    quality, 292
    summary, 56
data mining, 251

Declaration of Helsinki, 368, 369
decryption, 276
demand characteristics, 302
democratic model, 138
demographic development, 341
demographic information, 284
denial of service, 152, 339
destatis, 46
diabetes, 64
diabetes distress, 201
Diabetes Hands Foundation, 212
diabetes management, 201
diabetes mellitus, 211
diabetes mellitus 2, 209
diabetes nurses, 204
diagnostic logging, 181
diary, 126, 194, 203, 209, 212
diet, 197, 209
    recommendation, 194
dietitian, 56
digital divide, 102, 137
diligence, 376
dilution scenario, 43, 46, 49
DIMDI, 131, 349
disaster, 152
disaster relief, 143
Discern, 75
discharge management, 90
disclaimer, 115, 121–124, 158, 353
discontinuation of service, 153
disparity, 29
    ethnic, 289
dose adaptation, 111
dose-response effect, 199, 201
driving activity, 212
DTC, 71

E

e-mail, 84, 104, 136, 228, 345
    reminder, 207
eating, 208
    habits, 196
eating habits, *see also* nutrition
EDS, 106
education, 62, 63, 66, 102, 113, 200, 206, 232, 238
educational material, 266, 285
eHEALS, 179
EHR, 202, 274, 281, 291
elderly, *see also* older adult, 62
electronic mail, *see* e-mail
electronic signature, 184, 276
embarrassing condition, 110, 120

emedicine, 78
emergency, 148
emergency contact information, 285
empowerment, 92
ENABLE, 246
encouragement, 127
encryption, 275–277
Epic®, 283
Epic® systems, 282
EPP, 88
equity, 176
ethics, 158, 250
    clinical, 342
    descriptive, *see* empirical
    empirical, 371
    nonnormative, 371
    normative, 371
    public health, 342
Ethikkommission, 340, 369
ethnic minority, 166, 178
EU, 351
European Union, *see* EU
evaluation apprehension, 302
evangelism, 66
exacerbation, 128
exercise, 201
    recommendation, 194
exercising
    habits, 196
expert system, 110
exposure, 105

F
face validity, 76, 77, 151
face-to-face, 162, 208
fallback solution, 153
false negative, 129
familiarity bias, 178
family, 166, 251
family health history, 286
family physician, 71, 157, 159
family tree, 286
FAQ, 200
FD&C, 343
FDA, 71, 347
Federal State Medical Association, 47
feedback, 195, 198, 200, 201, 212, 295
FEV, 97
finance, 166
financial savings, 127
Fire OS, 148
firewall, 277

First Amendment, 344, 347
fitbit®, 290, 332
fitness for use, 344
Flesch Reading Ease, 172
Flesch-Kincade Grade Level, 172
flow measurement, 128
foreseeable reliance, 353
forum, 119, 212
    moderated, 208
    un-moderated, 104
free speech, 344, 347, 349, 351, 353
Fuelband, 332
functionality, 344
funding model, *see also* business model, 131
fundus camera, 211

G
GDP, 40, 55
Gesundheitsberichterstattung des Bundes, 47
gender, 178
general education, 161
genetic disposition, 190
Georgia Breast Center, 263
German Federal Statistical Office, 48
German unification, 42, 46, 48
goal, 198, 208
Google Health™, 283
Google Play™, 148
Google™, 77, 78, 148, 263
GPS, 17, 18, 58, 96, 148
Greek, 179
Group Health®, 229
Group Health® Cooperative, 282
growth, 55
growth scenario, 43, 46, 49
Grundgesetz, 349
Guardian Angel "Manifesto" Proposal, 282
guardianship, 129, 169
Gunning fog formula, 172

H
H.E.A.L.T.H., 195
habits
    eating, *see also* diet
hacking, 276
hand fingerprint, 185
hard of hearing, 170
harm, 72, 149
hash function, 276
Hawthorne effect, 192, 198, 301
HbA1c, 200, 201, 203, 206, 208, 212

health care
   delivery, 48, 52
   industry, 131
   material assets, 41
   spending, 132
   system, 52
   workforce, 39
      nursing, 48
      physician, 44, 45
   workload, 40, 131
health care provider, 207
health goals, 286
health history, 285
health literacy, 204
health myths, 124
health plan, *see also* insurance
Health Vault™, 260
heavy load work, 165
heuristic, 151
HIE, 291, 292
HIP, 368
Hippocrates, 158, 375
Hispanic, 230
HITECH, 287
home delivery
   drug, 125, 353
HON, 76, 77, 131, 151
hotel personnel, 56
human subjects, 368
hypnosis, 127
hypoglycemia, 204
   prevalence, 212
hypoxia
   perception of, 256

I

ICD, 316
IDEATel, 190
identity
   client, 85
   physician, 85
image, 129
imagination, 174
IMIA, 368
immigration, 44, 47
immigration policy, 49
immunization, 285
implantable cardioverters defibrillators, 316
in-person, 344
incentive, 218, 219, 232
independence, 245
indeterminacy, 66
Index Medicus, 337
informal caregiver, 52, 231

information, 123, 201
information broker, 77, 119, 124
information toxicity, 158
informed consent, 250
Informed Patient, 10
infotainment, 119
insulin
    dosage, 129, 202, 203
    pump, 285
insurance, 183, 289
integration, 207
integrity, 275
Internet café, 103
Internet pharmacy, *see* online pharmacy
Internet security, 228
interpersonal contact, 345
Interstate Nurse Licensure Compact, 343
intrusion detection system, 277
invisibility, 252
IOM, 36, 288
iOS, 148
iOS™, 79
IRB, 340, 342, 369
    exempt, 196
Italy, 91
IVR, 229

J
JAMA, 77
Jawbone®, 290, 332

K
Kaiser Permanente®, 229, 282
Kassenärztliche Vereinigung, 47
kiosk, 102, 132, 262
knowledge, 112, 192, 206, 208
    accurate, 344, 349, 351, 368
    timely, 344, 349, 351, 368
Komen®, 336

L
laboratory, 202, 285
Latin, 179
left handed, 170
legal maxim
    caveat emptor, 123, 158, 362, 365
    noli nocere, 158, 375
legal notice, 79, 123, 151
legal principle, *see* moral principle
liability, 158
    waiver, 158, 199

life expectancy, 39, 47
lifestyle, 58, 189, 199, 260
    change, 191
Likert scale, 179, 210
literacy, 102, 161, 206, 209, 290
    computer, 288
    digital, 179
    eHealth, 179, 180
    functional health, *see also* health literacy, 173
    health, 179, 288
        prediction, 178
    Internet, 181
    marginal, 173
Livestrong, 336
LMIC, 217
local language, 236
locator, 129
    function, 124
    service, 125
logistics support, 77, 112, 113, 124
Lorenz, Konrad, 73
loss, 166
lost in cyberspace, 77
Low and Middle Income Countries, 217

M

mail order pharmacy, 115, 351
maintenance effort, 132
majority vote, 66
mammography, 262
Mayo Clinic, 151
MedCertain, 75
Medicaid, 177, 179
Medical Association, 348
medical device, 98
    class I, 33
    class II, 33
    class IIa, 33
    class IIb, 33
    class III, 33
    software, 34
medical outcome, 197, 208
medical progress, 39
medical record, 121, 122
medical school, 44, 49
medication, 157, 201, 209, 285
    dosage, 202
medication change, 95
medication compliance, 117
Medicinal Products Act, 351
MEDLARS, 337
MedlinePlus, 77, 78
MEMS, 235

General Index 407

mentor, 141
MeSH, 19, 20, 32, 83
messaging, 207
metabolic syndrome, 261
metabolic testing, 192
Microsoft® HealthVault®, 283
military base, 194, 195
mobility restriction, 171
Model Professional Code, *see* professional code
moderator, 348
Molière, 132, 193
monitor
    blood glucose, 200
monitoring, *see also* monitor
    blood glucose, 202
        fasting, 203
    functional, 249
    physiological, 249
    safety, 249
    security, 249
    social interaction, 249
moral principle
    autonomy, *see* respect for autonomy, 169
    beneficence, 341, 375
    distributive justice, 53, 341
    impossibility, 368
    integrity, 368
    justice, *see* distributive justice, 341
    nonmaleficence, 341, 375, 376
    respect for autonomy, 341, 373–375
motion sensor, 58
    infrared, 246
motivation, 194, 198
MSM, 221
MU, 28, 281, 287, 288
MU stages, 287
multimedia, 206
Musterberufsordnung, 348
My HealtheVet, 283, 286
MyChart®, 282, 283

N
NABP, 347
National Institutes of Health, 77
navigation, 181
NCI, 263
negative obligation, 376
negligence, 376
NHS, 124, 337
NICE, 95
NIH, 336
NLM, 67, 76, 151
NLP, 103, 173

non-inferiority, 220
non-native speaker, 209, 289
non-repudiation, 275, 276
numeracy, 172, 173
    medical, *see also* literacy, 173
nutrition, 201
nutrition label, 177

O

obligation, 376
observer bias, 302
observer expectancy effect, 303
obtrusiveness, 250
off-label use, 143
Office of Disease Prevention and Health Promotion, 336
old age dependency ratio, 39, 46, 49
older adult, 289
oligopoly, 328
ONC, 287
online pharmacy, 72, 115, 117, 158, 346
online prescribing, 345, 346
open market, 52, 337, 342, 347, 354, 382
opinion leader model, 138
optometrist, 56
orthography, 178
outcome
    patient-reported, 111, 140, 295
over-utilization, 129, 192

P

PANDIT, 203
paper and pencil, 267
paramedical profession, 56
parent, 129
parental leave, 50
PatCIS, 282
pathology, 285
patient, 5
patient account, 286
patient autonomy, 103, 250
patient blog, 65
patient empowerment, 6, 190
Patient Portal
    Cerner, 283
    eClinicalWorks, 283
patient portal, 183, 281, 291
patient safety, 183
patient workflow, 290
patient-physician relationship, 344, 353
PatientSite, 282
payment, 353
payment of services, 346

PCHR, 283
pedometer, 194, 198
peer review, 75
peer support, 135, 137, 141
PEFR, 111
people finder, 140
Perfect Forward Secrecy, 276
perseverance, 202
person-to-person, 158
personal analytics, *see* quantified self
personal communication, 353
personality, 193
personalization, 77, 105, 132
pharmaceutical industry, 68
Pharmaceutical Substances Bill, 349
Pharmacies Law, 351
phone call, 208
PHQ-9, 109
PHR, 88, 274, 281, 289, 291
physical activity, 194, 198, 208
physical examination, 157
physician
   age pyramid, 44, 49
   early retirement, 44
   female, 44
   maternal leave, 44
   part-time work, 44
   working hours, 45
physiotherapist, 56
PIN, 276
Planned Parenthood®, 336
population pyramid, 45
practice of medicine, 116, 123, 343, 345, 350, 353
pre-screening, 120
prescription, 115, 121, 125, 184, 351, 353
   paper, 184
prescription drug, 158, 346, 351
prescription refill, 286
prevention, 354
primary care physician, 108
primary care provider, 201, 202
privacy, 87, 103, 291
problem-solving, 141
   strategy, 208
Professional Code, 348, 349
professional conduct, 343, 349, 351, 354, 371
professionalism, 344
pronunciation, 178
PROSAFE, 246
psychologist, 56
psychology sophomore phenomenon, 261
psychosocial outcome, 208
psychotherapy, 64
public health, 102, 218

public health outreach, 77
public institution, 74
PubMed, 19, 262
pulse oximetry, 97
purchasing power, 58
Pygmalion effect, 303

Q
quality improvement, 54
quality of life, 93, 210, 245
quantified self, 31, 88, 140, 290, 332
questionnaire, 103, 107
quiz, 208, 218

R
radiation exposure, 165
radiology, 285
rating, 127, 151
rationalization, 54
rationing, 53
    age, 53
RCT, 94, 105, 107, 108, 219, 220, 227, 233, 235, 237, 239, 251, 267, 307
RE-AIM, 207, 323
Reach to Recovery, 336
readability formula, 172
reading level, 102
readmission, 90
REALM, 176
rebound, 209
Recht auf freie MeinungsäuSSerung, 351
recommendation, *see also* advice, 129, 285
recording device, 129, 148
registration, 290
relapse prevention, 227
release form, 292
religious community, 169
reminder, 125, 126, 285
remote monitoring, 290
reproduction rate, 50
retinal scan, 185
retirement age, 42, 52
rhetoric, 66
risk
    of inaction, 205
    technological, 205
risk assessment, 208
risk awareness, 192, 193
risk factor, 202, 260
    cardiovasular, 207
Robert-Koch-Institut, 48
ROI, 89, 336
Roman Catholic Church, 170

General Index 411

Rosenberg Self-Esteem, 258
RTMM, 238
rule engine, 111

S
S-TOFHLA, *see also* TOFHLA
safe sex, 103
safety, 203
sales, 132, 332, 334
sampling bias, 261
Sanitas, 260
scalability, 114, 131
schizophrenia, 250
scientific journal, 22
    medical specialty, 22
screening, 191
search, 77, 79, 181
second life persona, 183
secure algorithm, 276
    AES, 276
    RSA, 276, 278
secure messaging, 286, 291
security
    appliance, 277
    architecture, 277
    audit, 277
    certification, 277
    hardware security module, 277
    VPN-device, 277
sedentary, 198
seed post, 199
selection bias, 178, 258
self diagnosis, 70
self rewarding, 127
self support, 212
self-efficacy, 105, 206, 207
self-efficacy theory, 227
self-help group, 74
self-management, 206, 208
self-tracking, 290, 332
semiotic triangle, 174
sensitivity, 258
service effort, 132
session authentication, 153
sex, 212
sexual contact, 103
Shakespeare, 194
Shared Decision Making, 10
sleep monitor, 285
smart home, 245
Smart Medical Home, 246
smart phone, *see also* app, 209
smoking, 261

SMS, 217, 219–221, 223, 224, 226–228
SNP, 165
social desirability bias, 302
social desirability effect, 192, 198
social media, 136
social network, 70, 86, 103, 139, 198, 348
social network persona, 162
Social Security Number, 285
social support, 198
specialty language, 89, 182
specialty language term, 172
specificity, 258
Statistisches Bundesamt, 46
step count, 198
stigma, 195
structure quality, 151
subject, 6
subject expectancy effect, 106, 194, 302
success story, 106
suicidal ideation, 106, 107, 168
surgery, 90, 174
survey, 64
symbols, 174
systematic review, 206

T
taboo, 225
tailored, 195, 353
TAN, 184
Techniker Krankenkasse, 192, 337
technology acceptance, 288
telemanagement, 84
telemedicine, 6, 56, 83, 345, 350
telemedicine service, 211
telephone, *see also* phone, 83, 120
temperature monitor, 246
temptation, 208
text readability, 172
Text to Change, 218
theory of science, 6
TLS, 276
toxic substance, 165
tracking, 208
tracking service, 88
triage, 339
trial
    clinical, *see also* RCT, 113
    non-randomized, 91
    pre-post, 207
truism, 66
trust, 73, 74, 87, 92, 94, 148
trustworthy provider, 202
two factor authentication, 276

U

ubiquity, 57, 148, 252
under-served community, 166
under-served population, 58, 114, 217, 321
under-served sub-population, 178
URAC, 75, 131
usability, 203, 206, 288, 290
user profile, 139
utilitarianism, 340
utility, 340
UV exposure, 129

V

VA, 201, 283
vaccination
    adverse effect, 376
validity approach, 76
value, 340
Viagra, 116
video, 91, 266
video telephony, 148
videoconferencing, 190
violence, 166
virtual private network, 275
virtual reality, 105
visual impairment, 170
visual loss, 210
visualization, 285
voice pattern recognition, 185
voice recognition, 176
volunteer, 14, 298

W

wearable device, 290
weight, 196
    control, 194
    loss, 196
    reduction, 197
well-being, 120, 127, 354
wiki, 138
Wikipedia®, 78
workforce, 42, 44, 48
workplace, 166
worst case scenario, 44

Y

Yahoo™, 77

Z

zero knowledge protocol, 276

Index of Services

A
Accu-Chek 360 from Google play, 333
AERIAL, 256

B
Bing®, 67

C
CoaguGame from App Store, 333

D
DASH for Health, 335
DrishtiCare, 211

E
everydayhealth.com, 123, 330

G
Google™, 64, 67, 70

H
H.E.A.L.T.H., 335
http://adultmeducation.com/AssessmentTools_1.html, 176
http://amazon.com, 195
https://answers.yahoo.com, 137
http://deprexis.com/, 338
http://ecoach.tk.de/coaches/, 337
http://experiencejournal.childrenshospital.org, 138
http://familyhistory.hhs.gov/, 259–261
http://health.gov, 336

http://healthy.kaiserpermanente.org/health/care/consumer/my-health-manager, 338
http://patientdave.blogspot.com, 138
http://TuDiabetes.org, 212
http://wikileaks.org, 268
http://ww5.komen.org, 336
http://www.activeliving.info/, 195
http://www.appsundco.de/iphone/apps/medizin/gesundheits-irrtuemer-wissenswertes-aus-gesundheit-medizin/, 152
http://www.breastcancergenescreen.org, 263
http://www.breastcancertrials.org/bct_nation, 378
http://www.cancer.gov/cancertopics/factsheet/detection/mammograms, 263
http://www.carepages.com, 139
http://www.dimdi.de/static/en/amg/var/index.htm, 349
http://www.dipexinternational.org, 138
http://www.diygenomics.org, 143
http://www.dr-bob.org/babble, 108
http://www.dred.com, 122, 164
http://www.drugs.com, 68
http://www.euroclinix.de, 116
http://www.facebook.com, 139
http://www.familyhealthware.com/, 259, 260
http://www.fda.gov/MedicalDevices/DeviceRegulationandGuidance/Overview/default.htm, 33
http://www.galaxyzoo.org, 143
http://www.healthcaremagic.com, 123, 367
http://www.hon.ch, 75
http://www.impact-information.com/impactinfo/readability02.pdf, 172
http://www.jameda.de, 119, 120
http://www.linkedin.com, 139
http://www.livejournal.com, 137
http://www.mbc.ca.gov/Breeze/License_Verification.aspx, 120
http://www.MedlinePlus.gov, 77, 336
http://www.myhealth.va.gov, 283
http://www.ncbi.nlm.nih.gov/pubmed/, 337
http://www.ncbi.nlm.nih.gov/pubmedhealth/, 77, 336
http://www.netdoctor.co.uk/, 119
http://www.nlm.nih.gov/bsd/disted/pubmed.html, 181
http://www.oncolink.com/oncolife/, 112, 262
http://www.oncolink.org, 336
http://www.patient.co.uk/, 337
http://www.patientslikeme.com, 137, 139, 143
http://www.plannedparenthood.org, 336
http://www.plannedparenthood.org/, 224
http://www.quantifiedself.com, 140
http://www.revolutionhealth.com, 122
http://www.twitter.com, 138
http://www.webMD.com, 119
http://www.wikicancer.org, 138
http://www.wikipedia.org, 138
https://answers.yahoo.com, 137
https://www.dimdi.de/static/en/amg/var/apotheken/index.htm, 367

J
JoHo Dortmund Innere Medizin I from Google play and App Store, 96, 333

Index of Services

L
LinkMedica, 256

M
Mayo Clinic from Google play and App Store, 96, 333
Mayo Clinic on Pregnancy from Google play and App Store, 96
My Health Manager, 338

R
Rauchfrei Pro from Etago, 328

W
WebMD, 64, 70, 348
Wikipedia, 68, 70
www.apo-rot.CountryCode, 122
www.dred.com, 330
www.getflorence.co.uk/, 291
www.healthcaremagic.com, 330
www.site.coagucheklink.com/, 333
www.virtuallybetter.com, 105

Y
Yahoo!^{TM}, 64, 67